PRAISE FOR JOE FRIEL AND
THE TRIATHLETE'S TRAINING BIBLE

"One of the most trusted coaches in triathlon."

—*LAVA* MAGAZINE

"Joe Friel is one of the world's foremost experts on endurance sports."

—*OUTSIDE* MAGAZINE

"Joe Friel's wealth of knowledge in triathlon is astounding, and he has a wonderful way of sharing that knowledge with all athletes from beginners to elite professionals."

—SIRI LINDLEY, TRIATHLON WORLD CHAMPION

"As a multiple triathlon world champion, I would consider Joe as one of the leading figures in triathlon coaching today. Joe's professional approach and practical understanding of sports physiology has helped many endurance athletes of all abilities reach their full athletic potential."

—SIMON LESSING, FIVE-TIME TRIATHLON WORLD CHAMPION

"*The Triathlete's Training Bible* is a fantastic guide. You can't go wrong using the advice in this book."

—SCOTT "THE TERMINATOR" MOLINA, TRIATHLON WORLD CHAMPION

"Joe Friel has spent most of his life in devotion to the understanding and teaching of sport. Joe has managed to focus on the key components to athletic success while weeding out the noise. This book will play a substantial role in helping you take the next step as a triathlete."

—JUSTIN DAERR, PROFESSIONAL TRIATHLETE

"As a triathlon coach, 2004 Olympian, and former top-ranked triathlete in the world, I've used *The Triathlete's Training Bible* as one of my key references. Joe Friel's training books have made the once 'crazy' sport of triathlon accessible to the public while also guiding seasoned athletes to their full potential. Joe does the hard work for the beginning triathlete by condensing, prioritizing, and simplifying all the science and practical experience, which he has mastered over decades of coaching."

—BARB LINDQUIST, 2004 OLYMPIAN

"*The Triathlete's Training Bible* combines scientific research with the experience of a top endurance coach to provide the best training resource book available."

—GALE BERNHARDT, 2004 TEAM USA OLYMPIC TRIATHLON HEAD COACH

"*The Triathlete's Training Bible* can help you train for any distance and is most useful to newbies and self-trained athletes who want traditional training advice."

—LIBRARY JOURNAL

"As an athlete with the unique ability to race multiple Ironman races every season, I have always been trouble for any triathlon coach. To coach myself successfully, I needed a reliable and strong tool. I searched all sources carefully until I found the one—*The Triathlete's Training Bible* by Joe Friel. Whatever my problem, there is always a solution in this book. This book makes my understanding of training, racing, and recovering more complete with every page."

—PETR VABROUSEK, PROFESSIONAL TRIATHLETE

"*The Triathlete's Training Bible* is an invaluable tool for every triathlete looking to improve."

—CLAS BJÖRLING, PROFESSIONAL TRIATHLETE

"*The Triathlete's Training Bible* is a 'must read' for both athletes and coaches. . . . It captures the essence of multisport training by outlining both the science and the art of the sport in a detailed, yet practical format. It is one of the most valuable resources I have on my bookshelf."

—LIBBY BURRELL, FORMER USA TRIATHLON NATIONAL PROGRAM DIRECTOR

"Any author who includes the word 'bible' in the title risks comparison to a very high standard. The original was divinely inspired, after all. Those with some tri experience who lack the time or the budget to hire a coach should find this book just what is needed to improve performance. Do I hear a chorus of hallelujahs?"

—IMPACT MAGAZINE

"Friel has combined scientific and technical information with his considerable experience as an athlete and coach of novices, elite amateurs and professionals, to create this very useful reference for triathletes of all types. It would be very surprising if you did not find something useful in *The Triathlete's Training Bible*."

—TRIATHLON MAGAZINE CANADA

"Friel explains the science of training in a language you can understand."

—AMATEURENDURANCE.COM

"What Friel is best at is reverse engineering how top athletes perform and then explaining it to the reader in simple, easy-to-use terms."

—BREAKINGMUSCLE.COM

THE TRIATHLETE'S
TRAINING
BIBLE

4th EDITION

THE TRIATHLETE'S
TRAINING
BIBLE

THE WORLD'S MOST COMPREHENSIVE TRAINING GUIDE
4th EDITION

JOE FRIEL

VELO
press

Boulder, Colorado

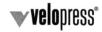

3002 Sterling Circle, Suite 100
Boulder, Colorado 80301-2338 USA

Distributed in the United States and Canada by Ingram Publisher Services

Library of Congress Cataloging-in-Publication Data
Names: Friel, Joe, author.
Title: The triathlete's training bible: the world's most comprehensive training guide / Joe Friel.
Description: Fourth edition. | Boulder, Colorado : VeloPress, [2016] | Includes bibliographical references and index.
Identifiers: LCCN 2016034831 (print) | LCCN 2016040894 (e-book) | ISBN 9781937715441 (pbk.: alk. paper) | ISBN 9781937716844 (e-book)
Subjects: LCSH: Triathlon—Training.
Classification: LCC GV1060.73 .F74 2016 (print) | LCC GV1060.73 (e-book) | DDC 796.42/57071—dc23
LC record available at https://lccn.loc.gov/2016034831

For information on purchasing VeloPress books, please e-mail velopress@competitorgroup.com or visit www.velopress.com.

This paper meets the requirements of ANSI/NISO Z39.48-1992 (Permanence of Paper).

Cover design by Kevin Roberson
Cover photo by Nils Nilsen
Illustrations by Charlie Layton
Art direction by Vicki Hopewell
Composition by Jessica Xavier

Text set in DIN and Warnock

17 18 / 10 9 8 7 6 5 4 3 2

To "Team Friel"
Joyce, Kim, Keara, and Dirk

CONTENTS

PREFACE

This is a love story. I fell in love with triathlon at my first race in June 1983. It was a bit shorter than what later would be called the Olympic or standard distance. That day, I swam 1,000 meters in a pool, biked 20 miles, and ran 10 kilometers. It was more fun than running a marathon, which was the type of racing I had done before that life-changing day. In fact, marathons were what led me to triathlon in the first place.

I had frequently been injured as a runner. Whenever an Achilles tendon, a balky knee, an aching hip, or some other overworked body part broke down because I was running too much, I would ride a bike to maintain fitness. That happened all too often. One day, while I was cycling my way through yet another injury, I crashed on a high-speed descent in the Colorado Rockies and ended up with some broken bones in my shoulder. Oh, great. Now what? My doctor told me the best thing I could do for the shoulder after it had healed would be to swim (there was no injury rehab back in those days). I followed his advice, and one day in the pool, it dawned on me that I was now swimming, biking, and running, which sounded a lot like a strange new sport I had heard of—triathlon. So, heck, why not give it a try? I did, and my life changed. I was in love.

Back in the early days of triathlon, athletes came to the sport much as I had come—from another sport. Most of the early triathletes were runners, but a few cyclists and swimmers also crossed over. Now that triathlon is part of the sports mainstream, most participants simply start their athletic careers as triathletes. The sport has also changed in many other ways. In the early days, training for triathlon was haphazard. We tried all sorts of things to see what would produce the best race performances. Because I had a running background, I applied what I knew about running to swimming and biking. Others, with backgrounds in swimming and road cycling (there was no mountain biking yet), applied their original sport's way of training to the other two. Triathlon in those early days was a melting pot of training ideas. It was an exciting time.

Given my strong interest in sports science, I was fascinated by what I was learning from other triathletes, whose perspective of their new sport was often different from mine. I experimented with various types of workouts in each of the three sports. Sometimes they worked, sometimes they didn't. I began to develop a personal triathlon training methodology based on what I was learning.

I was also new to coaching in the early 1980s. I owned a running store called Foot of the Rockies in a small town in northern Colorado, and I coached many of my customers on the side—only runners at first. But that changed after I fell in love with triathlon. I was so infatuated with my new sport that I bought the bike shop next to my running store, took down the wall between them, and had what was probably the first triathlon store in the world. (I soon discovered that the world was not ready for a triathlon store in 1984.)

After that change, my store's customers and coaching clientele began to shift from runners to triathletes, and also cyclists. I was also becoming aware that I enjoyed coaching much more than retailing. So I sold the store in 1987 and got a day job while spending nights and weekends doing what I was passionate about—coaching. It took 6 years before I had enough clients to be able to quit my day job and focus on coaching.

By the mid-1990s, I thought I had figured out how to train for a triathlon. And so I wrote a book about what I had learned in my 15 years in the sport—*The Triathlete's Training Bible*. I didn't write it for the reader. I wrote it for myself. I wanted to see if I could clearly explain what I had learned not only from my firsthand experience as a triathlete and coach but also from my other love—sports science.

I didn't expect the book to be around for very long. Perhaps a few hundred copies would be sold, but I would have put on paper what I had learned. Its only purpose was to help me grow as a coach. As it turned out, though, *The Triathlete's Training Bible* became the best-selling book ever written on training for triathlon. I learned a lot more in the years that followed, so I revised the book twice as new training concepts came along.

It's now coming up on two decades since I wrote the original. In the last couple of years, I began to realize that I couldn't just revise the old book a bit to bring it up to date. Too much had changed in 20 years. The book needed more than a revision. It needed a complete rewrite. So I threw out the entire manuscript and started from scratch. The only thing that remains today is the general layout of the book. If you have an older version, you can compare the tables of contents and see a similarity. But that's as far as it goes. Everything else in this book is new.

If you seriously studied the original book, you may well find some significant changes and even contradictions in this edition. I've rethought everything. Very little is exactly the same as it was 20 years ago. The sport has changed. Sports science has changed. I have changed. This newest book reflects where the sport, the science, and I are now.

And it's not just "all new"—it's also improved. I know that sounds like a marketing ploy. But it's true. As you start reading, I think you'll see what I mean.

Sometimes people don't like change. I've often been taken to task by someone who has read my blog and realizes that what I say there is different from what I said on the same topic two decades back, when I wrote the first edition of *The Triathlete's Training Bible*. That's fine with me; I believe the changes in what you now hold in your hands (or read on your screen) are for the better. If you've been following the guidelines from the original book, you'll be challenged to rethink what you know. That's a good thing. Change is the cost of improvement.

This book is about high performance. As such, it is not for novices. If you are new to triathlon, I encourage you to read an introductory book, such as another of my books—*Your First Triathlon*. Once you've learned firsthand, through your training and racing, what the sport is about, come back to this book. It will help you produce better race results once you start thinking of yourself as a high-performance triathlete.

High-performance training means becoming the best triathlete possible. But that isn't revealed only in race results. High performance is more than simply where you finish in your races. It's also an attitude grounded in the belief that you can always get better. I've never coached an athlete who couldn't perform at a higher level. Not one. Each of us has plenty of room for improvement between our current level of performance and our potential.

You are fully capable of racing faster and of achieving higher goals as a triathlete. I have no doubt about it. What I want to teach you in this book is how to go about achieving high-performance racing. You may learn only one thing from this book, but that one thing will make a difference. On the other hand, the book may cause you to rethink your training, racing, and athletic lifestyle completely. I've seen such things happen with athletes I've coached over the years, and it led them to better results.

Obviously, however, I am not going to be there to make daily training decisions for you, as I do with my clients. You're going to be your own coach. If you don't think you're up to that, I strongly suggest that you hire a smart coach and work with him or her on your chosen program. There are thousands of coaches around the world today.

One of the biggest changes in coaching since the early 2000s is the advent of coaching web sites, such as TrainingPeaks (www.training peaks.com). With one of these services, it really doesn't matter where you and your coach live. You can be on opposite sides of the world. If you are in your first 3 years of the sport, however, I strongly suggest that you hire a local coach. Some things, such as learning new skills, are best accomplished in a hands-on coaching relationship. But if you're an advanced tri-athlete—the athlete for whom this book is intended—there is much less reason to meet face-to-face with your coach.

So what's an "advanced" triathlete? We could probably come up with a long list of defining characteristics. But for now, let's just say that an advanced triathlete is someone who's been in the sport for at least 3 years. That's long enough to understand the sport, one's body, and training quite well.

This book, therefore, is intended for the advanced athlete who strives for high-performance racing. It is divided into six parts. Part I examines both mental and physical fitness. Part II is about the fundamentals of training, with an emphasis on basic concepts and on the most important element of physical training for the advanced, high-performance athlete: intensity. Part III lays the groundwork for purposeful training. This is perhaps the most critical topic for the self-coached athlete. In Part IV, we finally get into preparing to race by looking at the details of how to plan your season and drill, all the way down to planning a workout. I consider this the core of the book. Having a solid plan is essential for high performance. Part V examines what is perhaps the most neglected aspect of training for serious triathletes: balancing stress and rest. Many self-coached triathletes get this wrong and, as a result, never experience anything even close to their potential in the sport. And finally, in Part VI, I introduce topics that are often overlooked by athletes that can have a big impact on their triathlon performance—improving skills, becoming stronger, and effectively using a training diary.

Why do you do triathlons? What got you started? If you are like most in the sport, you took up triathlon because it looked like fun, or perhaps as a way to get in shape, or maybe for the challenge of competing against others or yourself. Or possibly you came to it as I did, from another sport, such as swimming, cycling, or running, and saw triathlon as a way to break the monotony of single-sport training and try your hand at something different. These are some common reasons I've heard from triathletes over the years, and I suppose there are many other possibilities. Whatever your reason, you must remind yourself of it frequently as you read this book.

In the coming chapters, we will take a serious look at what it takes to become a high-performance triathlete. And I do mean serious. You will read about stuff that only coaches usually think about. This book is essentially an advanced course in the philosophy and methodology of training for triathlon. It will get pretty deep at times. You may need to ground yourself occasionally by considering the answer to the question above: Why do you do triathlons? Some of what you will read in this book works best for athletes who are driven to compete at a high level. That may not be your thing. You may be reading this book just to get an idea of what you might do to improve your training a bit. You may not be looking to win your age group, make a national team, or qualify for Ironman® Hawaii. Nevertheless, most triathletes still want to race faster than they've done before, even if it only means shaving a few minutes off a personal best at a local race. Whatever your goals, stay grounded throughout your reading by reminding yourself of why you do triathlons.

And be prepared to be the best triathlete you can be. If you absorb the principles in this book, you will find yourself on the path to high-performance training and racing. So let's get started.

—*Joe Friel*
Boulder, Colorado

ACKNOWLEDGMENTS

Much of the credit for the content of this book is due to the hundreds of athletes I have coached for more than 30 years. Their comments, questions, thoughts, and feelings provided valuable feedback as my training philosophy and methodology evolved over many years. Athletes continue to ask great questions at my camps, at seminars, through social media and e-mail, and on my blog. Their curiosity has no limits and is contagious. Without their inquisitive interest in and wonderment about training, my approach to coaching and this book would never have been possible. I am greatly indebted to each and every one of them.

I also am indebted to several others who have directly contributed to the writing of this book. Especially instrumental were Rob Griffiths, owner and operator of Training Bible Coaching in the United Kingdom, for providing feedback on Chapter 1; Nate Koch of Endurance Rehabilitation for reviewing my physical exam suggestions in Chapter 5; and Josh Sutchar, chief experience officer of TrainHeroic, for reviewing and making suggestions for Chapter 13. My thanks to all of them.

As always, the editing and design of the VeloPress staff have made this book much more readable and enjoyable. Thanks to Connie Oehring, Vicki Hopewell, and Barbara Gormise. Thanks also to Charlie Layton for taking my rough sketches and turning them into the excellent figures found throughout the book. I especially want to thank publisher Ted Costantino, who encouraged me to put my thoughts on paper once again and who hung in there with me as the writing dragged on for more than 18 months.

And finally I want to thank my wife, Joyce, who put up with my daily 4 a.m. writing schedule as I researched and wrote about things that fascinate me. Without her encouragement, commitment, and support over more than 50 years, the pursuit of my dream would never have happened.

MIND AND BODY

In Part I, you will learn about the underlying foundations of fitness for your mind and your body as we examine the mental and physical components of triathlon training. The basics will ultimately determine how well your training and racing go.

Chapter 1 starts us off by examining what I have found to be the three most important mental skills for success in endurance sports: commitment, confidence, and patience. Taken together, they form what we typically call *mental toughness*. Mentally tough athletes are hard to beat. They seem always to find a way, even when things are not going right.

In Chapter 2, you'll read about the most basic elements of physical training for endurance sports. Here, you will learn of the philosophy of training I've used with athletes—at all levels of performance— for more than 30 years. We will also examine the three pillars of endurance fitness: aerobic capacity, anaerobic threshold, and economy. All of your workouts are intended to make you more fit in these areas. We will also delve into the technology you may already have and how it can be used to improve your training. And finally, we'll take a look at what successful training involves.

MENTAL FITNESS

TRAINING BOOKS commonly begin with an overview of the fitness program and lay out a few rules for how the program is to be followed. There's often a discussion of equipment, and usually a brief review of training principles. But I am not going to start that way. Instead, I want to begin with what I consider to be the most important asset every athlete must develop and nurture before beginning a training program. That asset is mental fitness. No athlete will ever reach his or her goals without a sound mental strategy and a commitment to success. So before we talk about anything else, let's look at why you want to take on the challenge of triathlon and how you can develop a winning approach to your training. Master the principles in this chapter and you will be on the path to a triathlon season marked by high achievement.

The common denominator for all of the high-performance triathletes I have known is a "can-do" attitude. It's a sure thing that they will succeed. They're convinced of it. This leads me to believe that mental fitness is at least as important as physical fitness—perhaps even more so. A mentally fit athlete always figures out a way.

High achievement always starts with a dream. And triathletes are big dreamers. They dream of what may be achieved in the coming season—finishing an Ironman, taking a podium placing at a favorite race, achieving a top-10 national ranking, qualifying for a world championship, or some other big dream.

I really don't know which comes first—the big dream or the will to achieve. I suspect it's the latter. But they go hand in hand. Because of this, I believe it is imperative that triathletes develop mental fitness along with their physical fitness. And just like physical fitness, mental fitness can be trained. In fact, physical fitness and mental fitness are similar in that both must be trained consistently.

Training, whether mental or physical, is a task you must attack every day. There are hard training days and easy training days for both. On some days your mind says, "I can't do this." That's a hard mental-training day. You must train your mental fitness to get through this. These are the days that ultimately determine your success as a triathlete.

Athletic success is not instantaneous or guaranteed. Achieving big dreams demands the best of you. Excellence isn't easy. If it were, everyone would be excellent. Most people do not dream big. For them, ordinary is OK. Some talk about dreams. Excellence sounds nice. But few have the will to achieve their dreams.

What is your dream?

DREAMS, GOALS, AND MISSIONS

Excellence is rare. It involves having big dreams. Unfortunately, most people have dreams that seldom become goals. Their dreams are actually wishes. Someone who really has a dream, a goal, *and* the will to pursue it is on a mission. That person has a purpose. If that person is an athlete, he or she will find a way to make the dream come true regardless of obstacles and setbacks.

Ryan's Dream

In December 1997, a young triathlete called me. His name was Ryan Bolton. He was new to the sport. But he had a dream—a big one. The International Olympic Committee (IOC) had recently announced that triathlon would be a sport in the 2000 Games in Sydney, Australia. The inclusion of triathlon as an Olympic event was something all of us in the sport had wanted for years. Ryan's dream was to qualify for the Olympics and represent the United States. There would be only three American men on the team. He needed a coach to help it happen. Would I coach him?

Right after the IOC announcement, I received several such contacts from athletes looking for a coach to help them make the team. Most were just wishing and knew little about what it would take. Most also had little or no background in the sport. Ryan was different. He not only had been an All-American distance runner in college but also had done some triathlons after graduation and understood what it would take to achieve his dream. He was very businesslike during our phone chat. Could I help him? I don't usually make snap decisions, but his tremendous desire and will to succeed convinced me that he could pull it off. I agreed to coach him.

To be eligible for the U.S. Olympic triathlon qualifying trials in the spring of 2000, Ryan would have to be ranked in the top 125 in the world. He made great progress throughout the first two years we worked together, moving up to 25th place in the world rankings. Things were going great. But in the spring of 1999, we started encountering setbacks that continued into the winter of 2000. Ryan had frequent upper respiratory infections that often interrupted training. His doctors could not determine the exact problem. We kept cutting back on his training to allow his body to fight the infections. His world ranking gradually slipped. By the fall of 1999, with only a few months remaining until the U.S. Olympic Team Trials qualifying race, he was ranked 75th in the world. Things only got worse that winter. We never did determine why he had so much illness, but we had to reduce his training considerably for most of the year. By the following spring, however, he was healthy again and ready for the trials.

Excellence involves having big dreams.

Throughout all of those pivotal months, when he was sick and the dream seemed to be slipping through his fingers, Ryan remained calm and confident. He never expressed any doubt that he'd make the team. He was always determined and optimistic. I had never coached anyone who was so committed to a goal and so mentally tough in working to achieve it. Finally, at the Olympic Trials race in May, in an amazing come-from-behind effort on a hot and steamy day in Dallas, Texas, he pulled it off. He qualified for the Olympics. The dream he had held for 3 years became a reality. He was a member of TeamUSA for the very first Olympic triathlon.

Ryan is a rare athlete who went on to have more big dreams, goals, and missions, including winning an Ironman triathlon. He did so in 2002, capturing the Ironman U.S. Championship in Lake Placid, New York.

Very few people allow themselves to do what Ryan did—dream big. Even fewer have the will to do what it takes to achieve big goals. They seldom make it a mission. At the first sign of a setback, they are likely to throw in the towel.

Ryan continues to have an impact on triathlon. He's now a coach who shares his wealth of knowledge about training and racing, as well as his drive for accomplishing high goals, with athletes from around the world.

Allow yourself to dream. What would you like to accomplish as a triathlete? Take your dream to the next level by setting a goal. (We'll take an in-depth look at goal setting in Chapter 5.) Once you have a goal, it must become your mission. The more challenging the goal, the more you must focus your life on it. It must be your mission every day. For the mission to become a reality in the face of setbacks, it takes one more thing—total commitment.

Commitment

Accomplishing big goals requires unwavering commitment. Commitment is simply doing what you said you'd do well after the mood you were in when you said it has passed. Carrying on with your goal for weeks and months—perhaps years—demands unwavering dedication and discipline. Total commitment to your goal, which is what a mission is, eventually produces passion. But dedication and discipline precede passion. In other words, you may not be passionate about your goal initially, but the more dedicated you become to it and the more disciplined you are in working toward it, the greater your passion will become. Passion for his goal is what kept Ryan going when reaching it seemed hopeless.

When it comes to achieving high goals, the greatest limiter you face is not the many miles you train, but rather the few inches between your ears. You are fully capable of achieving much more than you think you can. You must have commitment, dedication, and discipline. Is training for the goal hard? The best athletes I've coached for more than 30 years were dedicated and disciplined, and they thrived on hard workouts. Will you experience setbacks along the way? Most certainly. It's never easy when you are training near your physical and mental limits.

So success starts with a commitment that requires the dedication and discipline of a mission before your commitment eventually becomes your passion. Once passion sets in, goal attainment in the face of setbacks becomes easier. But there is an uneasy period of time when the passion isn't quite great enough and only dedication and discipline keep the mission going. During this time, you must remain fully committed.

> You are capable of achieving much more than you think you can.

Are you fully committed to your goal? What does that mean? It obviously means hard training. Wishing won't make you more fit. It's hard work. Blue-collar labor. Every day.

You must also be smart about training. The hard days must be balanced with easy ones if you are to be successful. Athletes are more likely to mess up the easy days than the hard ones. We'll get into that later.

The more challenging the mission, the more your life must be focused on it. That means not only your training, but also your eating and sleeping, the support of your family and friends, and much more. It's 24 hours each day for 365 days a year. Total commitment. This book will help you get the physical training part right. The mental part is every bit as important.

TRAINING YOUR HEAD

Preparing to achieve a high goal goes well beyond training your body to swim, bike, and run fast. There is also a very important mental-training component. This is where many athletes fall short in their race preparation. They are physically ready, but not mentally ready. Athletic success requires confidence, mental toughness, and patience. These three mental skills are every bit as important as your physical skills, perhaps even more so. What can you do to improve your mental skills? This is often more of a challenge than the physical training. Let's take a look at what mental training requires.

Believe to Achieve

There are bound to be setbacks in your race preparation, but they must be taken as stepping-stones on the path to success. All successful athletes at every level experience setbacks. When they occur, you must remain confident, be patient, and continue to be mentally tough. Anything less leads to failure.

At the start of training, before the passion is realized, the key to commitment when setbacks occur is self-confidence. You won't achieve your goal if you don't believe you can. You must believe to achieve. Can you do it? Do you really believe in yourself? Are you confident even when things aren't going well? Self-confidence is that wispy, soft-spoken voice in the back of your head that says, "I can do this." Unfortunately, that positive voice isn't always there when you need it. You're more likely to hear a negative voice in your head that always speaks to you in an angry, authoritarian way, saying loudly, "You *can't* do it!" That stern voice will be heard often in the preparation for your race, especially on race day, when everything is on the line. You need confidence at these times to remain focused and determined.

You were born to be confident. As a child, you did lots of risky things because you were sure you could do them. Why would you think otherwise? In fact, risk was fun. Unfortunately, along the road of life, most people lose their self-confidence. Early failures, magnified by especially negative people, drain it out of them. The good news is that you can overcome a lack of confidence about your goal. Here are two easy things you can do to build confidence. You must do these daily, without exception.

Saving successes. To promote self-confidence, open a *success savings account*. It's easy. Every night, after you've gone to bed and turned out the lights, you have the only time in the day when there are no external interruptions. This is

Athletic success requires confidence, mental toughness, and patience.

a good time to run a quick check of how training went that day. Review your workouts. Find one thing you did well. It does not need to be a big deal. Maybe you climbed one hill well, or had one good interval. Or you finished a hard workout. Or maybe you had one of the best workouts of the season. Relive today's successful moment repeatedly until you fall asleep. You just made a deposit into your success savings account.

Some of the deposits will be big and some will be small. But your account needs to grow every day. You can make a withdrawal whenever the negative, angry voice speaks to you. The week of a race is an especially good time to make withdrawals as you begin to question your readiness. Whenever you feel a bit of anxiety about the upcoming race, go back and pull up one of those success memories from your savings account. Relive it vividly. When the authoritarian voice in your head says, "You can't," make another withdrawal immediately. Drown out the voice with a success. When someone casually expresses doubt about your chances of success, make a withdrawal. When you step to the starting line, make a withdrawal. At these critical times, pull up the biggest successes in your account. Say to yourself, "Remember that time when I . . . ."

Never deposit the bad experiences or unwelcome moments in training. Never. Let them go. They're rubbish. Don't relive them. Stay focused on the positive experiences. Deposit only the positive experiences in your account. Withdraw only them. It works.

Fake it 'til you make it. The second thing you can do to boost confidence is to "act as if." That means always assuming the posture and disposition of a confident athlete. Always. Act as if you are confident even if you don't feel that way. You'll be amazed at what that does for your self-perception.

How should you express your confidence? Look around at a race or group workout and find athletes who exude confidence. How do *they* act? Study them. What you will probably find is that they stand tall and proud. Their heads are up. They look people in the eyes when talking. They don't denigrate others in order to elevate their own self-esteem. They move adeptly and fluidly—as good athletes always do. They don't look anxious or nervous. They're calm. They make it obvious they are confident by their demeanor.

Now you may not feel that way all of the time, especially on race day, but act confident anyway. Fake it until you make it. It's remarkable how taking on the posture and demeanor of confidence breeds confidence even when you're not feeling that way inside. It's not possible to be confident with a slumping posture and defeated demeanor. It's like saying no while nodding yes. The two don't go together. Simply *acting as if* will get you through those moments when your confidence is waning. Try it.

Mental Toughness

There comes a time in every race when success and failure are on the line. You sense that you are at your limit. Fatigue is setting in. Your mind is beginning to accept compromises—perhaps the goal that you've worked toward for so long isn't really that important. This is the key moment of the entire race. The mentally tough athlete will get through it. Others will let go of their dreams and settle for something less. They lack the race-day passion for their goals, and their efforts will fade.

The posture of confidence breeds confidence, even when you're not feeling that way inside.

There comes a time in every race when success and failure are on the line.

What are the details? What is it that mentally tough athletes have that the others don't have?

A few years ago, Graham Jones, PhD, a professor of elite performance psychology, published a paper in the *Harvard Business Review*. He studied Olympic athletes in order to learn what psychologically set those who medaled apart from those who didn't medal. Dr. Jones discovered that unlike the nonmedalists, the Olympic podium-placers did these things:

- Paid meticulous attention to their goals
- Had a strong inner drive to stay ahead of the competition
- Concentrated on excellence
- Were not distracted by other people or athletes
- Shrugged off their own failures
- Rebounded from defeat easily
- Never self-flagellated
- Celebrated their wins
- Analyzed the reasons for their success
- Were very confident of their abilities

There were other findings in Dr. Jones's study, but these give us a good idea of what it takes to be mentally tough. These are some of the same things we've been discussing throughout this chapter: excellence, big dreams, goals, a mission, commitment, dedication, discipline, and confidence.

As you can tell from the list, mental toughness isn't just something that mysteriously appears on race day in the lucky few. It's an everyday state of mind in the preparation for your race. It's every thought you have; it's everything you do day in and day out. Mental toughness just happens to show up during hard races.

To be mentally tough, you need one more thing that Dr. Jones alluded to in his paper, but didn't precisely address—patience.

Patience

Success does not come quickly. Just because you have a dream, a goal, and a commitment, it doesn't mean that success is imminent. Triathlon is a patience sport. And the longer your race, the more patience it takes. An Ironman triathlon, for example, is not so much a race as a test of your patience. I go to several Ironman races every year. It never ceases to amaze me that there are always athletes who are obviously anaerobic— they're breathing hard—only 1 mile into the bike leg. And they still have 111 miles to go! What are they thinking?

It takes supreme patience to be a good triathlete, not only in races but also in your approach to training. A true peak performance requires months and years, not hours and days. Patience is necessary. You must be ready for a long and often uphill battle.

How patient you are is evident even in your workouts. An impatient athlete starts a workout or a set of intervals much too fast, then fades as the session continues and finishes weakly. In a race, the impatient athlete does the same thing— starts much too fast and then limps to a whimpering finish. This is often the result of being on a passionate mission—the very thing you must do to succeed. Only now, your dedication and determination are working against you.

Commitment must be held in check by patience if you are to succeed. Your high goal won't be accomplished in the first few minutes of a key workout session or race. The first interval won't achieve your goal. It's what happens late in

It takes supreme patience to be a good triathlete.

the workout, interval set, and race that makes the difference. This is when success occurs. It takes patience to hold yourself in check and save your energy for when it really matters later on. We usually call this asset *pacing*, but it's actually emotion control. Patience means controlling your emotions in the early stages of anything you do.

How do you become patient? There is no easy fix. It's just something you must do every day with everything in your life. When I coach athletes who show signs of impatience, such as doing the first interval too fast, I have them repeat the workout again and again until they get it right. If they start a race too fast and then fade, we have a long conversation afterwards about the reason why they didn't achieve what they are capable of accomplishing. Helping athletes learn patience is the hardest thing I have to do as a coach.

As you learn to be your own coach, be aware of your impatience. Keep it in check. Remind yourself before a hard workout or race that you must contain your emotions early on in order to finish strongly. Remind yourself at the start of the season that patience means making small gains toward your goal every day for months, not forcing it to happen immediately in a single workout. If you can learn to do all of this, you can become patient. Patience is a mental key to success in triathlon. If you can't develop patience, then you are doomed to struggle and fail in achieving your goals. It's that simple.

YOUR TEAM

Let's shift gears. I want to propose something that is related to the above discussion but that is not a mental quality. It's something else in your program that will certainly add confidence that you can achieve your goal while increasing your commitment.

Early in my career, I learned that building a "team" for the athletes I coached increased their chances of achieving their goals while elevating their motivation. I suggest you do this also. It's a big step toward making your goal more achievable.

The purpose of your team is to provide professional and other sports-related assistance to help you train. Of course, a very important part of that team is already assembled—your family and friends. I strongly suggest adding training partners—a coach or knowledgeable training mentor, a physical therapist, a sports medicine doctor, a masseuse, and a bike fitter—to your team. Additional professionals to consider are a personal trainer for gym workouts, a swim instructor, a nutritionist, a chiropractor, and a sports psychologist. The higher your triathlon goal, the greater the benefit of having such a team behind you. Because of their individual ways of assisting, each will help you successfully navigate the many challenges you'll face in the coming season.

Describe your goal to each member of your team and then discuss how he or she can help you achieve it. You may never actually use some of your team members; for example, you may not need a doctor if you don't have any breakdowns throughout the season. But knowing that they are ready to help will boost your confidence and get you through rough patches when something isn't going right.

In addition to their contributions to your success as an athlete, the members of your team must be happy, positive, and successful people who are fully aware and supportive of your goal.

Building a team will make your goal more achievable.

If any of them don't fit that description, then replace them with people who do. Surround yourself only with positive people who believe in you. Avoid those who don't.

SUMMARY: MENTAL FITNESS

We have talked about several mental characteristics that I strive to develop in every athlete I coach. They are critical to success at the highest level. These include commitment to a high goal, the confidence that it can be achieved, and the patience to view the goal as a long-term project. Lumped together, these make up a big chunk of what may be called mental toughness. Athletes with these qualities have already taken a big step toward achieving their goals before the serious physical training even begins.

Just as I need to know the current level of physical fitness of the athletes I train, I also need to know their current level of mental fitness as we start working together. To discover these mental fitness markers, I ask lots of questions. A starting point is how they got started in the sport and why they continue to do it. Are the words *fun* or *enjoyment* ever used? They should be. Do they talk about the challenge of the sport? That evolves into telling me about their season's biggest goal and how it came to be. We talk about the goals of previous seasons and how well they did in working toward them. Did the goals

SIDEBAR 1.1 Evaluating Mental Toughness

Learn about your mental toughness by frankly answering the following questions:

Why do you do triathlon?

Why not do something else instead?

Do you have other important hobbies or activities in your life besides triathlon?

What would you most like to achieve in the sport this season?

What is the most important thing you must accomplish to achieve that goal?

What stands between you and success this season?

How confident are you that you can achieve your goal?

What was your biggest goal last season? Did you achieve it?

What obstacles did you overcome to achieve last year's goal? Or why did you not achieve it?

If you don't achieve your goal this season, will you try again in the future?

Were there other people who were supportive of your goal last year? If so, who were they?

Do you commonly start workouts and races too fast and then fade later?

How often do you miss workouts, and for what reasons?

Do you prefer to train with others or alone?

How often do you train with other athletes?

How supportive of your triathlon goal are your family and friends?

seem easy to accomplish, or were they difficult? This discussion reveals something about their patience and persistence. I ask what it will take to achieve the new goal and how that matches with their current physical abilities. This is an opportunity to find out their level of confidence.

I also ask about their training. Do they ever miss workouts? Is this common? What sorts of situations interfere with workouts? Training consistency is an indicator of commitment. Does the athlete train with other athletes? How often? I've learned that athletes who have a training partner for nearly all workouts—they seldom do one solo—often have a low commitment to their goals. External motivation for such an athlete is necessary to get out the door. As you can imagine, this is a long and in-depth conversation.

From such a discussion I get a good sense of an athlete's potential for goal achievement and what mental skills need further development. The blueprint for a training season starts to take shape before I've even seen the athlete swim, bike, or run.

How goal-committed, confident, and patient are you? Sidebar 1.1, "Evaluating Mental Toughness," lists the questions I use to learn what makes an athlete tick. Read those questions and think your way through the answers. Be honest and sincere. There is no one here to impress. It's just you. If you determine there is a chink in your mental toughness armor, go back to the pertinent section above and reread it to learn what you can do to strengthen it. Or read a book on mental toughness in sports. Better yet, if you have a coach, wise training mentor, or sports psychologist on your team, arrange a meeting to discuss the mental aspects of training and racing.

There's no denying that mental fitness is necessary for success in sports. It's at least as important as anything you do in workouts, if not more so. The rest of this book is about physical training. But that doesn't mean that you should consider mental training as done. It never is. You must work at it daily, as suggested earlier in this chapter. Your physical fitness will never allow you to realize your potential as a triathlete without sound mental fitness.

PHYSICAL FITNESS

IN CHAPTER 1, you read about dreaming big and believing in yourself. That culminates with setting a challenging goal. We'll come back to goal setting in Chapter 5. It will give a focus to your training and help determine what types of workouts you should do. Even though you may have high aspirations for triathlon, your goal can't be so great that you must change your entire life for it. After all, you do have a lot going on aside from triathlon. Most of your day is undoubtedly spent focused on stuff other than swimming, biking, and running, such as your family, friends, home, and career. All of these and more have to be balanced along with training.

What does *balanced* mean? It has to do with your priorities, so only you can answer that question. But I can tell you this: The more challenging your triathlon goal becomes, the more all of the stuff in your life needs to center on it—within reason. For most triathletes, a goal of finishing a sprint-distance triathlon doesn't require much lifestyle focus to achieve. But qualifying for the Ironman World Championship in Kona, Hawaii, is a huge goal and will demand that nearly everything in your life be aimed at this achievement.

Even a huge goal such as racing in Kona must still be reasonable, however. You aren't going to abandon your family and quit your job to accomplish it (although I've known that to happen). But within obvious boundaries, such a high goal will still test your limits.

In this chapter, we will explore what it will take physically to realize your triathlon goal. I'll describe a philosophy of training that will make your goal highly achievable. We'll also examine how to train to get the most out of your workouts and the equipment that will help you pull it off. The starting point for all of this is something you've probably pondered many times before: What are you capable of achieving in triathlon?

YOUR TRIATHLON POTENTIAL

So far, we've explored only the mental determiners of triathlon success, such as commitment, confidence, and mental toughness. The remainder of this book, starting now, is about your physical determiners of success. In this and the next three chapters, we'll lay the groundwork for understanding how to train. Then we'll examine the critical topic of your physical limiters in great detail in Chapter 6. They will become a central focus of your training throughout the season as you work toward your goal. Limiters, and how you go about training them, have a lot to do with what you can hope to accomplish.

That brings us back to the key matter at hand—your potential. Setting a reasonable triathlon goal for the season always raises the issue of what you are capable of achieving. When an athlete considers this matter, what is really being asked is, *Given my core lifestyle, which isn't going to change, what is my physical potential for performing at a high level? Am I capable of achieving more than what I've done in past seasons?* These are tough questions for anyone to answer short of using a crystal ball. Even if you were tested in a sports science lab with the best equipment and the most experienced and scientific minds available, you really couldn't get a definitive answer. There simply are far too many variables—mental as well as physical—that can't be measured. But you can probably resolve such questions about yourself better than any scientist. Instead of by gazing into the future with lab testing, the answer can be found by looking backward in time.

If your training routine for the past few years has been physically challenging and highly structured while based on the best sports science methods available, and if you've also been fully dedicated to following it without missing workouts, then you likely have little room for improvement. The same goes if you've had a smart coach and followed his or her schedule religiously. You're at or very near your potential. But if your recent training hasn't been well structured or very scientific, if you've missed a lot of workouts, or if the training hasn't been all that challenging, then you have a lot of potential left to realize.

You likely are somewhere between these two extremes. That means you still have room to grow as a triathlete. Most do. How much room separates you from your top-end potential we simply don't know with any degree of certainty. We do know for certain, however, that growing toward your potential in the sport will demand the most of you. The two keys that are necessary to do this are mental toughness and training with a purpose. Being purposeful starts with your philosophy of training.

PHILOSOPHY OF TRAINING

Whether you know it or not, you have a philosophy of training. You just may never have thought about it. But everyone has one. Based on what they do, rather than what they say, the training philosophy of many triathletes is "never enough" or "more is always better." The sport attracts many type-A overachievers who often take their training to their absolute limits. As a coach, I've come across many such athletes who pushed themselves to the point of collapse. They are often tired and sometimes become completely burned out. Overtraining is not a pretty sight. (We'll return to the topic of overtraining

Being purposeful starts with your philosophy of training.

You still have room to grow as a triathlete.

in Chapter 10.) Massive amounts of physical exercise are not necessary to achieve high goals. Don't get me wrong; your training won't be easy if you follow the guidelines in this book. It will require mental as well as physical toughness. But it can be accomplished without overtraining to the point of breakdown if you simply think the right way about training. This is where a training philosophy can pay off.

I propose a way of thinking about your training that is probably very different and also much more effective when it comes to race performance than what you've done in the past. It has to do with training consistently. I know that sounds overly simple. Training consistently doesn't sound like a big deal. But if you accept and follow the philosophy I'm about to describe here, I can assure you that your triathlon performance will improve if there is still unclaimed potential. If you have room to grow, you will definitely get better by training consistently. I've seen it happen many, many times with athletes I've coached over the years.

Consistent Training

Highly motivated athletes often train too frequently, too long, and too intensely. "Never enough. More is always better." Such thinking inevitably leads to overtraining, burnout, illness, or injury. Over the last 30 years, I've helped many athletes get out of these training ruts they've dug for themselves by teaching them to train consistently. What does consistent mean? "Relentless, regular, and resolute" is the best catch phrase for success at the highest level in sport. This comes down to doing the *least* amount of training that still achieves your goal—the least, not the most, training. Doing more than is necessary is just

another way of saying "overtraining." That will ultimately lead to a setback. It's only a matter of when, not if.

If your race performance is spotty and you are unable to perform at what you believe your potential is at A-priority races, then inconsistent training is possibly the cause. In fact, I've found this usually to be the reason for lackluster performance among serious athletes. If you are frequently tired when it's time to do a long or high-intensity session, then inconsistent training is certainly the cause. If illness, injury, or burnout is common, then you are not training consistently. You must learn to harness and direct your desire to succeed. That's mental toughness. How can you do that? Being relentless, regular, and resolute starts with something that may seem out of place in training for triathlon—moderation.

Moderation in training means that you seldom explore your physical limits. Athletes often attempt the hardest workouts they can do. Long workouts are much too long, and intensity is often way too high. Most seem to believe that peak fitness comes from pushing their limits several times each week, and rest is viewed as something for sissies. That way of thinking is a sure way to derail your training frequently. Moderation in workout duration and intensity is what you should seek.

Figure 2.1 shows how inconsistent and consistent training look for a real athlete. In the first 22 weeks of the season illustrated in this figure, the athlete had several high-training-load weeks that were the result of workouts that were frequently too intense and too long. As a result, she often experienced extreme fatigue, developed a nagging knee injury, and had a couple of head colds. These were enough to derail her weekly

Being relentless, regular, and resolute starts with moderation.

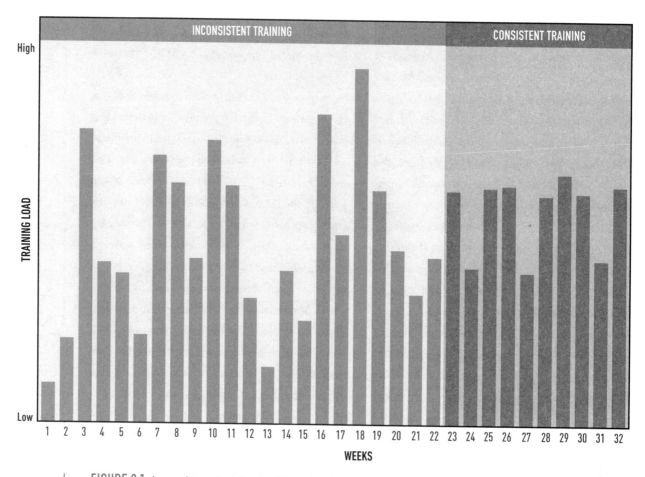

FIGURE 2.1 Inconsistent training for 22 weeks, followed by 10 weeks of consistent training with a more moderate approach

Sometimes you have to hold back to move ahead.

workout plan repeatedly, resulting in little progress in performance to show for nearly 6 months of training. That's what zeroes in your training log do. They set you back. When this athlete realized that she wasn't making progress toward her race goal, she hired a coach. Smart move. For the next 10 weeks, the coach had her doing workouts at a more moderate level of intensity and duration. This resulted in much more consistent training and a marked improvement in her fitness and race performances. Sometimes you have to hold back to move ahead.

The strange thing is, though, that while moderation produces steady improvement, it's also

a moving target. Fortunately, it moves in a good way. As your fitness improves, what a few weeks ago would have been a hard workout becomes moderate. So within the same season, your definition of moderation rises relative to how long and hard your workouts are. You're becoming more fit and capable of training at a higher level.

The same sort of thing is going on from season to season. If you are training moderately, your capacity to handle a high training load gradually increases over the long term. What was a hard workout last month is a moderate workout this month; what was hard last year is moderate this year. All of this has to do with a critical mental toughness skill you read about in Chapter 1—patience. You must be patient to train consistently.

Consistent training is a result of moderation. Consistent training means that you never miss workouts. Well, hardly ever. Let's face it: Everyone misses a session now and then. That can't be avoided. You've got a lot of stuff in your life. But frequent zeroes in your training log are a huge problem for high goals. Missing scheduled workouts is often the result of too much: too much intensity, too much duration, too much working out, and too much to do in your life. If you train (and live) moderately, you will be consistent. If you are consistent, you will race faster. It's not how hard the workouts are. It's how consistently you train. Consistent trumps difficult every time.

A couple of weeks after I start coaching an athlete, I ask whether the training is harder or easier than it was when the athlete was self-coached. The answer is usually that it's easier. I almost always have athletes do less than they did before, and guess what happens? They become fitter and faster. I focus attention on their weaknesses that must be improved for success in the next A-priority race.

If you want to improve as an athlete, you must know your race-specific weaknesses, and then you must train moderately and consistently with your focus primarily on them. That is where success starts—not from doing lots and lots of random training. The path to success involves a patient commitment to relentless, regular, and resolute training in moderation.

What Is Moderate Training?

So what is moderate training? First of all, *moderate* means doing a workout that you know you can complete because you've done it recently (or something very close to it). By "close to it," I mean it's within about 10 percent of the duration or intensity of a workout you've done previously. Avoid big increases in workout difficulty.

Second, a moderate workout is one that you know you can bounce back from quickly in time to do the next scheduled and demanding workout.

Third, if you aren't fully recovered in 48 hours, then the workout was probably too hard. You weren't ready for it—yet. You will be, but you have to get there gradually. Patience.

This doesn't mean you should *never* do workouts beyond the 10 percent limit. I'll propose some to you in later chapters, but they will be rare. They will certainly test your limits, but they must be done at just the right times. They aren't something you will do frequently.

Moderation also involves paying close attention to your body. It can't be forced to adapt and become more fit on some artificial schedule just because you have a race coming up. Your body has its own natural schedule that you must follow if you are to make progress toward your race goal. The body's schedule is slow, or at least it seems that way to most athletes. It's best to do harder-than-usual workouts when your body says it's time, and that's not necessarily when you'd like it to be. But your body will always tell you when the time is right. In later chapters, we'll look at some of those biological "messages" you should watch for when specific workouts are described.

PURPOSEFUL TRAINING

After you have given thought to your training philosophy, the next step in becoming good at coaching yourself is establishing a methodology for training. Your workouts must follow a proven

If you want to improve as an athlete, you must know your race-specific weaknesses.

Moderation involves paying close attention to your body.

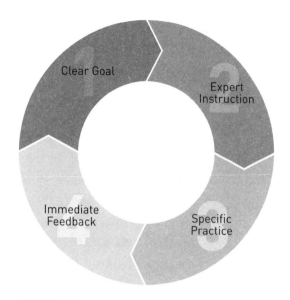

FIGURE 2.2 The process of purposeful training

process with structure and purpose if you are to succeed at the highest level. Haphazard sessions may work when your goals are not very challenging, but not when you are focused on high performance. There are four steps I want you to follow in your daily training process to help make your training more purposeful and effective. The steps are illustrated in Figure 2.2.

Step 1: Clear Goal

Purposeful training starts with having a clear goal for the season. That defines the principal outcome you are seeking—the reason you train. If the goal is vague, then the entire process of purposeful training collapses. For the goal to be clear, it must meet several criteria. We're not going to get into those now, but we'll return to them in Chapter 5. By then, you should be ready to determine your season's goal exactly.

Every workout should also have a goal. I call the workout goal a *purpose* so that the two types of goals don't become confused. The workout purpose can be something such as this: Run 20

minutes at zone 3 for muscular endurance. Or this: Ride easy in zone 1 for 1 hour to recover. (We'll get into specific workout types in Chapter 6.) The purpose doesn't always have to be hard-core training. On occasion, it could even be something such as riding with friends just to have a good time. After all, fun is probably why you started doing triathlon in the first place.

The primary reason for the workout purpose is to avoid haphazard training. Frequently heading out the door with no idea of what you will do is a sure way to accomplish little and show up at races unprepared. Training without purpose ultimately means poor performance. Before starting any training session, always ask yourself the key question: What is the purpose of this workout?

Step 2: Expert Instruction

Your workout purpose should ultimately point at your season's goal. In fact, your goal is nothing more than the accumulation of daily purposes achieved over the course of several weeks. The purposes should follow a pattern that leads from where you physically are at the start of the season to your goal. This can be rather complex because it involves understanding a lot about sports science (which we will get into in the next chapter). At this point, it helps to have someone who is an expert give you clear directions on what you should do. That person could be a coach or trusted mentor who designs a training plan for you. Most triathletes improve exponentially by having such a person in their corner. At the other extreme, you could simply purchase a training plan online and follow it. Realize, however, that such generic plans are not designed specifically for you but for a rather large category of athletes who have similar characteristics. If those char-

Purposeful training starts with having a clear goal for the season.

acteristics happen to match yours, then the purchased training plan may be your "expert."

The expert could even be you, if you're a knowledgeable student of training. Unfortunately, most athletes aren't, and they don't have the time or inclination to study sports science the way coaches do. Self-coached athletes typically make a lot of mistakes; the learning curve for them is quite steep while the goal-progression curve is shallow because of frequent interruptions and setbacks. That's not to say you can't be your own coach. You can. I've known many good self-coached athletes. This book will give you a lot of guidance in becoming one.

Without some sort of expert instruction, however, your chances for success in achieving your challenging goal are greatly decreased. The expert should have a good understanding of what you want to achieve and then provide instructions for getting there. The type of instructions you need on a daily basis are such things as how long the intervals should be; how to vary the intensities within a workout to develop the various energy systems; how to move to improve skills; when to schedule strength workouts relative to swim, bike, and run sessions; and on and on.

If you're new to the sport, almost anything you do will bring rapid improvement. But for advanced athletes preparing for high performance, training requires more than simply raising your heart rate and breathing hard during workouts.

Who is the expert you will rely on?

Step 3: Specific Practice

Once you know the workout purpose and supporting details provided by the expert for a given session, everything you do must be specific to them. You must stay focused on doing the workout as planned. An exception is made when you decide to make the session easier because you discover you aren't ready for it; you need more recovery time, for example, or the timing may not be right for some other reason. Going the other way—making the workout harder than its intended purpose—first requires consulting with the expert who designed it. There could be a good reason for its seemingly low level of difficulty. I tell the athletes I coach that if they feel the need to make the workout easier, they can always make that decision and tell me about it later. But I discourage them from making the session more challenging without talking with me beforehand.

It's important that you know exactly what is to be accomplished in every workout. If the workout is fairly complex, write it down and take your notes to the pool, road, track, or indoor trainer so you can check from time to time to make sure you're doing things right.

Perhaps the greatest impairment of purposeful practice comes from other athletes. For most workouts, it's very difficult to follow the session purpose and details specifically if your training partner wants to do something different. When training with others, it's a good idea to talk about the purpose of your session for that day. If the other athlete is unwilling to follow it, you are better off training on your own. With the possible exception of swim workouts, triathlon is largely a solo sport anyway. You are generally better off doing bike and run workouts by yourself.

The bottom line is that what you do in any given workout must be specific to the intended purpose of that workout if you are to reap the planned benefits.

It's important that you know exactly what is to be accomplished in every workout.

You are generally better off doing bike and run workouts by yourself.

Step 4: Immediate Feedback

Without doubt, the most effective way to make progress is to have your coach (the expert) with you throughout your training. That way, you can get immediate feedback from him or her regarding what adjustments need to be made if things are not going as they should. A perfect example of this is refining your swim skills. Having someone on deck to tell you how to adjust your "catch" when it's done incorrectly will bring about much greater progress than if the coach views a video and tells you a day later. But even a day later is better than never at all. The same goes for doing an interval session. Reviewing workout data immediately after a workout is much more effective than reviewing the data several hours later. Immediate pointers from the coach are vital to your progress. The sooner you get feedback, the better.

It's unlikely, however, that a coach will be able to attend all of your workouts. The most common exceptions for triathletes are masters swim sessions with a coach on deck or a weekly group track workout led by the coach. These are perfect for getting expert feedback. But usually the coach's feedback will be delayed. The sooner you can get it, the faster your progress will be. The feedback can be hands-on by the attending coach, or it can come through e-mails or text messages. A weekly telephone call to discuss how training is going is a perfect opportunity to ask questions of the coach to make sure you are achieving the intended purposes of your workouts.

If you are self-coached, you must stay mentally engaged with what your body is doing during workouts. If your mind drifts while you are working on swim skills or doing intervals on the track, then it's the same as if the coach leaves. The self-coached athlete must always be analyz-

> If you are self-coached, you must stay mentally engaged with your body during workouts.

ing what is happening. And that continues into the post-workout analysis. Data files from whatever devices you are using should be analyzed as soon as possible following each session. Video recordings of a skills session should also be viewed as soon as possible following the workout, but preferably immediately after the drill is done. The key question you should always be seeking the answer to is, *Did I accomplish the purpose of the workout?*

When you've followed all four steps in the training process for each workout, you've come full circle back to step 1 for the next workout. But before finalizing the purpose for the next workout, you need to assess your progress to date relative to your seasonal goal. If you're coming along as planned, then continue to the next workout. Otherwise, if you're seeing a trend where things aren't going as planned, you may need to reconsider your goal and adjust your training strategy appropriately.

TRAINING TECHNOLOGY

Step 4 in purposeful training calls for analysis. Many athletes don't like doing analysis. That's understandable because it's tedious work. This is where having an expert working with you can make a big difference. A coach knows what to look for and can explain it to you. But if you enjoy crunching data after a workout, then you just need to know what to look for.

The first objective is to determine if the workout accomplished its purpose, and secondarily to see how it contributed to your goal. So what are you going to measure and how can you do it? This brings us to training technology, the equipment commonly used for analysis.

There are only three things to measure in your training: frequency, duration, and intensity. In the next chapter, we'll take an in-depth look at all three. For now, though, we need only to take a brief look at two aspects of your workouts: duration and intensity.

It's helpful to have some sort of technology to measure the duration and intensity of your workouts. Duration is easy. A clock or stopwatch will do. But measuring workout intensity is quite difficult. This is where advanced technology can help make your workouts more productive, not only in terms of getting the intensity right during the session but also in getting immediate feedback in the form of workout analysis afterward.

The mention of technology often ruffles feathers. There have always been athletes who are adamantly opposed to technology in sports, no matter what it is. When rear derailleurs were invented for bicycles in the early 1900s, there were athletes who refused to use them. When bicycle speedometers came into use in the 1930s, many were opposed to them. When heart rate monitors were introduced in the 1980s, they were adamantly opposed by many. All were too "techie" for some. No matter what the technology is, some people will always be opposed. They think of themselves as "purists" who maintain the spirit of competitive sports. They dislike numbers.

And, to be honest, advanced, high-tech equipment is not necessary for everyone. Some experienced athletes are good at sensing how hard they are working. In fact, there are runners who can tell you their running pace to within a handful of seconds based on nothing more than experience and how they feel. They do indeed have a great sense of what they are doing. And if they are self-coached, not having any intensity-measuring technology seldom presents a problem. But if the athlete has a coach or mentor, that person can't know what happened in the workout. Not having data also means the athlete must accurately remember the sensations of each workout for weeks at a time in order to compare them, gauge progress, and determine how best to train. It's not very precise, but some can manage it, I've found.

However, intensity-measuring equipment will definitely help feel-based athletes analyze, gauge progress, and design future training, even if they never look at the device during a workout or race. Am I improving or not? How am I doing compared with this time last year? Am I getting enough racelike intensity in my training? How could I better pace my race? How did I pace the race the last time I did it? How did I manage the hills and wind? Technology will help you answer such questions by eliminating your reliance on memory and guesswork.

There are three intensity-measuring devices I require the triathletes I coach to have: a heart rate monitor, a speed-and-distance device for running (usually a Global Positioning System, or GPS), and a power meter for the bike. As I write, power-measuring devices have just been developed for runners. If they prove to be accurate and reliable, I will require my athletes to have running power meters, too. The power meter for running has the potential to change training for running the same way the power meter revolutionized cycling.

Why do I require these devices? Because the athlete and I will have much better data with which to make decisions. Not having accurate measurements puts the competitive athlete at quite a disadvantage. If you have a high-performance goal,

Accurate measurements give you a competitive advantage.

you should have the technology to help realize it. Training and racing without these devices greatly limits the athlete's development.

I understand that triathlon is an expensive sport and that having such devices adds to the cost. But prices are coming down for each of the devices I suggest you get. Sure, you can still buy top-of-the-line technology and spend a small fortune. But even the least expensive of these products are accurate at providing what you most need—a repeatable measurement of how hard you are working. Any money you spend beyond that basic information is for bells and whistles you don't really need, but perhaps want. If you are on a tight budget, check around with sporting goods shops and clubs for used equipment for sale. Athletes often upgrade to new technology and want to sell their old stuff.

Heart rate monitors, GPS devices, and power meters are not perfect. You need to learn how to use them, and that can take some dedicated study time. This, again, is where working with an expert makes life easier. Of course, it's also possible to become too focused on device numbers, especially when the equipment is brand-new and you're still learning how to use it. For example, there is a safety issue. Riding in traffic while focusing intently on the numbers displayed on your power monitoring device is not wise.

There can also be a loss of "feel" for the athlete who becomes overly dedicated to numbers. From what I said above, it may seem that I'm opposed to training and racing based on the sensations you are experiencing in your body, but that is not the case at all. I often have athletes put a piece of tape over the display on their device and train based only on feel. It's a good way to learn the art of training and racing. If you had a bad race

because the battery on your device died, then you haven't learned the art of endurance sport. This "art" has to do with something called the rating of perceived exertion (RPE). We'll get into the details of how to use the high-tech equipment in Chapter 4. I will boil down all of the information there on how to use the equipment, as well as on how to use RPE.

The intensity for the workouts in this book is described in terms of RPE (all three sports), pace (swim and run), heart rate (run and bike), and power (bike). A few of the workouts require comparing different measures of intensity, such as heart rate and pace, or heart rate and power. You can do the workouts without one of the devices, but the feedback is greatly lacking without both.

SUMMARY: PHYSICAL FITNESS

You should now have the basic components necessary to organize a training program for high-performance triathlon. The starting place is determining your triathlon racing potential by looking back at how you've trained in the past. The less structured your training has been and the more inconsistently you've trained, the greater your potential for performing at a high level. That can be good news. Of course, to make that happen, we have to assume that going forward you will give greater structure to your exercise program and do your best to complete every workout. For best results, the structure of your program should be based on purposeful training. That starts with having a goal-oriented purpose for every workout, having the workout expertly designed, paying close attention to carrying out the details of the session, and getting

I often have athletes put tape over the display and train based only on feel.

For best results, your program should be based on purposeful training.

feedback on how it went as soon as possible after the session is over.

Your ultimate success as a triathlete depends on incorporating all of these purposeful training steps and then evaluating how you're doing on a frequent (at least weekly, although more often is even better) schedule.

To get the details of the workout right while you're doing it and to get feedback afterward require measuring both the duration and the intensity of the session. While duration is easy to measure, intensity is much more complex and at least as important as duration—perhaps more

so (we'll get into this issue in the next chapter). Intensity is best measured with devices that keep the workout on track in real time and provide feedback after it's over. The most common intensity-measuring devices are heart rate monitors, GPS devices, and power meters. To truly perform at the highest level possible, given your potential, all three of these devices are beneficial depending on the workout's sport. Some unique athletes can get by without them, but they are rare. Most of us will improve much more rapidly with such technology. I think you'll see why in Part II.

TRAINING FUNDAMENTALS

What is fitness? That seems like a simple question that is easy to answer. After all, you and your training partners use that word a lot. How about fatigue? I'm sure you've been there, but what is it really? Then there's form. That's a bit vaguer than the others, although serious athletes seem to understand the concept.

Are you familiar with aerobic and anaerobic thresholds? Do you have a sense of when you are experiencing these levels of intensity and how they can be used to optimize your training?

Fitness, fatigue, form, thresholds, and intensity are all fundamental training concepts that are drawn from the science behind training. They are more complicated than they may first appear to be. But don't worry—I'm not going to try to make you into a sports scientist in this part of the book. There is a lot that we can learn from science, however, about how and why we should train in certain ways. That's what I want to introduce to you in the next two chapters.

We'll start in Chapter 3 by digging, although not too deeply, into the science of training. By the time you've finished this chapter, you'll have a well-grounded understanding of how training works. Then, in Chapter 4, we'll delve into what is perhaps the most critical aspect of training for the high-performance athlete—intensity.

Let's get started learning about the fundamentals of training.

BASIC TRAINING CONCEPTS

THIS CHAPTER introduces concepts that are fundamental to training for high performance. Each of the topics that we will explore has grown from an understanding of how the human body operates, especially for endurance sports. Most of what you read here will probably make a lot of sense. You may already understand many of these concepts, but you've probably never given them much thought because they seem to be so basic. They are so critical to your success, however, that we need to ensure that you have a handle on each and every one of them. You'll learn here what they are about, and in later chapters I'll show you how to apply them so that your training produces the desired results. Once you understand how to use these concepts in the real world of triathlon training, you will greatly improve your fitness and race performance.

TRAINING PRINCIPLES

Preparing for an important race involves getting many different things right in your training. But the starting point is developing a thorough understanding of four bedrock principles of training: overload, specificity, reversibility, and individuality. You must adhere closely to these principles to prepare effectively. While these principles are the products of academia and science, they are superficially obvious to most serious athletes, and I'm sure you will be nodding your head in agreement throughout this chapter. Occasionally, however, we make a mistake in training because we do not fully understand them. Yet everything in training boils down to them, and much of what you will read in the rest of this book is ultimately based on them. Therefore, as you read this chapter, consider how you've trained in the past to see if you have always appropriately applied these principles in your workouts and planning. Later in the book, you'll learn how to use them in order to grow as an athlete.

The Principle of Progressive Overload

Training load is a measure of how demanding your workouts are. If the training load stays the same week after week, your body will adapt to it and no longer grow stronger and fitter. That means your race performance will stabilize. There are times when that is a good thing, such as shortly before a race when you are tapering to get rid of fatigue. But most of the time, it's good to see positive fitness changes taking place.

For your fitness to improve steadily over time, your training load must gradually increase. That's where the word *overload* comes in. You make the workouts more challenging. You do that by training more frequently, by doing longer workouts, or by doing workouts with a higher intensity.

Progressive is the other key word here. The increases you make in training difficulty can't be overly great and rapid or your body will soon break down, especially if you've also been limiting rest and recovery in order to train harder. To train *progressively*, the training increases should be small. Increases of 10 percent are managed quite well by the body. If the workouts are made a great deal harder than that—especially if you increase the training load well beyond 10 percent and continue that way for a few weeks (or even a few days)—you greatly increase your risk for injury, illness, mental burnout, or overtraining. You'll certainly stop making fitness gains and most likely will take a huge step backward.

The take-home message of the principle of progressive overload is that you should be quite conservative in how quickly you ramp up the difficulty of your training. Remember *moderation* from Chapter 2? If you pay close attention, your body will tell you when the time is right to turn up the difficulty knob by one small click. In later chapters, we'll explore how to listen to your body effectively so that the overload is gradually progressive.

The Principle of Specificity

There are two broad, physiological categories of fitness changes that take place in your body when you exercise. Sports scientists refer to one category as *central* and the other as *peripheral*. *Central* changes are those that occur primarily in the heart, lungs, and blood. It doesn't make much difference which endurance sport you participate in for these changes to happen. The heart, for example, doesn't know the difference between running and biking. It simply pumps oxygen-rich blood regardless of what type of exercise is being done. So the cross-training benefits of triathlon workouts for the central systems are excellent.

Peripheral fitness has to do with the muscles. You can't fool a calf muscle. It knows the difference between running and biking. Although it's used in both, the ways in which it's used in these two sports are completely different. So you can't train your calf muscle to be fit for running by riding your bike. The same goes for all other muscles that are the primary movers in the three sports. They must be trained in a way that is very *specific* to the sport. The cross-training benefit is largely ineffective for the muscles. The possible exception is strength training with weights and doing other forms of gym exercises to increase the

Training load is a measure of how demanding your workouts are.

power of the muscles. But even here, the exercise movements in the gym must closely mimic the way the muscle is used in the sport. It isn't enough simply to load a working muscle with a lot of weight; you must move it under this load in a way that is very specific to the way the muscle is used during swimming, biking, or running. You'll see how this principle is applied to muscles in Chapter 13.

So which is more important, central fitness or peripheral fitness? As you've probably guessed, both are important. You'll never be a high-performance triathlete without both systems being well trained. Generally, the training season starts with an emphasis on the central systems and then gradually moves toward an emphasis on the muscular system. So we might say that the closer in time that you get to your most important race, the more your training emphasis should be placed on muscle fitness, which therefore means increasing training specificity. The demands of your workouts become increasingly like those of the race.

I've noticed that when athletes talk about training their muscles, they sometimes consider only what they do in the weight room. While muscle fitness can certainly be developed there, training the muscles by doing each of the three sports is much more important. The muscles must be taught to contract effectively and efficiently by making the movements of the sport *in* the sport. In Chapter 6, we'll get into swim, bike, and run workout categories called *muscular force* and *muscular endurance*. These have a lot to do with achieving your race potential through specific peripheral exercise.

Ultimately, your muscles are responsible for how fast you go in a race. They produce the power that propels you through the water, drives the pedals, and pushes you off the ground when you are running. The role of the heart, lungs, and blood is to respond to the demands of the muscles and supply what they need to contract forcefully. In that regard, we might conclude that the muscles are in charge, while the heart, lungs, and blood are only doing what is asked of them.

Of course, the more powerful your endurance muscles become, the greater the demands they place on the central systems. The bottom line here is that one without the other won't get the job done. You must have both operating at a high level to be a high-performance triathlete. But note that they can be trained differently. The central systems respond well no matter which sport is being done at the time. But the muscles, which may be the most critical system—and the most often overlooked by endurance athletes—demand specificity in training. You must train them by doing the sport in which you want to improve at the time, not by cross-training or by doing any other activity that raises your heart rate but doesn't stress the triathlon muscles in a *specific* way.

In Chapters 7 and 8, you will see how this principle of specificity plays out in the planning of your season and how the types of workouts you do change over time as a result.

The Principle of Reversibility

Reversibility has to do with losing fitness. There will be many times during the season when that happens (some of them intentional, as we'll see). Whenever your training load decreases, there will be negative consequences for your fitness. That's why I emphasized consistent training in Chapter 2.

Ultimately, your muscles are responsible for how fast you go in a race.

A zero in your training log means a loss of fitness. The loss from one missed workout is likely to be quite small, probably much less than 1 percent, but regaining it usually means doing two or more workouts for every one missed.

It can also be acceptable and even good to give up some fitness. One instance of this occurs in the days immediately following your most important and stressful race of the year. There aren't too many of these post-race periods, and the reduced training load (typically *not* a bunch of zeroes) will last only a handful of days. The most significant loss of fitness, assuming you aren't injured or sick for several days at a time, comes at the end of your season when you take a long—and necessary—break from focused training. We'll get into that in greater detail in Chapter 7.

The basic idea here is that fitness is always changing—sometimes positively and sometimes negatively. You have complete control over the direction. Moderate workouts lead to consistent training that results in greater fitness.

The Principle of Individuality

You are unique. I'm sure that's not a great revelation for you. Just as you're taller than some athletes and shorter than others, how fast you can swim, bike, and run is also unique to you. You may be a great runner, a poor swimmer, and a mediocre cyclist—or some other combination. That helps to define who you are as a triathlete. And just as your height and performance in each sport help to define who you are, your physiology is also unique in many more ways. You may deal with the heat well or suffer more than most when it's hot. You may be good at going up hills, but not so good when the course is flat. It could be that your body processes food well during a long

race while others would become nauseous eating the same thing. Yes, you are certainly unique in many ways.

Because you are unique, it therefore follows that your training must also be unique. You can't simply do what your training partner does and expect the same results. Even though your favorite pro triathlete does a certain workout, that doesn't mean it's a good one for you. The training program you follow must match *your* capabilities if you are to achieve your potential. Starting in Chapter 5, you will discover your unique characteristics, and in Chapters 7, 8, and 9, you'll learn how to design a training plan that is effective for *you*.

FREQUENCY, DURATION, AND INTENSITY

Let's take a look at another core concept you probably understand but may not have given much thought. This one has to do with what defines exercise. It is basic for understanding how to plan your training.

No matter how experienced you are as a triathlete, the only three things you can change in your training are frequency, duration, and intensity. Whether you are a seasoned triathlon veteran or a brand-new novice makes no difference. The three training variables you can change to improve your fitness are how often you work out, how long your workouts last, and how intense they are.

Actually, there is one more thing triathletes have to consider—the sport you do in the workout. But that's sort of a given, so we'll not consider it a variable here. We will, of course, get into which sports to do as workouts and how to do

A zero in your training log means a loss of fitness.

Because you are unique, your training must also be unique.

them in later chapters. For now, let's get a deeper understanding of the three basic training variables: frequency, duration, and intensity.

Frequency

How often do you work out? It's common for pro triathletes to do two or three workouts on most days, or about 18 to 20 sessions per week. Novice triathletes are more likely to do one workout per day—about seven in a week. There are obvious reasons for this. The pros must do a lot of frequent training to reap the small gains available because they are so near their fitness potential. For the novice triathlete, though, this certainly would be disastrous. Doing only a few workouts in a week will produce significant improvement for the athlete who is new to the sport.

How often do *you* train? How many workouts do *you* do in a week? For most of us, the answer depends on our lifestyles. While training to race is a pro's "job," it's more than likely not yours. You undoubtedly have a career, a family, and lots of other important stuff going on in your life every day. Yet somehow, you manage to shoehorn a couple of workouts into your very busy day. It's common for serious, age-group triathletes to do about two workouts daily, fitting in 10 to 12 in a week. That isn't easy by any means and places great physical and emotional demands on the athlete.

So the key for age-group triathletes is to make the best use of their quite limited and valuable "free" time. That implies doing the right workouts at the right times. There is no room for training mistakes. You can't be sloppy. Every workout must count. That's why I strongly suggest you have a detailed plan for your training. I know, planning doesn't sound like fun. But it's necessary if you want to reach your high-performance triathlon potential. Part IV will help you with planning.

Duration

Duration is a measure of the time length of a workout, not its distance. Athletes tend to think in terms of distance because races are designed that way. But a successful triathlete will prepare for a race by determining how much time it will take to complete. The point I want to make with you here is that it's the race time, not the race distance, that is critical to your success. So you need to think in terms of duration, not distance, in training. I'll explain that.

With rare exceptions, the workouts you will read about in this book are based on duration, not distance. The reason is that the intensity of a workout is specific to its length in time, but not necessarily to its distance. For example, if there are two runners in a 10-km race and one finishes in 30 minutes while the other, also working as hard as he can, finishes in 60 minutes, their intensities were not the same. The 30-minute finisher was working at a much higher intensity as a percentage of VO_2max (more on VO_2max in the next chapter). If they were both to run as hard as they could for 30 minutes, they would be at about the same intensity; one would simply cover more ground than the other. But races aren't designed that way.

Here's another example to help you understand why I suggest you use duration for your workouts. Let's say you're going to do a half-Ironman-distance race. The bike leg is a flat 90 km long, so you've trained to do it at a given intensity. But it just so happens that on race day it's extremely windy. The bike leg will probably take an additional 30 minutes to complete. What should you do about how intensely you'll ride the

> Duration is a measure of the time length of a workout, not its distance.

bike? Should you keep it as planned? After all, the race is still 90 km long. That hasn't changed. Or should you reduce the intensity because the duration will be longer?

The answer is to reduce the intensity. Intensity is *always* directly related to duration, not distance. If you keep the intensity the same but the bike portion takes an additional 30 minutes, you will fade badly in the last few kilometers and have a terrible run as a result.

The underlying rule here is that intensity is *inversely* related to time. This means that as one increases, the other decreases. As the time of a race or workout gets longer, the intensity you are capable of maintaining is reduced. It's obvious. You can't run a marathon at your 5-km pace. You run more slowly in the marathon because you have to run for a longer time. A 30-minute 10-km racer and a 60-minute 10-km racer are essentially not doing the same race, and they shouldn't train the same way either. If the race will take longer than planned because of environmental conditions such as wind, then you need to reduce the intensity. This is a long way of simply saying that the intensity of your workouts and races is more closely tied to their durations than to their distances.

Now let's take a closer look at the intensity of your training.

Intensity

Frequency and duration are very easy to measure. All you need is a calendar and a clock. Intensity is much more complex and difficult to measure. In Chapter 2, I told you that I require the advanced triathletes I coach to have a heart rate monitor, a GPS device, and a power meter. Why? Because intensity becomes increasingly critical to race performance as an athlete becomes more experi-

> The underlying rule is that intensity is inversely related to time.

enced and fit. Novices need to focus only on the frequency of training by getting into the pool and onto the road often. If they do this with no concern for how long the workout is—short is fine—or how hard it should be—easy is best—they will make great improvement in their first year in the sport. The intermediate triathlete in the second and third years in the sport should focus on increasing the durations of swims, bike rides, and runs. Year 4 is the time when a triathlete should begin to give greater emphasis to workout intensity. By then, he or she has made most of the gains possible from frequency and duration. That doesn't mean those two training components should be ignored. They're still important. However, for someone to continue growing as a triathlete after the first few years, intensity must become the training focus. Research has repeatedly shown this to be true.

Unfortunately, many advanced triathletes continue to believe that long-duration workouts are the key to their success. That, in part, is because duration is easy and cheap to measure, and athletes became hooked on it early in their sports careers. Accurate intensity measurement is neither easy nor cheap. Study is required if you are to become good at using it. And such equipment is certainly more expensive than a stopwatch.

In Chapter 4, we'll take an in-depth look at intensity and how it can help you become a high-performance triathlete once you know how to use it properly.

VOLUME

Volume is the combination of frequency and duration. Simply add up your hours for the week and you have volume. If you do 10 workouts in a week and each is 1 hour long, your weekly volume is 10 hours. Most triathletes think of their training progress in terms of volume. When asked how their training is going, most reply with how many weekly hours they are doing. Why? Because this number is easily measured and understood. And yet, as you read above, for the seasoned athlete intensity is the key to success. It's very difficult to quantify intensity, however.

This does not mean that volume is *unimportant* to the advanced triathlete. It's just less important than intensity. For the experienced, high-performance triathlete, volume accounts for roughly 40 percent of fitness, while intensity produces the remaining 60 percent.

So it's obvious that your focus should be on the intensity of your training. This doesn't mean that your workouts must be at the highest possible intensity. There are varying degrees of intensity, called *zones*, that we'll address in the next chapter. All of the zones are used in your training. How much time in each depends on the event for which you are training, your unique needs, and the current seasonal period. We'll come back to this concept several times in the remaining chapters because it's so critical to your success.

DOSE AND DENSITY

To produce the best possible race performance, you must get the emphasis on volume and intensity right in your training—somewhere around the ratio of 40 percent volume to 60 percent intensity explained above. This brings us to the concepts of dose and density.

Dose has to do with how hard a workout is. A very hard workout is called a *high dose*. This could be a long-duration workout, such as a very long swim, ride, or run. Or it could be a very high-intensity workout, such as intervals or hill repeats. It could also be a combination of duration and intensity—a long-duration workout with lots and lots of moderate intensity—such as training for an Ironman-distance triathlon. On the other hand, a low-dose workout is typically of short duration and low intensity.

Density has to do with how closely spaced the high-dose workouts are. High-density training means that your hardest workouts are very close to each other—perhaps separated by only 1 day or even done on back-to-back days. In the same way, low-density training would mean there are several low-dose days between the hardest sessions.

Dose and density aren't the same for all athletes. Given the principle of individuality, they are unique to your specific needs and capabilities. The dose of each workout must be chosen based on your current needs. But all advanced athletes must do high-dose workouts specific to their goal race from time to time. The durations and intensities of those workouts will vary based on the type of race for which you are training. Long-course triathletes do high-duration, moderate-intensity workouts in the last few weeks before a race. For short-course triathletes, the workout durations are not as long, but the workout intensities are greater.

Within those race-specific parameters, the dose is quite similar regardless of who the athlete is. Density, however, varies considerably among athletes training for the same types of events. Typically, younger and fitter triathletes train with high density—their hard workouts are closely spaced. The older or the less fit you are, the lower the density of your training. In other

Volume accounts for roughly 40 percent of fitness, intensity for 60 percent.

The older or the less fit you are, the lower the density of your training.

words, there are more easy, low-dose workouts between the high-dose sessions.

This concept of dose and density may be new to you, but if you've been around the sport and training seriously for a few years, you should readily understand it because you've undoubtedly trained that way—even if you never thought about it this way. Later on, when we get into training periodization, you'll give dose and density a lot of thought because they ultimately have a lot to do with how fit you become.

TRAINING LOAD

When volume and intensity are combined, the result is something called *training load*. Some triathletes can handle an extremely high training load. They may put in 20 hours in a week that includes high-intensity intervals and several other sessions that are equally challenging. Their dose and density are quite high. Others can manage only a handful of hours a week along with one or two high-dose sessions. The reason again often has to do with the individuality principle. But there are other factors that determine training load, the most common of which is available time.

If your career is demanding, especially with long work hours, then your training load is likely to be at the low end. In the same way, family and home responsibilities determine your available time and therefore training load. Such lifestyle factors have a lot to do with volume. Whenever workout duration is decreased below what you would be capable of handling were there no such time constraints, then training intensity must be increased to produce an adequate training load for achieving high-performance racing. That's

a conundrum many age group triathletes must deal with. We'll get into how all of this is done in Chapter 7 as we study periodization.

SUPERCOMPENSATION

The training load should be great at times. As a result, you will often be tired. That's why we include rest-and-recovery days between hard workouts. It's during these easy days that the body actually becomes more fit. That's because a high-dose workout produces only the potential for fitness. Fitness is realized in the subsequent low-dose day, which may be either a day off from exercise or a short and low-intensity session. This process of alternating stress and rest is necessary to become more fit.

If you apply only high-dose and high-density stress and do not recover frequently, you will likely experience overtraining (see Chapter 10). This is not just a little fatigue. It's much more serious than that. Overtraining is very much like having a severe illness, such as mononucleosis or chronic fatigue syndrome. You must avoid it. I've seen it end triathlon careers. On the other hand, if you rest only by doing low-dose workouts and frequently take days off from training, you will not produce a positive change in fitness. The principle of progressive overload is violated, and race performance will suffer.

The process of building greater fitness by alternating stress and rest is called *supercompensation*. The human body is an amazing organism that can be molded through consistent training to produce an athlete capable of achieving great things in sports. Supercompensation can't be forced on the body. You cannot make it happen at a faster rate than nature intends. Nature has endowed some lucky individuals with a fast response time. Others respond slowly. This is just the principle of individuality showing up again. The difference between a slow and a fast responder is likely genetic in origin. This is why in order to avoid overtraining while trying to improve fitness, you must pay close attention to how your body is responding and not try to speed it up artificially.

FITNESS, FATIGUE, AND FORM

So far, I've used the words *fit* and *fitness* quite a bit in talking about your training. I've assumed that those words make perfect sense to you. In endurance sports, we commonly talk about fitness without ever thinking about what it means. In Chapter 6, we'll get into a deeper understanding of fitness for triathlon. For now, let's think of fitness as meaning readiness to race. In what follows, I will introduce a way of thinking about race readiness that is rather novel, but again something you probably already fully understand even though you've never given it much thought. I'll also introduce two other concepts that are directly related to race readiness: fatigue and form.

Fitness

There are four common ways triathletes determine changes in their race readiness. The one we are most interested in has to do with race results. That's the ultimate measure for the serious athlete. Did you achieve your targeted race goal? If so, then you were very fit on race day. So we can deduce that your training before the race must have gone quite well. Race results don't lie.

While hitting your goal may be the ultimate gauge of race readiness, it comes a bit late. You are likely to sleep better the night before a race if there were indicators during the previous weeks that your fitness was making steady gains. So how do you do that? Here are three other common ways of determining fitness.

Along the way, as you're preparing for the race, you will frequently take note of how your workouts are going and how you feel while doing them. This information will often indicate the direction of your fitness—increasing, stable, or decreasing. It can be quite subjective, especially judging how fit you are feeling, yet this is still good information about your progress. You can't take it to the bank, however.

If you want to get *objective* feedback about your fitness progress, you can go to a clinic for testing. The technician will hook you up to high-tech equipment and put you through your paces for several increasingly grueling minutes. And when it's all over, you'll be given a printout with a set of numbers that tell you how fit you are. This is good information, and if the testing is done a few times in a season, it reveals your fitness progress as you prepare for the race. Although an excellent and objective way of actually measuring fitness, however, such testing can become rather expensive.

A fourth way is to measure your daily training load and determine its progress over time. This method merely applies numbers to the "how you feel" method described above. As explained earlier, training load is the combination of volume and intensity. If training load is increasing over time, your fitness is also increasing because you're able to handle a greater dose and also perhaps a higher density. That's an

Race results don't lie.

TABLE 3.1 Sample 60-Minute Workout "Score" Based on Time in Each Training Zone

A. ZONE AND VALUE	B. TIME IN ZONE (TO NEAREST MINUTE)	ZONE SCORE (A × B)
1	30	30
2	8	16
3	5	15
4	15	60
5	2	10
	Total: 60 minutes	Workout Score: 131

Intensity
plus duration
gives you a
workout score.

indirect measure of increasing fitness. So measuring and keeping track of your training load over time reveals a great deal about how fit you are becoming.

The problem, of course, is combining workout duration, which is easy to measure with a clock, and intensity, which is much more challenging to measure. Even if you can easily measure intensity, how do you combine it with duration? One way, which has been around for a long time, involves the use of a heart rate monitor, a clock, and software to produce a workout "score" every day. The daily scores are then added together at the end of the week to come up with a training load number that can be compared with other weekly training loads going forward. If the training load is increasing, you can assume that your fitness is improving because you're now capable of handling more physical stress than you were earlier in the season.

Here's how it works. At the completion of your workout, download your heart rate monitor to your software. Your software should already be set up to show how much time you spent in each heart rate training zone. (Chapter 4 will help you set up zones.) Assuming you use a five-zone system, which is the most common method, a numerical value is automatically assigned to

each zone. For example, zone 1 is assigned a value of 1 and zone 5 gets a value of 5. The other, in-between zones are assigned values of 2, 3, and 4, respectively. Then you multiply each zone's value by the time spent in each zone in minutes. Add all of the resulting numbers and you have the workout score. You can also do this with a power meter or a GPS device, or anything that measures intensity for which you have zones. Table 3.1 provides an example of how a workout may be scored with this system.

The athlete's 1-hour workout shown in Table 3.1 produced a total workout score of 131. In the same way, each workout would be scored over the course of a week, and then at the end of the week all of the individual workout scores would be added together to result in the week's training load. While this way of producing a training load number is simple, it is quite tedious and time-consuming to produce.

An easier way is to use software that calculates a workout score for you after you've downloaded your heart rate monitor (or power meter or GPS device) to it. Perhaps the most powerful such system was developed by sports scientist Andrew Coggan, PhD, and is found on the web site TrainingPeaks (www.TrainingPeaks.com). His system, called the *training stress score*, is widely used by athletes in many endurance sports. The software does all of the number crunching for you.

Keeping track of your training load through such a scoring system week after week gives you a good idea of how fit you are becoming. If you are able to increase your training load gradually over time, you can conclude that you are becoming more fit. The TrainingPeaks web site provides another tool, called the *performance management chart*, that shows your training load progress over the course of the season. In a similar way, it also reveals your fatigue.

Fatigue

When training load increases, you can surmise that fitness is increasing. We can also assume that fatigue is increasing. And with good reason. If you are training with greater volume and intensity, you are bound to be tired. On the other side of the coin, if your training load is decreasing, you are losing fitness, but you also aren't as tired. So fitness and fatigue trend in the same direction relative to training load. When one is rising, the other is also rising. When one falls, the other also falls.

Fatigue always appears before fitness. If you do a hard workout today, you will be tired tomorrow. It will be quite evident by the way you feel. But we won't be able to measure a change in fitness tomorrow. Fitness changes very slowly, while fatigue changes rapidly. This is a good thing and something you will learn in Chapter 9 to use as you taper for an important race. The purpose of the taper is to produce form on race day.

Form

You may hear the word *form* a lot, especially when listening to TV announcers describing how well an athlete is performing. They may say, "He's on form," or "He's lacking form." What exactly does form mean?

The concept of form in sport is thought to have originated in the late 1800s with horse racing in Europe. If you went to a race and wanted to place a bet, you would find a "bookie"—a bookkeeper who keeps the records on bets. The bookie would provide a sheet of paper—a form—with a list of all of the horses racing that day and how they had raced recently. You would then pick one to put your money on because *on the form* that horse appeared to be racing well. Bike racing, which was starting at about the same time in Europe, also was a betting sport with similar forms. So bike racing adopted the word. Over the next century, other sports also began to talk about form.

So what exactly does *form* mean? From the above, you can tell that it means race-ready. That can be taken to mean that the athlete is fresh, rested. If fatigue is high, you can't be on form no matter how great your fitness is. Fatigue will stifle your performance. The only way to be fresh on race day is to rest in the preceding days by doing what we commonly call a *taper*.

Recall that I explained above that fitness and fatigue trend the same direction. When one is rising, the other is also rising. And when one falls, the other falls. So if fatigue is falling, what is happening to fitness? It's also falling. I know that sounds scary when you are tapering for a race. How will you race well if your fitness drops? The key to understanding this is also found above: Fatigue changes more rapidly than fitness when you are resting. So while a pre-race taper will shed a lot of fatigue quickly, fitness will be lost very slowly. On race day you will *feel* as if you had gained fitness, even though that feeling is

When training load increases, you can surmise that fitness is increasing.

The only way to be fresh on race day is to taper in the preceding days.

actually the result of having less fatigue. It doesn't matter—you'll be *on form*. In Chapter 9, I'll show you how to pull this off so that you lose only a tiny amount of fitness while getting rid of all the fatigue. Understanding and applying this concept is key in high-performance racing.

SUMMARY: BASIC TRAINING CONCEPTS

Whew! That was a lot of what you've probably thought of before as simple ideas about training. If you've been around endurance sports for a few years, there may not have been any new training concepts for you here—but I believe you may now have new ways of thinking about them. I hope you also have a deeper understanding of each of them. We'll return to these concepts frequently in the following chapters as you read about how to apply them to your training. Thoroughly understanding them gives you a deeper appreciation of the many subtle nuances of training.

Training is nothing more than the interplay of all of these concepts. It isn't just how long

the workout is or how many hours you do in a week; it's how intensely you work out. It isn't merely how hard the workouts are, but also how closely spaced they are. Putting in lots of hard training hours isn't the goal; supercompensation through well-timed rest is. Fitness must be thought of in relation to fatigue and form, not as an independent, stand-alone objective. And all of this is blended together through the principles of training: overload, specificity, reversibility, and individuality. Getting all of this right is what will lead you to high performance and goal achievement.

Note that many of these concepts involve understanding the intensity of training. As noted above, intensity is the key component for the serious and experienced athlete. If you have a high goal for the coming season, how well you manage your workout intensity will have a lot to do with your success. It accounts for roughly 60 percent of your race performance, while workout duration makes up the remainder. So you need to have a deep understanding of training intensity. That's where we're going next.

TRAINING INTENSITY

IN THIS CHAPTER, we're going to take a hard look at a topic that age-group triathletes, including those who are very serious about the sport, don't fully appreciate. Why do I think that? When I ask any athletes about how their training is going, they almost always answer by telling me the volume of their training—how many weekly hours they are putting in. It's rare to find someone who doesn't answer this basic question that way. And yet, research study after research study tells us that the most important element of training for the advanced athlete is intensity. Sure, serious triathletes sometimes (perhaps too often) do hard and even very hard training sessions. Who hasn't? And they know it has an effect on their fitness. No question about that. The sticking point is that intensity is difficult to explain briefly when you are answering the question of how training is going.

In this chapter, we'll start down the road toward being able to talk about training in a broader context by coming to understand a bit more about the intensity of your training. It's a huge topic that will continue into many subsequent chapters.

MEASURING INTENSITY

In Chapter 3, I introduced the three variables you can change around to produce your weekly training schedule. The first was the frequency of your workouts—how often you do workouts. This is easy to measure. All you need is a calendar. Merely count how many times you swam, rode your bike, and ran in a week and you have frequency. Duration is also simple to measure. All that's needed is a stopwatch. How long was your workout? If we add up the times of all your workouts for a week, we have your training volume, which is nothing more than the combination of frequency and duration.

Intensity is different. It's much more difficult to measure. Special tools or skills are required. Currently, there are four ways a triathlete can measure workout intensity, depending on the sport: rating of perceived exertion, pace, heart rate, and power. For the experienced triathlete—someone who has been in the sport for more than 3 years—intensity is the key to high performance. To achieve your potential, you need to understand and be able to use these common measures of intensity.

Rating of Perceived Exertion

The most basic way to measure intensity, and one that all triathletes need to master, is called *rating of perceived exertion* (RPE). For this, you simply assign a level of intensity to a workout with a numeric scale. The most common scale is from 0 to 10. At the low end, 0 means no exercise intensity at all, and 1 indicates you're moving really slowly at a low level of effort. At the high end, 10 means as hard as you can go given the duration. Table 4.1 shows the entire scale.

Becoming skilled in the use of this scale is an art that is learned by using it frequently. While you are swimming, biking, and running, give some thought to how hard the level of intensity feels at the moment and use the scale to assign a rating. By doing this frequently, you'll eventually become very good at using RPE. You'll probably discover it's more difficult to rank your effort when you are training with partners than when you are alone. It's common for athletes to assign a lower RPE to any given level of intensity when they are with others.

TABLE 4.1 The Borg 10-Point Scale for RPE

RATING	PERCEIVED EXERTION
0	Nothing at all
1	Very light
2	Light
3	Moderate
4	Somewhat hard
5–6	Hard
7–8	Very hard
9	Very, very hard (almost maximal)
10	Maximal

RPE is highly subjective. In fact, that's all it is—your opinion of how you feel while exercising. To be more precise, you need to use tools for measuring intensity that are objective. The most common ones to use are a heart rate monitor, a speed-and-distance device such as a Global Positioning System (GPS), and a power meter. In Chapter 2, I suggested that these tools are very beneficial for training. Measuring intensity accurately is so important that I require the athletes I coach to have all of these tools. Later in this chapter, I'll give you a quick tutorial in how to set training zones for each of them. Each measures intensity in a unique way, providing information that is not available from the other two.

Pace

Pace, or how fast you're going per mile or kilometer, has been around as long as athletes have been swimming, biking, and running. Well into the late 20th century, it was the only way intensity in endurance sport could be measured precisely. Every athlete had access to a stopwatch for this purpose and described workout intensity by expressing pace. "I ran 3 miles at a 7-minute pace," or "I swam 1,000 meters at 1 minute 30 seconds per 100," was how workout intensity was explained. That didn't work so well for cyclists because outside factors such as wind, hills, and drafting made pace (or speed) quite imprecise. As a result, training for cycling was the least scientific of the training for the three sports and depended heavily on RPE for gauging intensity. So bike training was strictly subjective.

Today, pace is still commonly used in swimming and running. And because swimming in a pool means the distance of the workout is well controlled and there is typically a clock on the wall, pace is easily measured and therefore still the primary way of conveying intensity. Pace is a little less meaningful for a runner because there are seldom mile markers on the roads where running takes place. So heart rate has become the common intensity metric for runners. In recent years, runners have also started using GPS devices to measure pace. As you will learn later in this book, both pace (or speed) and heart rate are valuable information to have when training. I'll eventually teach you how to combine these to train your aerobic endurance fitness.

Heart Rate

Heart rate monitors have been around since they were invented in the late 1970s in Finland. It wasn't until the early 1990s that the tipping point was reached for their common use by endurance athletes. It took about 15 years for the vast majority of runners and cyclists to adopt this technology. Triathletes were among the first to use heart rate monitors but found that they didn't work very well when they were swimming.

Heart rate tells you how intensely you are working. It does not tell you anything about performance. The last finisher in a race can have the same average heart rate as the winner. There are no podium positions for high heart rates. Your heart rate doesn't tell you how fast you are going; all it tells you is how much effort is going into the workout. But when it comes to precisely measuring effort, it's the best tool we have. In that regard, heart rate is very much like RPE, only more objective.

Power

The mobile power meter was invented in the late 1980s by a German engineer turned cyclist. It took about 20 years for cyclists and triathletes to adopt it widely as a tool for measuring intensity. Since riders' acceptance of the power meter, cycling has moved from being the least to the most scientific of the three sports. The power meter has revolutionized bike training. As of this writing, there are companies working on developing power meters for running. It's not known yet how accurate and reliable they will be, but if they live up to the standards created by bike power meters, then run training is also in for a dramatic change.

A bike power meter measures two things: the force that's applied to the pedal and the speed at which the pedals are turned. Pedal force is called *torque*. Pedal speed is called *cadence*. The combination of the two is expressed in *watts*. Suffice it to say for now that learning how to use a power meter has the potential to improve your training and racing greatly. (It's beyond the scope of this book to go into the details of power meter use. To learn more about how power meters work and how to train with them, see my book, *The Power Meter Handbook*.)

Heart rate tells you how intensely you are working.

A bike power meter measures the force at the pedal and the pedaling cadence.

INTENSITY REFERENCE POINTS

I should warn you that in this section on intensity I'll get a little "sciency." Bear with me as I try to explain the meaning of the terms I use throughout the book when talking about intensity. I'll try to keep it as painless as possible.

Sports scientists often use RPE when gauging the intensity of exercise because it tells them what the athlete is experiencing. But they also like to have physiological markers of intensity that serve as the athlete's fixed reference points for the effort. Two of the most commonly used markers are called *aerobic threshold* (AeT) and *anaerobic threshold* (AnT). I'll refer to each of these many times in the following chapters, and they will also have a lot to do with your workouts. For now, we'll take a ten-thousand-foot view to get a general idea of what they mean. Later on, we'll dig into them more deeply.

Figure 4.1 compares these markers with RPE to give you an idea of how intense each is. With this figure in mind, let's get a general overview of these intensity reference points.

Aerobic Threshold (AeT)

There are various ways sports scientists measure intensity during exercise in the lab. A common way is to capture a drop of the athlete's blood by pinpricking a finger or an earlobe and then analyzing the blood in a machine specially designed for this purpose. The blood contains something you've undoubtedly heard of—lactate. Lactate in and of itself is not the "problem child" we've been told it is. It has nothing to do with fatigue or muscle soreness. It is, however, a good predictor of how intensely an athlete is exercising. The

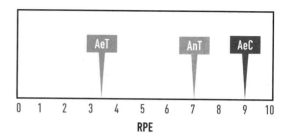

FIGURE 4.1 Intensity reference points compared with RPE

more lactate in the blood, the greater the exertion. Scientists measure lactate in millimoles per liter (mmol/L). At rest (0 RPE), lactate is about 1 mmol/L. This is a very tiny amount. As the exercise intensity increases to around 3 or 4 RPE and lactate in the drop of blood rises to 2 mmol/L, the athlete is often said to be at aerobic threshold.

AeT can also be determined in other ways. In the lab, another common way is to measure the oxygen and carbon dioxide the athlete breathes in and out during exercise. This "gas analysis" method predicts changes in lactate levels. It's noninvasive—no blood is drawn. But it still requires an expensive test.

That's a lot of scientific gobbledygook. You don't really have to understand all of it or have lab testing done to find your AeT. A much simpler and far less expensive method you can use simply requires a heart rate monitor, which you probably already have. AeT typically occurs at a heart rate of around 65 percent of max heart rate. You don't even have to know what that is, for another method places your AeT at roughly 20–40 beats per minute (bpm) below anaerobic threshold (note the *an-*, meaning "not" aerobic). We'll come back to that reference point next. So, short of going to a lab to be tested, you can watch your heart rate while exercising and assume that at 30 bpm below anaerobic threshold, you are close to your AeT.

Lactate in and of itself is not the "problem child" we've been told it is.

Later on, I'll teach you how to use this critical intensity level in training to fully develop your aerobic system. It makes for a great workout that, as you'll see, I suggest you do frequently.

Anaerobic Threshold (AnT)

Anaerobic threshold is the higher of the two intensity reference points. Here, you begin to "redline" during exercise. The effort is high on the RPE scale, at about 7. When you reach this level of exertion in a workout or race, you're working hard and realize that you won't be able to maintain it for very long because "suffering" is just beginning. The general intensity at which you reach AnT is also referred to as *lactate threshold*. From a sports scientist's perspective, the lactate and anaerobic thresholds aren't exactly the same thing because one is determined by using a gas analysis test (AnT) while the other is determined by measuring the lactate in a drop of blood (lactate threshold). But for our purpose we'll use the terms interchangeably.

You read above that when lactate reaches a level of 2 mmol/L in the blood you are at about your AeT. When it reaches 4 mmol/L you're at AnT. At the lower level, the body removes the lactate-associated acid flooding the muscles as quickly as it's produced. But at 4 mmol/L and higher, the acid in the form of hydrogen ions (and perhaps other chemicals, such as inorganic phosphate) begins to accumulate and so restricts muscle contraction. That's why you start to suffer and can maintain this level of intensity for only a limited amount of time. An athlete in good physical condition can maintain an intensity at AnT for about an hour, whereas intensity at AeT can be sustained for several hours.

With the right type of training, your AnT can be raised so that you go faster before it's reached. But note that your heart rate will remain about the same when you are at AnT despite changes in fitness. That's an important lesson we'll examine more closely later in this chapter. It has to do with what we call *fitness*.

Most triathlons are raced at intensities between AeT and AnT, as shown in Figure 4.2. In an Ironman triathlon, you will be near your AeT and the RPE will be on the low end of the scale. At the other end of the RPE scale, when doing a sprint triathlon, you're likely to be a little below or above your AnT, around an RPE of 7. In other words, there is an inverse relationship between intensity and duration. The harder you work, the shorter the duration of the race. And the lower the intensity, the longer the race duration. This should be obvious—you know you can't race an Ironman at sprint-distance intensity. We'll return to this basic concept in several of the following chapters.

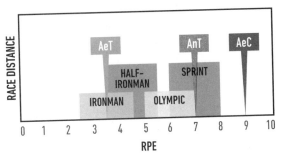

FIGURE 4.2 Intensity reference points compared with RPE and standard triathlon race distances

Aerobic Capacity (AeC)

Aerobic capacity, also known as VO$_2$max, defines your ability to use oxygen to produce energy. In general, the higher your AeC, the greater your potential power or speed. Aerobic capacity isn't important to our discussion here;

Intensity at AnT can be maintained for about one hour; at AeT for several hours.

instead, we'll look at it in Chapter 6, as we learn how to build fitness.

Functional Threshold (FT)

Between AeT and AnT, the more critical for your training and racing is AnT because if you know it, you can roughly estimate AeT by subtracting 30 bpm from AnT heart rate. The AnT is also more easily recognized by the athlete because there is a very definite sense of suffering that accompanies it. Once you know this critical reference point, it's easy to set up training zones, which we'll get to shortly.

The downside of all of this is understanding the science behind AnT, the lab test needed to identify it initially, and then the periodic tests in the lab to measure what's happening to it over time in order to gauge changes in fitness accurately. Although testing provides good information, it is not cheap. This is where a sports scientist by the name of Andrew Coggan, PhD, comes in.

Dr. Coggan is also a cyclist who came up with an idea in the early 2000s that revolutionized the whole process of setting zones. He not only simplified the concept of AnT but also greatly reduced the need for lab testing to identify it and gauge fitness progress. His thinking went something like this: If we know that a well-conditioned endurance athlete can maintain AnT for about an hour, why not just do a 1-hour time trial and assume that the average heart rate, average pace, and average power for that hour represent AnT? Brilliant! This is easily understood by everyone, and there is no cost for expensive testing. Anyone can do it anytime. He called this new reference point the *functional threshold.*

So FT is a simple stand-in for your AnT. This means that you have a functional threshold heart rate (FTHR), a functional threshold pace (FTPa), and a functional threshold power (FTPo). Each is simply the average of that metric from a 1-hour time trial. And just like AnT, they all vary by sport. For example, FTHR is not the same for cycling and running. It tends to be a bit higher for running than it is for cycling, and higher for cycling than for swimming.

The downside of Dr. Coggan's idea, of course, is that a 1-hour time trial done as a workout is extremely painful. Most people could never come up with the motivation to go as hard as possible alone for an hour. We always feel sorry for ourselves and so we slow down after the first few minutes of suffering. The results of such a field test would be too low to predict something close to AnT.

If there are frequent stand-alone (not triathlon) swim, bike, or run races where you live that take you about an hour to complete, then those races provide the perfect opportunity for field testing. That's unlikely, however.

To solve this dilemma, Dr. Coggan came up with a simple field test you can do anytime that doesn't take an hour of suffering. For cycling and running, it takes only 20 minutes. You still suffer, only not as long. The swim test is a bit different. We'll come back to it shortly. Once you know your FTHR for cycling and running, FTPa (running), and FTPo (cycling), you can set your intensity zones and you're ready to train. Let's see how that is done.

SETTING TRAINING ZONES

The reason you don't use a triathlon to set zones is that in a multisport race, you must hold back just a bit for each portion so you have enough energy to finish the entire race. To get usable data

Set intensity zones with FTHR for cycling and running, FTPa (running), and FTPo (cycling).

The field test effort must be as hard as you can go for about 20 minutes.

to set your zones, the field test effort must be *as hard as you can go* for about 20 minutes. If you have to hold back on the effort in order to finish the entire triathlon—which you should—then the data you get will be too low for setting accurate heart rate, pace, and power zones. In other words, you could have gone harder—meaning a higher heart rate, faster pace, and greater power output—had it been a stand-alone swim, bike, or run race. With that in mind, let's get on with setting your training zones.

Swim Pace Zones

For the swim test, we're going to deviate a bit from Dr. Coggan's 20-minute protocol because this is the one sport in which distance is generally easier to work with than duration. A measured pool provides a standard that can be used anywhere and anytime to test FT.

There are many ways of conducting a swim-pacing test. The standard field test I use is based on a 1,000-meter (or yard) time trial. What you want to find in this time trial is called your *T-time*, which is your average pace for 100 meters (or yards). After warming up, swim 1,000 meters (or yards) as if it were a race. It may help to have someone on deck counting laps because it's easy to lose track. To determine your pace zones, use Table 4.2. Find your 1,000-meter (or yard) finishing time in the left-hand column. Read across the table to the right to find your swim pace training zone T-times. These zones are then used to determine pacing for swim workouts, as suggested in Appendix B.

Bike and Run Heart Rate Zones

To set run and bike heart rate zones, we go back to Dr. Coggan's 20-minute test. Before getting into the details of this, however, I want to make a point about not using formulas to set your training zones. If you search the web, you will find many formulas that rely on your personal data, such as age, gender, and other variables, to determine your max heart rate. Once you have that number, you're often encouraged to take a percentage of it and call that your AnT or some other name referring to the same high RPE. The most common of these formulas for finding max heart rate is 220 minus your age. None of these work across the board for all athletes because we're unique individuals. (Remember the principle of individualization from Chapter 2?) Such a formula will work for a few athletes but not for most. When it comes to graphing the actual max heart rates for a large group of people, such as all of the triathletes reading this book, a bell-shaped curve results. For those athletes in the middle of the curve, a formula such as 220 minus age produces results that are quite accurate. But for those to the left or right of the curve's middle, the formula provides increasingly inaccurate results. And because you don't know where you are on the curve, the zones you come up with are likely to be off by quite a bit—perhaps by as much as 20 bpm—either high or low. That's a 40-bpm range! You might as well simply guess your max heart rate as to do it this way. So the take-home message here is, don't use a formula. Do a field test to find your FTHR. Here's how.

The test is done the same way whether you are cycling or running. So I'll describe the standard way it's done, which can then be applied to either sport. Determining zones, however, is unique to each sport so they are set up differently, which we'll come back to a little later.

Do a field test to find your FTHR.

TABLE 4.2 Estimated Swimming Zones

TIME 1,000M/YDS	ZONES (BY 100M/YD PACE IN MIN:SEC)						
	ZONE 1	ZONE 2	ZONE 3	ZONE 4	ZONE 5A	ZONE 5B	ZONE 5C
9:35–9:45	1:13+	1:09–1:12	1:04–1:08	1:01–1:03	0:58–1:00	0:54–0:57	0:53–max
9:46–9:55	1:15+	1:11–1:14	1:06–1:10	1:02–1:05	0:59–1:01	0:55–0:58	0:54–max
9:56–10:06	1:16+	1:12–1:15	1:07–1:11	1:03–1:06	1:00–1:02	0:56–0:59	0:55–max
10:07–10:17	1:17+	1:13–1:16	1:08–1:12	1:04–1:07	1:01–1:03	0:57–1:00	0:56–max
10:18–10:28	1:18+	1:14–1:17	1:09–1:13	1:05–1:08	1:02–1:04	0:58–1:01	0:57–max
10:29–10:40	1:20+	1:15–1:19	1:10–1:14	1:06–1:09	1:03–1:05	0:58–1:02	0:57–max
10:41–10:53	1:22+	1:17–1:21	1:12–1:16	1:08–1:11	1:05–1:07	1:00–1:04	0:59–max
10:54–11:06	1:23+	1:19–1:22	1:13–1:18	1:09–1:12	1:06–1:08	1:01–1:05	1:00–max
11:07–11:18	1:24+	1:20–1:23	1:14–1:19	1:10–1:13	1:07–1:09	1:02–1:06	1:01–max
11:19–11:32	1:26+	1:21–1:25	1:15–1:20	1:11–1:14	1:08–1:10	1:03–1:07	1:02–max
11:33–11:47	1:28+	1:23–1:27	1:17–1:22	1:13–1:16	1:10–1:12	1:05–1:09	1:04–max
11:48–12:03	1:29+	1:24–1:28	1:18–1:23	1:14–1:17	1:11–1:13	1:06–1:10	1:05–max
12:04–12:17	1:32+	1:26–1:31	1:20–1:25	1:16–1:19	1:13–1:15	1:07–1:12	1:06–max
12:18–12:30	1:33+	1:28–1:32	1:22–1:27	1:17–1:21	1:14–1:16	1:08–1:13	1:07–max
12:31–12:52	1:35+	1:30–1:34	1:24–1:29	1:19–1:23	1:16–1:18	1:10–1:15	1:09–max
12:53–13:02	1:38+	1:32–1:37	1:26–1:31	1:21–1:25	1:18–1:20	1:12–1:17	1:11–max
13:03–13:28	1:40+	1:34–1:39	1:28–1:33	1:23–1:27	1:20–1:22	1:14–1:19	1:13–max
13:29–13:47	1:41+	1:36–1:40	1:29–1:35	1:24–1:28	1:21–1:23	1:15–1:20	1:14–max
13:48–14:08	1:45+	1:39–1:44	1:32–1:38	1:27–1:31	1:23–1:26	1:17–1:22	1:16–max
14:09–14:30	1:46+	1:40–1:45	1:33–1:39	1:28–1:32	1:24–1:27	1:18–1:23	1:17–max
14:31–14:51	1:50+	1:44–1:49	1:36–1:43	1:31–1:35	1:27–1:30	1:21–1:26	1:20–max
14:52–15:13	1:52+	1:46–1:51	1:39–1:45	1:33–1:38	1:29–1:32	1:23–1:28	1:22–max
15:14–15:42	1:56+	1:49–1:55	1:42–1:48	1:36–1:41	1:32–1:35	1:25–1:31	1:24–max
15:43–16:08	1:58+	1:52–1:57	1:44–1:51	1:38–1:43	1:34–1:37	1:27–1:33	1:26–max
16:09–16:38	2:02+	1:55–2:01	1:47–1:54	1:41–1:46	1:37–1:40	1:30–1:36	1:29–max
16:39–17:06	2:04+	1:57–2:03	1:49–1:56	1:43–1:48	1:39–1:42	1:32–1:38	1:31–max
17:07–17:38	2:09+	2:02–2:08	1:53–2:01	1:47–1:52	1:43–1:46	1:35–1:42	1:34–max
17:39–18:12	2:13+	2:05–2:12	1:57–2:04	1:50–1:56	1:46–1:49	1:38–1:45	1:37–max
18:13–18:48	2:18+	2:10–2:17	2:01–2:09	1:54–2:00	1:50–1:53	1:42–1:49	1:41–max
18:49–19:26	2:21+	2:13–2:20	2:04–2:12	1:57–2:03	1:53–1:56	1:44–1:52	1:43–max
19:27–20:06	2:26+	2:18–2:25	2:08–2:17	2:01–2:07	1:56–2:00	1:48–1:55	1:47–max
20:07–20:50	2:31+	2:22–2:30	2:12–2:21	2:05–2:11	2:00–2:04	1:52–1:59	1:51–max
20:51–21:37	2:37+	2:28–2:36	2:18–2:27	2:10–2:17	2:05–2:09	1:56–2:04	1:55–max
21:38–22:27	2:42+	2:33–2:41	2:22–2:32	2:14–2:21	2:09–2:13	2:00–2:08	1:59–max
22:28–23:22	2:48+	2:38–2:47	2:27–2:37	2:19–2:26	2:14–2:18	2:04–2:13	2:03–max
23:23–24:31	2:55+	2:45–2:54	2:34–2:44	2:25–2:33	2:20–2:24	2:10–2:19	2:09–max
24:32–25:21	3:02+	2:52–3:01	2:40–2:51	2:31–2:39	2:25–2:30	2:15–2:24	2:14–max

Based on a 1,000-meter or 1,000-yard time trial.

TABLE 4.3 **How to Determine Your Bike Heart Rate Zones**

BIKE HEART RATE ZONES	MULTIPLY YOUR bFTHR BY	YOUR BIKE HEART RATE ZONES	
1	81%	Lower than _____	
2	81%–89%	_____	– _____
3	90%–93%	_____	– _____
4	94%–99%	_____	– _____
5a	100%–102%	_____	– _____
5b	103%–106%	_____	– _____
5c	106%	Higher than _____	

To find your bike training zones, use the percentages shown of bike FTHR (bFTHR) as determined by a 20-minute field test.

The venue you choose for the test is critical to getting good data. It should be a course you can come back to for future tests. For a run test, a track works well because it's flat and safe. A good bike test course is a bit more difficult to find. Look for a stretch of road with a wide bike lane, light traffic, no stop signs, and few intersections and corners and that is flat to slightly uphill (grade of less than 3 percent). You will probably need 5 to 10 miles like this depending on how fast you are. This test is especially risky on a bike, so having a safe course is critical. Keep your head up so you can see ahead throughout the test while being especially mindful of traffic. Do not take risks to get good data. Always be careful when you are riding, but especially when doing an all-out test such as this.

To ensure that you get good data, the test should be done on a day when you are well rested. Treat it much as you would a race by backing off your training for the last two or three days prior. Do short workouts only.

Whether it's a bike or a run test, warm up well before starting the 20-minute field test. For most athletes, the warm-up is usually at least 20 minutes of building intensity from a very low and steady RPE to progressively longer accelerations done at increasingly higher efforts that take you above RPE 7 (Table 4.1) for a few seconds at a time. After the last such high effort, recover for about 2 minutes at a very low RPE before starting the 20-minute test.

Begin the test at a high but somewhat conservative effort. In other words, you should feel as if you could go much faster. The most common mistake athletes make when doing this test is starting out too fast because it feels so easy for a few minutes. The more times you do the test, the better you will become at pacing it. The first 5 minutes should feel relatively easy. After every 5 minutes, decide whether you should go somewhat faster or more slowly for the next 5 minutes. These 5-minute changes in RPE should be slight.

At the end of the 20-minute test, begin an easy cooldown, allowing your heart rate and breathing to return to resting levels. After recovering from the exertion, you are ready for the fun part—analyzing the data.

Upload your heart rate data to your favorite software and find your average heart rate for the 20-minute test. Subtract 5 percent and you have a good estimate of your bike or run FTHR. Then

Do not take risks to get good data.

TABLE 4.4 How to Determine Your Run Heart Rate Zones

RUN HEART RATE ZONES	MULTIPLY YOUR rFTHR BY	YOUR RUN HEART RATE ZONES
1	85%	Lower than _____
2	85%–89%	_____ - _____
3	90%–94%	_____ - _____
4	95%–99%	_____ - _____
5a	100%–102%	_____ - _____
5b	103%–106%	_____ - _____
5c	106%	Higher than _____

To find your run training zones, use the percentages shown of run FTHR (rFTHR) as determined by a 20-minute field test.

use Table 4.3 (bike) or Table 4.4 (run) to compute your training zones.

Bike Power Zones

If you have a power meter on your bike or use an indoor trainer that has a power meter, you can determine your power training zones by doing an FTPo test. In fact, if you do the 20-minute test for heart rate described above, your FTPo can be found in the same test data. There's no need to do a separate test. All you do is subtract 5 percent from your average power (not "normalized" power) and you have a good estimate

of your FTPo. Then use Table 4.5 to set your power training zones. As with FTHR testing, the more times you do this test, the more accurate the results will become because there is a learning curve associated with such a solo race-like effort.

Run Pace Zones

Just like your bike power, your running pace can be determined from the same test you used to find your run FTHR. From the 20-minute test data, find your average mile (or kilometer) pace from your downloaded GPS. Then compute your

TABLE 4.5 How to Determine Your Bike Power Zones

BIKE POWER ZONES	MULTIPLY YOUR FTPo BY	YOUR BIKE POWER ZONES
1	55%	Lower than _____
2	55%–74%	_____ - _____
3	75%–89%	_____ - _____
4	90%–104%	_____ - _____
5	105%–120%	_____ - _____
6	120%	Higher than _____

To find your bike power training zones, use the percentages shown of FTPo as determined by a 20-minute field test.

Source: Adapted from Allen and Coggan, *Training and Racing with a Power Meter.*

TABLE 4.6 How to Determine Your Run Pace Zones

RUN PACE ZONES	MULTIPLY YOUR FTPa BY	YOUR RUN PACE ZONES
1	129%	Lower than _____
2	114%–129%	_____ - _____
3	106%–113%	_____ - _____
4	101%–105%	_____ - _____
5a	97%–100%	_____ - _____
5b	90%–96%	_____ - _____
5c	90%	Higher than _____

To find your run pace training zones, use the percentages shown of FTPa as determined by a 20-minute field test.

pace zones by using Table 4.6. This is best done by converting average time to minutes and 10ths of a minute. For example, 7 minutes, 30 seconds would be 7.5 minutes. *Add* (notice that you don't *subtract* when using pace) 5 percent to determine your FTPa. For example, if your average pace for the 20-minute run test was 7.5 minutes, multiply 7.5 by 0.05 to get 0.375. Adding 0.375 to 7.5 produces your FTPa. In the example, it would be 7.875 minutes (7 minutes, 52 seconds).

Zone Agreement

If you use both a power meter and a heart rate monitor when riding your bike and a GPS device and heart rate monitor when running, you'll soon discover that the zones you set up above don't always agree. When you're in heart rate zone 2, you aren't necessarily in power zone 2 when cycling or pace zone 2 when running. This is not an issue regarding your heart, legs, or devices. It's just the way it is. And this is a good thing. Here's why.

For advanced athletes, heart rate zones change very little, if at all, throughout the season. On the other hand, power zones and pace zones change significantly. As you get into bet-

ter shape, your FTPa and FTPo rise. You become faster at running and more powerful on the bike. This means that all of your power and pace zones also rise. When fitness decreases, your FTPa and FTPo also decrease, and down come your zones. But all the while, heart rate zones remain constant. So there may well be large and small overlaps over the course of a season—or no overlaps at all at some times in the year.

Why does this happen? Look at it this way. If your power zones didn't change, you'd never get any faster at given heart rates. As you'll see later, riding with high power and running fast at a given effort or heart rate are the keys to measuring improvements in fitness. In other words, it never gets any easier; you simply go faster.

INTENSITY DISTRIBUTION

There is currently a great deal of debate among sports scientists on how your training time should be distributed over a season relative to AeT and AnT (Figure 4.1). Should most of your training time be spent below your AeT, between AeT and AnT, or above AnT? There are those who make the case that you should train either very easy below

> For advanced athletes, heart rate zones change very little throughout the season.

AeT or very hard above AnT, with very little in the middle. This is called *polarized training*. Others suggest that a great deal of training should be done at race intensity, and as you saw in Figure 4.2, that would mean much of your training time would be between AeT and AnT.

Where the scientists do agree is that most of your time over the course of a season should be below AeT. So it appears we can take that to the bank. This means that most of your training time—perhaps 70 to 80 percent—is very easy and below AeT. Your time distribution for the season then may look something like that shown in Figure 4.3, with a huge amount below AeT and the remainder spread between the other two segments. How much time is spent in each of these two more intense segments may well be an individual matter (there's that pesky principle of individualization again) based on how much training you do, the type of event for which you are training, and how you seem to respond to training. I don't think there's one way of distributing the remaining time that fits everyone. The most important point of this discussion is that a huge portion of your training will be at or below AeT.

Why should so much of your training time fall around or below AeT? Doesn't that make for quite easy workouts? Yes, and that's the key point: The easier your easy workouts, the harder your hard ones can be. An easy day of training ensures that the next hard day will be truly hard. If you shift a great deal of training time from the huge below-AeT portion shown in Figure 4.3 to either of the two higher ranges, especially the AeT-AnT segment, you'll create enough fatigue that your key weekly workouts will suffer each week. They won't be as challenging as they should be to pro-

> A huge portion of your training will be at or below AeT.

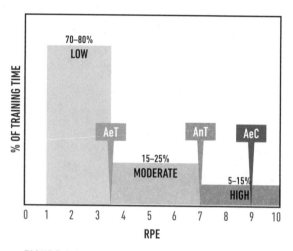

FIGURE 4.3 Seasonal training time distribution relative to the AeT and AnT reference points

duce a high level of fitness. This practice of making easy workouts (less than AeT) moderately hard (between AeT and AnT) and thus decreasing the amount of recovery time is undoubtedly the single biggest mistake serious athletes make. You need lots and lots of easy workouts if you are to perform at a high level. I know that seems contradictory, but it works.

Of course, all of this raises the issue of seasonal planning. It's not a good idea to train the same way, week after week, for an entire season. Not only is the risk of burnout increased, but there is also likely to be a plateauing of your physical gains in a matter of a few weeks that can't be overcome by continuing with the same training method. Change is beneficial in this regard. We'll get into the matter of planning a season in Chapter 7.

SUMMARY: TRAINING INTENSITY

Like most things, training for endurance sport is quite simple. Regardless of your experience or ability level, it is based on manipulating only three things—the frequency, duration, and intensity of your workouts. It doesn't matter whether you are a novice who is just getting started in triathlon or a professional triathlete—training boils down to these three. The ways in which you organize them, however, has a lot to do with how you progress. For the advanced athlete, the key to triathlon success is the intensity of the workouts. That doesn't mean going all out all the time, but rather training at intensities that are appropriate for the time of the season you are currently in and the goal race.

There are many ways to calculate intensity. Currently, the most common are subjectively rating perceived exertion (RPE) on a scale from 0 to 10, monitoring heart rate, computing power on a bike, and using a GPS device or stopwatch on a measured course to gauge running pace.

The key to understanding how to use intensity properly in your training comes down to understanding certain physiological reference points. The most commonly used are aerobic threshold and anaerobic threshold—AeT and AnT. AeT has the lower intensity of these two and occurs when you are training at a moderate effort. That's about a 3 or 4 on the RPE scale. You become very aware of AnT when exercising at an RPE of about 7—very hard. AeT is roughly 30 bpm below your heart rate when you are at your AnT.

AnT is probably the more important of these two reference points because we base all of your training zones on it, regardless of the measuring tool used. The only problem with AnT is the cost of determining it in a lab. A nice, inexpensive substitute for AnT that can be done with a field test is FT. In this chapter, you learned about FTHR in cycling and running, FTPa in swimming and running, and FTPo for the bike. And you learned how to do a field test for each of these in order to set your zones.

You also found out that the various types of zones you use in a given sport, such as heart rate and pace zones in running or heart rate and power in cycling, don't necessarily agree—and that they shouldn't. As your fitness improves throughout the season, the zones will move farther apart. This is because your pace gets faster at your FTPa while your rFTHR stays the same. The same goes for an increase of your FTPo during the season while bFTHR doesn't change. And the opposite is true as your fitness declines, which is common at the end of the season.

Once you have your training intensity zones set, you should monitor how much of your training time is spent below AeT, above AnT, and between the two thresholds. The bulk of your training should fall at and below AeT. In other words, most of your training—perhaps as much as 80 percent—should be at or below a moderate RPE in the 3 to 4 range. That will help to ensure that you are rested and ready when the next above-AnT or between-AeT-and-AnT workouts are done. Those are the high-quality training sessions that play such a pivotal role in how fit you are on race day. If you train this way, then your training has taken the first step toward being purposeful. In Part III, we'll dig deeper into this topic of purposeful training for high-performance racing.

As your fitness improves throughout the season, your zones will move farther apart.

PURPOSEFUL TRAINING

Training for high-performance triathlon racing is like everything else in your life at which you want to truly excel. It begins with having a purpose. Haphazard workouts may have worked when you were new to the sport, but once you have become an advanced athlete, that approach just wastes valuable time and leads to frustration when you are racing. If you've not been racing up to the level you think you are capable of achieving, you probably need to consider how purposeful your training has been.

Purpose starts with having a goal. More than likely you already have one—or several. But is your goal driving your training to make it purposeful? We'll explore that question in Chapter 5. In Chapter 6, we'll get into how your goals are tied to your workouts by examining your abilities and limiters.

Training with purpose is perhaps the most important aspect of striving for high performance in triathlon. By setting appropriate goals, closely aligning them with your limiters, and then training with a well-defined purpose, you will improve your race-specific fitness.

GETTING STARTED

IN THIS CHAPTER, I'm going to take you step by step through the process I use to get an athlete started on a new season. We follow this process—all of it—*every* season, regardless of how many times we may have done it previously. This may seem excessive, but we do it because things change over time. Lots of things. The most important changes take place in your body; it is never static. All of your physiological systems are in a relentless state of makeover. Your body is constantly rebuilding itself. Some of the changes may be so slight from year to year that you are not even aware of them. But trust me, they are happening and affecting your race performance. Others are more significant. We'll get into those shortly.

Much of what I suggest you do on the following pages may seem pointless right now. You'll be tempted to skip over them. But I can say with great certainty that in the long run you will appreciate having done them. You not only will learn a lot about how you function as an athlete but also will have historical markers of where you were at the start of every season. This record of your fitness will prove invaluable over time as you progress as an athlete.

In the previous season, you may have been injured. If so, I hope you are fully healed now and ready to start afresh. If not, the transition from the end of one season to the start of the next is the time to fully recover from the injury while taking steps to prevent its recurrence. Starting to train for a new season is pointless if you are nursing a nagging injury. There is nothing to be gained from this, but a lot to lose. You should start the new season with a well-rested and healthy body. You also need to make a strong commitment not to become injured again. Some of the suggestions in this chapter will help with this.

There are other reasons for going through the start-up procedure. You may have purchased a new bike or a new component, such as a saddle, at some time in the last season. We need to make sure that these are right and ready for your new season. The same goes for the running shoes you are currently using. Also, some muscles may have become stronger while others grew weaker during the course of the past year. Your ranges of motion in various joints may have increased or decreased. You may have gained or lost weight. Your movement skills for each of the three sports may have changed slightly.

At the start of the season, you also need to know how fit you are and how your current fitness compares with that in previous years. This benchmark will eventually help you make decisions about how to start your training plan, which we'll come back to in Chapter 7.

It's important to collect this information before your first serious workout of the new season. But what if you are coming to this chapter when it's not the start of the season? Perhaps you're well into it. What should you do if you have just a few weeks until a race? I'd strongly suggest you begin right now to start your season anew by following the guidelines here as if it were the actual start of the season. In many ways, it will be a new season if you follow the guidelines in the remaining chapters.

On the other hand, if you are currently in the midst of frequent racing, it may be best to delay all of the suggested start-up procedures until you have a break of a few weeks before your next high-priority race. Regardless of where you are in the season right now, you need to eventually incorporate the seasonal start-up steps described in this chapter. They will help you make gains in training right away and, as a result, significant gains in performance later.

Let's get started on your new—or ongoing—season with a more effective way to prepare to race than you've ever tried before. It all starts—believe it or not—with dreaming.

DREAMS, GOALS, OBJECTIVES, AND PURPOSES

When it comes to goals, some athletes believe that shooting for the stars is a good idea because if they fall short they may still make it to the moon. I've known athletes who set goals like that. But reaching a goal really doesn't work that way. Aiming well beyond what is a realistic challenge will produce just the opposite of what you really want. It's good to dream, but the dream can't involve wishing on a star with your fingers crossed.

In 1961, President Kennedy dreamed of putting a man on the moon and returning him safely to earth by the end of the decade. There were lots of reasons for this, of which the most important was probably a demonstration of technological dominance during the Cold War. Regardless of the reason, the dream soon became NASA's greatest goal—and arguably the biggest technological challenge in human history. Landing safely on the moon and then returning safely to earth was huge. But it started as a dream.

Note that NASA didn't start with the stated intent of putting people on the nearest star and then wishing and hoping down deep that somehow they would at least make it to the lunar surface. Goals don't work like that. A good goal is challenging but is not beyond belief. If you don't believe you can achieve a goal because it's too great, then it's not even a dream. It is just a wish.

A good goal is challenging but is not beyond belief.

Wishes are cheap. They are seldom realized. They have no substance. When you wish upon a star, nothing happens. Unlike wishes, though, dreams can and often do succeed. They're one step removed from becoming a goal. Just as with Kennedy, they are the starting place for your highest accomplishments as a triathlete. In early 1961, what would become NASA's all-encompassing goal was merely a dream. Nothing more. But it soon became a goal, and within a few years an accomplishment. What are your dreams as a triathlete? What are your goals?

Your Season Goals

Your goals are always the starting point for a new season. I've found that three seasonal goals are about the right number. When there are too many, something gets neglected. You can certainly have fewer, but I'd suggest no more than three. I've found it works best if these goals are performance outcomes—what you'd like to achieve in a race. They are not statements of what you would like to accomplish somewhere along the path to the race.

Just as with Kennedy, dreams are probably where your goals begin. You may have been dreaming for a long time of accomplishing something big as a triathlete, such as qualifying for Ironman Hawaii, making a national team, winning a local race, finishing your first 70.3, or whatever it is that lights your fire. How do you make your dream into a goal? You've undoubtedly heard all of what follows many times before, but I'm going to refresh your memory anyway. It's important that we get started on the new season correctly.

Each goal should be well defined by including one basic element: what it is, exactly, that you want to achieve in a given race. Supporting achievements, such as losing weight, improving power, and running faster, are actually the starting places for *training objectives*, not goals. We'll get to objectives shortly. If you are training to perform in a race at a high level, then state your goal exactly as what you want to accomplish in the race.

A goal should be measurable. It isn't enough to set a goal to "race faster." Your goal should be more along this line: Complete the XYZ triathlon on May 7 in less than 2 hours, 20 minutes. Note the inclusion of a goal race time. The more tightly you define your goal, the easier you will find it is to work toward its successful accomplishment throughout the season. In this regard, setting a time goal is better than setting an age-group placement goal, such as winning your division or finishing in the top 10. Such goals always depend to some extent on who shows up in your age group on race day. The only thing you can control is how well you perform relative to your own ability and training. If someone with greater ability and training than yours happens to be there on race day and wins, but you still accomplished your time goal, then you can and should be happy with your performance outcome.

Your Training Objectives

Can you achieve your goals? There should be at least a seed of doubt in your mind; otherwise, the goal is too easy and won't really be a challenge to achieve (or worth the time and effort invested when it's over). If there is no question at all about your potential for success, then the goal isn't going to challenge you, your training will have little purpose, and the outcome will be empty.

On the other hand, if the goal is so big that you can't even imagine accomplishing it, then

Your goals are always the starting point for a new season.

your training will likely be a waste of time. You are wishing. Wishing is no good. If you are to succeed, you must have a strong reason to believe that achieving the goal is within your grasp. Let me tell you a story about that.

I once had a brand-new client tell me that he wanted to win the national championship. OK, I thought, that's a great place to start talking about achievements. So I asked him if he'd ever raced in the national championship before. "No," he replied. I then asked how long he'd been racing. "I've never done a race," he told me. How much training have you done? "I've never done any serious training." Wow! I recall thinking that this was going to take a lot of discussions to set a challenging, but not *overly* challenging, goal. He had a wish, not a dream. He was shooting for the stars and hoping he'd make it to the moon. Maybe someday in the not-too-distant future, we could make it to the top step of the podium at nationals, but it was unlikely to happen in his first season in the sport.

Here's something else for you to ponder: Why can't you achieve your goal now? It's a matter of definition. If you could achieve it now, we'd call it an accomplishment, not a goal. But because there is some level of uncertainty about your capacity to perform at the level of the goal, there is obviously something that stands between you and immediate success—a *limiter*. The purpose of your training is to fix this performance limiter. The subgoals that define what's needed to make your limiters stronger are called *training objectives*. In Chapter 6, we will dig more deeply into this important concept of limiters.

For now, you need only understand that a training objective is a short-term subgoal to be accomplished along the way to achieving your overarching season goal. You will likely see these objective outcomes happen in training, showing that you are making progress toward your goal. An objective may, for example, be a time, power, or pace outcome that you achieve in specific workouts or tests throughout the season as you prepare for your goal race. They may also be lifestyle matters or even mental roadblocks that limit your performance. If they involve your lifestyle or mental skills, they will initially show up as accomplishments away from the pool, road, and track, but they will still play a critical role in your race performance. We'll come back to all of this shortly.

Your Daily Purposes

The achievement of high goals and objectives is never easy. It always takes determination, sweat, and patience. You must chip away at your goals and objectives every day—a little bit here, a little bit there. If you do, then the training objective—and eventually the goal—is within grasp. Step by step, you're steadily making progress. This means that every workout and every day must have a purpose. Each workout must focus on at least one thing that will help you improve—something every single day. Consequently, workouts must have a purpose. Where you focus on any given day can be something that is quite challenging, such as improving your bike power or swim skill. Or, on the other side of the coin, it can be something quite easy, such as recovering from the previous day's hard training sessions. For that too is critical for success. Whatever it is, you should wake up every morning knowing what you'll do that day to move closer to your objectives and your goals. High performance requires daily action. The higher your goal, the more important each day's decisions.

The purpose of your training is to eliminate performance limiters.

Every workout and every day must have a purpose.

The best athletes strive for small, daily gains knowing that they will eventually lead to the accomplishment of their season goals. Along the same line, the greater your goal is, the more important every decision in your day becomes. This includes daily choices ranging from nutrition to sleep to training partners, and even to such small things as what you think about. Making it to the moon is not easy.

For right now, you should be dreaming. What is it you'd most like to accomplish this season? Your goals, objectives, and purposes will eventually bloom from that. Later on, in Chapter 7, you will be called upon to write down your goals and objectives. Then we'll get into your daily purposes in Chapter 8 when we examine how to plan a training week.

ASSESSMENT

What will it take to achieve your goals? The higher your goals, the greater your objectives and the bigger the task at hand. It's much like driving through a big city you've never been in before. It will take some planning. It would be foolish just to hop in the car and take off without having a direction and route in mind. The most basic components of route selection are these: Where am I now and where do I want to go? Without knowing the answers to both questions, your trip is doomed to failure. Without answers, making the journey successfully will result only from luck.

While it's nice to have luck on your side, we can't count on it for a seasonal training strategy. As discussed above, you need to establish your season's goals. That's the destination for this trip. The other navigational component is knowing where you are right now. We'll determine this from three vantage points: your physical readiness to train, your mental readiness to train, and your current levels of fitness.

Physical Assessment

As I start athletes on their new seasons, one of the first things I have them do is to see a physical therapist (PT) for a complete physical exam. This is something you also should do. It's best if you can find a PT who specializes in the treatment of athletes and has experience working with athletes involved in endurance sports. Ask around, especially your training partners and the staff at sporting goods stores where you shop for equipment. The person you are looking for is someone who can do a comprehensive head-to-toe exam of your posture, strength, range of joint motion, muscular balance, dynamic function, and any other structural idiosyncrasies and asymmetries that may affect your physical health and your training consistency. The purpose is to determine your risk for injury and, most importantly, how to avoid injury in the coming season.

On discovering your unique areas of potential breakdown, the therapist should design an exercise program for you that may involve functional strengthening and mobility exercises. She or he may also make bike position suggestions for your bike fitter and recommend the types of running shoes that may be best for you. The therapist may also have suggestions for you and your coach, if you have one, on the types of workouts that may prove structurally beneficial, as well as exercises and movements that are best avoided.

The injury-prevention program designed for you is as important as your swim, bike, and run workouts and should be followed throughout

The best athletes strive for small, daily gains in pursuit of season goals.

the season with great care. A PT who is used to working with endurance athletes will understand that you have limited time and should streamline the corrective exercise program so that it provides maximal benefit in a reasonable amount of time. If you are found to have severe structural weaknesses, it's a good idea to schedule a follow-up with the therapist who examined you to gauge your progress and make adjustments to your exercise routine. Predicting future injury and reducing risk for injury through a good physical assessment is often the difference between a successful race season and a season of frustration and tears.

Mental Assessment

In Chapter 1, you read about the importance of mental fitness when it comes to high performance as a triathlete. Now it's time to assess your mental skills. Complete the mental skills profile in Sidebar 5.1. Be completely honest as you consider your answer for each of the questions found there. No one else is going to see your results (unless you decide to share them), so there is no reason to inflate your answers. When you're done, return to reading this section. I'll wait for you.

Because you're reading this book, I assume you scored high (4 or 5) for motivation. In general, triathletes are highly motivated people. Although being highly motivated to train and race is commonly accepted as a positive characteristic, it can also have a dark side. That happens when an athlete finds it difficult to reduce training in order to rest after a hard training period, or even to back off from training to taper before a race. I've known athletes who were so motivated that they avoided rest and recovery unless forced to do

so by overwhelming fatigue. Overtraining is often the result. Very few athletes understand how devastating overtraining can be. We will discuss it in greater detail in Chapter 10, but for now suffice it to say that you must learn to control your enthusiasm for training and high achievement if you are to race at your highest possible level.

Your confidence, thought habits, ability to focus, and ability to visualize also play key roles in your performance. If your score for any of these is low (1, 2, or 3), then you need to find a way to improve that mental skill. The most effective way, if also the most expensive, is to work with a sports psychologist. An inexpensive alternative is to read books written by sports psychologists. You can find a list of such books currently in print (as of this writing) in Sidebar 5.2.

Fitness Assessment

There's an old saying I put a lot of stock in when training athletes: "That which is measured improves." If you want something in your life to improve, start by measuring it to see where it is now. Then measure it again regularly and frequently to see how it's progressing. Its likelihood of improving is greatly increased if you do this. For example, if you want your bank savings account to grow, check it regularly and frequently. If you want to spend more time with your family, monitor how you allocate your time regularly and frequently. If you want to read more often, regularly and frequently keep track of how many books you're reading. If nothing else happens—and there are a lot of good things that can come from this simple concept—you will think more often about how you're doing relative to your goal. Thinking leads to action. You're more likely to do something to achieve your financial,

Your confidence, thoughts, focus, and ability to visualize play key roles in your performance.

If you want something in your life to improve, start by measuring it to see where it is now.

SIDEBAR 5.1 Mental Skills Profile

Read each statement below and choose an appropriate response from these possibilities:

1→ NEVER   2→ RARELY   3→ SOMETIMES   4→ FREQUENTLY   5→ USUALLY   6→ ALWAYS

_4_ 1. I believe my potential as an athlete is excellent.

_5_ 2. I train consistently and eagerly.

_3_ 3. I stay positive when things don't go well in a race.

_3_ 4. In hard races, I can imagine myself doing well.

_5_ 5. Before races, I remain positive and upbeat.

_4_ 6. I think of myself more as a success than as a failure.

_5_ 7. Before races, I'm able to erase self-doubt.

_5_ 8. The morning of a race, I awake nervous but enthusiastic.

_6_ 9. I learn something from a race when I don't do well.

_4_ 10. I can see myself handling tough race situations.

_4_ 11. I'm able to race at or near my ability level.

_5_ 12. I can easily picture myself training and racing.

_5_ 13. Staying focused during long races is easy for me.

_4_ 14. I stay in tune with my exertion levels in races.

_2_ 15. I mentally rehearse skills and tactics before races.

_3_ 16. I'm good at concentrating as a race progresses.

_5_ 17. I'm willing to make sacrifices to attain my goals.

_4_ 18. Before an important race, I can visualize doing well.

_4_ 19. I look forward to doing hard workouts.

_1_ 20. When I visualize myself racing, it almost feels real.

_3_ 21. I think of myself as a tough competitor.

_4_ 22. I tune out distractions in races.

_6_ 23. I set high goals for myself.

_4_ 24. I like the challenge of a hard race.

_4_ 25. When the race gets hard, I concentrate even better.

_6_ 26. In races I am mentally tough.

_4_ 27. I can relax my muscles before races.

_5_ 28. I stay positive despite late race starts, bad weather, etc.

_5_ 29. My confidence remains high the week after a bad race.

_4_ 30. I strive to be the best athlete I can be.

SCORING: Add up the numerical responses you gave for each of the following sets of statements and then determine your rating for each by using the scale at the bottom of the page.

MENTAL SKILL	STATEMENTS	TOTAL	RATING
Motivation	2, 8, 17, 19, 23, 30	4+5+	28
Confidence	1, 6, 11, 21, 26, 29	4 44345	24
Thought habits	3, 5, 9, 24, 27, 28	3 56445	27
Focus	7, 13, 14, 16, 22, 25	5 54344	25
Visualization	4, 10, 12, 15, 18, 20	3 45241	19

How to determine rating:	
IF "TOTAL" IS . . .	THEN "RATING" IS . . .
32–36	5
27–31	4
21–26	3
16–20	2
6–15	1

time management, reading, or other goals than if you never did any measuring.

It works the same way with your triathlon goals and objectives. If you measure their indicators of success regularly and frequently, they will become uppermost in your mind, and you'll find ways to improve them. If you never do any measurement, you won't find out until race day how you did in your training preparation. That's too late. With regular and frequent measurement of the right markers, your probability of goal success greatly improves.

So what will you measure, and when? There are a few things that serve as good markers of how your fitness is coming along. Some can be measured only in a clinical setting, while others are easily done as field tests. What's the difference between these?

SIDEBAR 5.2 Recommended Sports Psychology Books

Afremow, Jim. *The Champion's Mind: How Great Athletes Think, Train, and Thrive.*

Bell, Jonny. *Sports Psychology: Inside the Athlete's Mind.*

Cox, Richard. *Sport Psychology: Concepts and Applications.*

Gonzalez, D. C. *The Art of Mental Training— a Guide to Performance Excellence.*

LeUnes, Arnold. *Sport Psychology.*

Lynch, Jerry. *Spirit of the Dancing Warrior: Asian Wisdom for Peak Performance in Athletics and Life.*

Smith, Leif, and Todd M. Kays. *Sports Psychology for Dummies.*

Weinberg, Robert. *Foundations of Sport and Exercise Psychology with Web Study Guide.*

A clinical test, sometimes called a *lab test*, is usually done at a university, health club, sporting goods retail store (e.g., a triathlon, running, or cycling shop), or medical clinic (orthopedist, chiropractor, physical therapist, or sports medicine doctor). Endurance coaches often offer the same sort of testing service. Ask around to find out where such testing is done in your area.

A field test is something you do on your own in the pool, on the road or track, and in the gym. These are simple tests of performance that also measure progress, but in a different way than a clinical test. Both types of testing have their upsides and downsides.

A clinical test measures highly specific physiological markers of fitness. The accuracy of such testing is usually quite good. The downsides are cost—they can be expensive—and interpreting what the test results mean because they are so technical. The latter is usually resolved by having the technician explain what was found.

The field test has no financial cost. Field tests are also advantageous because they are quite similar to racing. Clinical tests are typically done on treadmills and bicycle ergometers, whereas field tests more closely mimic race conditions out on the open road or track or in a pool. Also, the outcome of such tests is generally quite easy to interpret because there are typically only one or two numbers, and those numbers are obviously related to your performance in the test. The major downside of a field test is that there is a greater possibility of error than with clinical tests. In the clinic, the technician will see to it that variables, such as equipment choices and warm-up, are the same from one test to the next. Athletes are less likely to do that in a field test, so they introduce variables that can easily interfere with outcomes that

SIDEBAR 5.3 Clinical Test Metrics

Commonly measured endurance markers in clinical tests using gas analysis and/or lactate analysis are listed here. Such testing, with few exceptions, is done only for the bike and run portions of triathlon. Swim test facilities are quite rare. Measurements of heart rate apply to the bike and run, measurements of pace to the run, and measurements of power to the bike.

Common Gas Analysis Markers

- Aerobic capacity (also called VO_2max): a measure of how much oxygen an athlete is capable of using when at a maximal aerobic effort
- Aerobic threshold (AT1) heart rate, pace, or power: a measure of the lowest intensity at which aerobic fitness progress may be made
- Anaerobic threshold (AT2) heart rate, pace, or power: the intensity at which an athlete begins to "redline," typically with labored breathing, a rating of perceived exertion of about 7 (on a scale of 10), and the sensation of burning muscles
- Calories burned at various heart rates, paces, or power intensities
- Your body's ability to use fat for fuel while sparing limited carbohydrate energy stores

Common Lactate Analysis Markers

- The first lactate threshold (LT1) heart rate, pace, or power is a measure of the lowest intensity at which aerobic fitness progress may be made.
- The second lactate threshold (LT2) heart rate, pace, or power is the intensity at which an athlete begins to "redline," typically with labored breathing, a rating of perceived exertion of about 7 (on a scale of 10), and the sensation of burning muscles. A closely associated metric is maximal lactate steady state (MLSS).
- Lactate levels at various heart rate, pace, or power intensities, which indicate how hard you are exercising, are closely related to race pace.

are often in the range of 1 to 3 percent improvement from one test to the next. Such small gains (or losses) in performance can be canceled out by an uncontrolled variable, such as weather, nutrition, warm-up, or course selection.

There are other considerations. A clinical test gives you lots of details about how your body works and therefore what you can do in training to improve performance. A field test, on the other hand, is more of a "black box" test: You simply put in a hard effort and see what the resulting performance number is. How that number is interpreted is up to you, unless you have a coach who can help you draw conclusions.

Both types of testing are valuable, and I use both with the athletes I coach in order to get a

A clinical test gives you lots of details about how your body works.

broad view of our seasonal starting point. Follow-up testing is easy to fit in (and inexpensive) with field tests, whereas clinical testing requires considerable scheduling (and cash outlay).

Sidebar 5.3 suggests what type of testing you may consider having done in a clinic. You can narrow this list—and reduce the cost—by meeting with the technician and discussing your race goals and previous training history. He or she can help you focus the list of what to test based on your specific needs. It would be great if you could test for both bike and run (swim testing is seldom available), but that's expensive and takes a lot of time. So I'd suggest testing on the bike only because it plays a greater role in your race outcome. The best times to do clinical testing are at the start of your season and again at the ends of the base and build periods (see Chapter 7 for period details). That's a minimum of three tests in a season, and likely two or three more, depending on your race goals. Assuming $150 per test (they can be significantly more expensive in some places), we're talking about $450 to $900 per season. I certainly couldn't blame you should you decide to use only field tests.

Field tests are easy to fit into your schedule. As before clinical tests, you need to cut back on training for a couple of days, much as you might dial back before a B-priority race. Going into either type of test fatigued will greatly skew the results. The part you must strive to get right when doing field tests is controlling the variables that can mess up the outcomes. In addition to your rest-and-recovery status, which is the most important variable, here is a short list of factors you need to keep much the same from one field test to the next (and should record in your training diary to help maintain consistency):

- Equipment choices (bicycle equipment and running shoes are especially critical)
- Course selection (the same for every test within a sport, if possible)
- Pretest food and drink
- Warm-up
- Initial test pacing

The last item, pacing, is especially critical for field tests. Athletes almost always start much too fast when doing the functional threshold field tests described in Sidebar 5.4. Because of poor pacing, they slow down dramatically in the latter portion of the test. It's better to start out too slowly than too quickly. I should emphasize that there is certainly a learning curve associated with each of these tests. The more times you do them, the better you will get at pacing.

I recommend doing the functional threshold tests for each sport right away. In addition to giving you good markers of your current fitness levels, they will also help to get your pace, power, and heart rate zones set up. If you don't have a power meter or GPS device, you should do the tests anyway with the focus only on setting heart rate zones. The decoupling and efficiency factor tests will be scheduled into your weekly training, as you will see in Chapters 6 and 8.

As mentioned above, the best times to do both types of testing during the season are upon the completion of a training period of several weeks' duration, such as at the ends of the base and build periods. And, of course, you should test just before you start a new season in order to establish baselines for comparison with later tests to see how you're progressing. Again, faithfully maintaining a training diary will help you keep track of all these baselines.

Test at the start of your season and the ends of the base and build periods.

Pacing is critical for field tests. Don't start too hard.

Field Test Metrics

Common field tests for swimming, biking, and running are listed below. Measurements of heart rate apply to the bike and run, measurements of pace to the swim and run, and measurements of power to the bike. Each of these field tests is described in greater detail in Appendixes B (swim), C (bike), and D (run). Strength field tests are described in Chapter 13.

Common Swim Field Tests

- Functional threshold pace (sFTPa): a 1,000-meter time trial to determine swim pace training zones and gauge swim fitness progress

Common Bike Field Tests

- Functional threshold power (bFTPo) and heart rate (bFTHR): a 20-minute "time trial" to determine bike power and heart rate training zones and gauge bike fitness progress
- Power–heart rate decoupling (Pw:HR): a "long" aerobic endurance ride done to determine when fatigue occurs on a given day
- Efficiency factor (bEF): a "long" aerobic endurance ride done at the aerobic threshold to gauge aerobic fitness progress over time for similar workouts

Common Run Field Tests

- Functional threshold pace (rFTPa) and heart rate (rFTHR): a 20-minute "time trial" to determine run pace and heart rate training zones and gauge run fitness progress
- Pace–heart rate decoupling (Pa:HR): a "long" aerobic endurance run done to determine when fatigue occurs on a given day
- Efficiency factor (rEF): a "long" aerobic endurance run done at the aerobic threshold to gauge aerobic fitness progress over time for similar workouts

TRAINING PREPARATION

The purpose of this chapter is to get you started on a new season in such a way that the possibility of your success is greatly improved. So far, we've looked at your goals to see where you want to go this season, assessed your physical and mental readiness to train, and started you on testing to establish a baseline for your fitness. Now is the time to focus even more closely on the multisport components of triathlon by making sure you have the right equipment and other resources to get the most from your training.

Swim

Among the three sports, swimming is unique in that performance is determined largely by technique. In fact, for most age-group swimmers, technique trumps fitness when it comes to performance. In Chapter 12, we'll examine the skills you need to master to improve your swimming. In developing your swim skills, the most important thing you can do is have a coach or swim instructor who frequently gives you feedback on your technique. This source can be a trusted training partner who has a good grasp of swim skills, an instructor you hire, your triathlon coach, or the feedback you get from a masters swim group that has an on-deck coach at workouts. A good masters swim program with a knowledgeable coach will do wonders for your swimming. Scout around to find one that is focused primarily on triathlon and that has sessions at times you can fit into your daily routine. Try to attend such sessions two or three times weekly.

If you can't find a masters program to swim with, then you'll need a swimming pool that is close to your home or work to keep travel time to a minimum. Triathlon is already a very time-intensive sport; you don't need to add lots of driving on top of training if it can be avoided. The perfect pool will have daily times and lanes dedicated to lap swimming, with few people and with lanes assigned by ability. It is also great if the pool has a moveable bulkhead so that it can be switched between a 25-meter and a 50-meter length. The longer distance is helpful for developing open-water swim endurance.

Speaking of open water, having access to a lake or ocean swim area is great for improving your race skills. Just a word of caution here: Don't ever swim solo in open water. Always arrange to have at least one other swimmer with you. There are some clubs that schedule group open-water swim sessions on a regular schedule throughout the summer. These offer a great opportunity to become more comfortable in conditions that mimic what you'll experience in a race.

As for equipment, I'm not a big believer in having lots of swim toys. But you may find that pull buoys come in handy when you are trying to master swim technique. Otherwise, all you need are good goggles, a cap, and a swimsuit.

Bike

I attend a lot of races every year. A depressing thing I often see is an athlete who I'm certain has spent hundreds of hours training for the event and probably thousands of dollars on equipment and travel, but who has a bike that doesn't fit correctly. What a waste! That poor athlete has no chance of even coming close to his or her potential.

Why is bike fit so critical? The bike is the key to the race. About half of one's race time is spent on the bike. A poor bike setup—saddle too high or low, saddle too far forward or aft, handlebar reach too long or short, handlebars too high or low, and lots more—means the rider can't apply optimal force to the pedals, is not appropriately aerodynamic, and is wasting energy and losing time. It's so sad to see to that. And yet it can be fixed so easily with a formal bike-fitting session.

I have every athlete I coach get a bike fit at the start of every season, even if it's the same bike that was used in the previous season. Let me repeat that: We do this *every year*. We always use a professional bike fitter. I strongly suggest that you do the same. Don't do the fit yourself. Don't ask a training partner, friend, or spouse to help you get set up. Go see someone with experience, especially a fitter who regularly works with tri-athletes. In Chapter 12, we will get into this topic a little more deeply because it has a lot to do with your cycling skills and performance.

Frequent feedback is critical to swim technique.

The bike is the key to the race.

When it comes to equipment, the bike portion of triathlon is the most expensive, as I'm sure you're quite aware. You can spend thousands of dollars getting the right bike. So it behooves you to do some serious shopping and pricing when looking for a new ride. If you're on a tight budget, check out used bikes. Bike and triathlon shops often have bulletin boards on which athletes post notes about bikes they are selling. Triathlon club members often sell their used bikes when getting a new one, and any difference in speed between last year's model and this year's is usually negligible. You can often find a great deal on a used bike. Just make sure it fits. A good price doesn't mean much if the bike is the wrong size. Be patient and shop around until you find one that is just right for you.

In addition to a good bike, you'll need a heart rate monitor, and I'd also strongly suggest purchasing a power meter. I require both of these for every athlete I coach. You probably already have a heart rate monitor, but you may have been holding off on a power meter because of the cost. I can't blame you for that. But the prices are falling fast. At one time, they cost about 25 times as much as a heart rate monitor. Now, some can be purchased for about the same price—and heart rate monitors have not become more expensive. If you simply can't afford a new one, check around for a used power meter. When athletes upgrade, they often sell their old ones.

The other confounding issue in getting a power meter is learning how to use it. The data that power meters collect are somewhat more complex than the data from a heart rate monitor and can seem overwhelming, but they are still easily mastered. I wrote a small book, called *The Power Meter Handbook*, that is intended to be a simple introduction. It will quickly teach you how to use your new power meter, and I wrote the book because I truly believe that a power meter will do more to improve your race performance than any other equipment you can purchase, including aerodynamic wheels. It's the "engine" that determines the outcome of a race, not the wheels, and you are the engine. A power meter will help you develop your full potential.

In most places, weather can be an issue when it comes to riding. Rain, snow, heat, cold, and wind may often interfere with riding on the road. For these situations, an indoor trainer is very useful. And this is where your power meter comes in handy once again. If you have one, you don't need an expensive trainer with a built-in analysis tool. All you need is something that provides resistance; your power meter will do the rest.

The last thing you need for bike training is an appropriate course. It's best if you have a flat to gently rolling course and also hills, both short and long, that you can ride. Steep gradients of around 7 percent and gentler ones of about 3 percent can be used for some workouts, which will be described later, to develop power. Of course, you may live where it is tabletop flat. Usually, when that's the case, strong winds can be used in place of hills to help you become a stronger rider.

Safety on the bike is paramount. Your greatest concern in this regard is traffic. It's best to ride where there is a bike lane and traffic is light. That may require driving some place away from the big city to train. I've known many athletes for whom that has become second nature; they think nothing of it. Small flashing headlights and taillights will help you to be seen out on the roads and are inexpensive.

A power meter will do more to improve your race performance than any other gadget.

Run

Running is simple. Running shoes are the most important gear. Be sure to purchase shoes that fit your unique running characteristics. Again, the running-savvy physical therapist who performs an evaluation of your body mechanics can make recommendations for shoe types. I'd also strongly suggest shopping for your shoes at a local running or triathlon store where the salespeople have a good understanding of running. It's generally a good idea to have a couple of pairs of shoes that can used for specific types of courses. For example, you may have different shoes for the road, track, and trails.

Replace your shoes at the first sign that they are breaking down. To gauge their changes in support over time, periodically set them on a flat surface and look at them from the heel end. If you see any signs of leaning to the inside or outside, replace them. It's less expensive and far less psychologically stressful to buy new shoes than to undergo treatment for an injury.

In addition to shoes, I'd strongly suggest getting a speed-and-distance device that also doubles as a heart rate monitor, such as a runner's GPS. There are some on the market that not only tell you instantaneous pace and distance covered but also provide feedback on running mechanics, such as vertical oscillation, time in contact with the ground, and more. We'll come back to such technique topics in Chapter 12 when we examine skills for the three sports.

As with cycling, it's good to have both a relatively flat course and some steep and gradual hills to train on. Use the hills to improve your running power. Also as with cycling, it's good if you have access to an indoor training facility, such as a treadmill or indoor track, that can be used on days when the weather is too nasty for running outside.

Strength

In Chapter 13, we'll get into the details of strength training to improve your triathlon performance. Having easy access to free weights, such as barbells and dumbbells, is especially valuable. But if your only available equipment is strength building machines, we can make them do. The ultimate gym would be one at your own home to cut out travel time when you are working on strength. It really doesn't cost much to set up a basic home weight room, but you may face a challenge in finding a place for it in your home. I've known athletes with multicar garages who turned one bay into their "gym." A set of dumbbells ranging from 10 pounds (5 kg) to 50 pounds (25 kg) in 10-pound increments is usually adequate for most triathletes. With a bench and sturdy backpack that can be loaded with smaller weights, you're all set for most of the basic exercises I'll show you in Chapter 13.

SUMMARY: GETTING STARTED

In this chapter, I have taken you step by step through the process I use in starting an athlete's season. Getting started is a rare opportunity to take a close look at those things that are likely to affect your training and racing. I'd strongly recommend that you return to this chapter at the start of every season. The triathletes I've coached over the years came to expect it annually. They knew it would pay off with better performances in the coming season. It will for you, too.

Replace your shoes at the first sign that they are breaking down.

The starting place for your new race season is the direction you want to go in the months ahead. That comes down to dreams, goals, objectives, and eventually the daily purpose of your workouts. In later chapters, I will give more structure to each of these and blend them into an annual training plan for your new season. For now, I just want you thinking about your dream-based goals. What have you dreamed of accomplishing as a triathlete? What high-performance goals do you most want to achieve in the coming months?

To accomplish those goals, I need to get you started down the path that will set you up for success. That involves an assessment of your mental strengths and weaknesses as an athlete and a plan to eliminate your weaknesses. You need to do the same for your body. What are your physical limiters? Do you have a structural weakness that is just waiting in the background to appear as an injury and upset your training in the coming season? Everyone has these. An hour spent with a physical therapist as the new season is just kicking off will help to diminish these weaknesses. By attacking your mental and physical weaknesses, you will start the season with greater potential for success than ever before.

Next comes an assessment of your fitness. That involves testing to establish a baseline for each sport. The start of the season is a great time to be tested in a clinic to determine precisely where your fitness is now. The technician administering the test can give you important feedback on what your physiological strengths and weaknesses may be as an athlete and suggestions for how to go about training your limiters. This is also the time to do a field test in each sport in order to get another view of what your fitness is like. In addition, such testing will allow you to set your heart rate, pace, and power training zones. Just realize that while your heart rate zones will stay relatively constant throughout the coming season, your pace and power zones will change to reflect your fitness. So you will need to repeat the field testing from time to time as the season progresses. We'll come back to this topic a little later.

Because the bike leg of a triathlon is so long relative to the swim and run, it's imperative that you give it great emphasis now. The single most important thing you can do to improve it is to get a position fitting done by a professional who has experience working with triathletes. The adjustments he or she makes have the potential to enhance your bike splits and therefore your overall performance greatly.

The last step in preparing for the new season is to be certain you have the equipment, facilities, and training venues needed to train effectively for each sport. Warning: This can be expensive, especially in regard to bike equipment. To cut costs, consider buying used equipment. Bikes, power meters, fast wheels, GPS devices, heart rate monitors, weights for a home-based gym, and other such training and racing aids can often be purchased secondhand. Shop around.

That's it. You're ready to start the new season. As you look back at the end of the year, you'll realize how much following all of the suggestions in this chapter did for your performance. Now it's time to get started building fitness for the coming race season. That's where we are headed in Chapter 6.

The starting place for your new race season is the direction you want to go in the months ahead.

BUILDING FITNESS

CHAPTER 2 explained why training must be purposeful. We made considerable progress toward establishing that purpose in Chapter 5 with testing to determine your current state of fitness. This chapter will add even more purpose to your training by introducing concepts for developing race readiness. We will examine the critical concepts of fitness, abilities, and limiters. By the end of this chapter, you will be ready to start focused training for race preparation. The starting place is developing a deeper understanding of what seems like a simple concept—fitness.

WHAT IS FITNESS?

In Chapter 3, I introduced a novel way of thinking about fitness. I started with the idea that fitness is simply a way of expressing your readiness to race. A great race is in part a result of great fitness. Poor fitness leads to a poor race. Then I took

you down the path of understanding fitness as a product of training load—a combination of the frequency, duration, and intensity of your training. As your training load steadily increases over time, your fitness is also assumed to increase. It increases because you are applying stress to your body, which then adapts and grows stronger.

I also described a couple of ways to measure this change in fitness based on training load. One involves adding up how many minutes in a workout you spend in each heart rate zone (or power zone or pace zone). That produces a score for the workout that can then be added to all of your other workout scores for a given week. As this training load score increases from week to week, we can safely assume that your fitness is also increasing. Doing this math for every workout is a rather laborious and time-consuming task, so I pointed out that software is available at TrainingPeaks (www.trainingpeaks. com) that uses a similar, but more precise, method to measure your training load. The software then displays the data in a performance management chart over the course of your season so you can easily see the progress of your fitness.

That's one way of measuring fitness while using your training load as a gauge. But what if you want a more precise way of measuring your fitness based on physiology, rather than arithmetic, in order to measure progress more precisely? That's where the clinical tests described in Chapter 5 come in. Such testing measures your fitness and gives you numbers that can be compared with previous fitness-related numbers to show how your physiology is changing.

So what exactly is being measured in these clinical tests? If you know what these are, then you know what fitness is in a much more accurate way than simply calculating changes in training load. Of course, the downside of such testing is the cost. Nevertheless, knowing what the clinical tests measure can give you a deeper understanding of fitness and therefore what you should do in training to get ready for a high-performance race.

What is being measured in a clinical test is actually quite simple. There are only three basic physical metrics that are representative of fitness as determined in testing: aerobic capacity, anaerobic threshold, and economy. Let's take a quick look at each of these and then get into how we can develop them through specific types of workouts.

Aerobic Capacity

Also referred to as *VO₂max*, aerobic capacity is your ability to use oxygen to produce energy. The more oxygen your body can process, the more energy you can produce and the greater your power or speed. It's common to find that the fastest athletes in a race have the highest aerobic capacities of all entrants. Typically, the farther down the race results you go, the lower the athletes' aerobic capacities. But don't take this to mean that knowing your VO₂max tells you how well you will do compared with others in your race category. The order of finish within your age group will not just be a ranking of aerobic capacities. The two other physiological factors—lactate threshold and economy—also play a major role in race outcomes. One of these three by itself does not constitute all of what it takes to race fast. And, of course, these factors don't include critical race components such as pacing, nutrition, heat adaptation, and more.

The effect of these race components doesn't diminish the need to boost your aerobic capacity to a higher level; aerobic capacity is literally at the heart of fitness for triathlon. Changes in aerobic capacity largely have to do with how much oxygen-carrying blood your heart pumps out to the working muscles with every beat. This per-beat measurement, called *stroke volume*, has a lot to do with how great your aerobic capacity is. One purpose of training is to improve your stroke volume.

There are basically two ways to increase stroke volume. The first is to focus on the hours, miles, or kilometers of your training. The heart responds positively to lots of time spent at higher-than-resting intensity—above 50 percent of VO₂max, approximately—by becoming more efficient and effective, which ultimately means pumping more blood per beat.

The other way to improve stroke volume (and therefore aerobic capacity) is by doing high-intensity intervals, especially doing them at about the power or pace associated with your VO₂max, as found in a clinical test. At that inten-

Aerobic capacity, or VO₂max, is your ability to use oxygen to produce energy.

sity, your heart rate is approaching its maximum, so these are very hard efforts. This method will produce a higher stroke volume sooner than will relying only on how great your training load is. Most experienced athletes employ both training strategies by having a high training load and by doing high-intensity intervals. Later in this and the following chapters, you'll learn how to incorporate both of these into your training.

Besides stroke volume, there are other physiological contributors to aerobic capacity, such as the aerobic enzymes found in the muscles, blood vessel diameter and ability to dilate, blood volume, and hematocrit or red blood cell count. All of these have to do with delivering massive amounts of oxygen to the muscles when you put the pedal to the metal.

Body weight also has a lot to do with aerobic capacity. The formula for determining VO_2max is expressed in terms of milliliters of oxygen consumed per kilogram of body weight per minute. What this means is that as you lose body weight—especially by shedding fat as opposed to sport-specific muscle—your VO_2max increases. You have undoubtedly experienced this phenomenon at both ends of your normal weight range. When you gain weight, you run or ride a bike uphill more slowly. Conversely, when your body weight has been low, the effort of exercise is decreased at any given power or speed. This is clearly the effect of body weight on aerobic capacity.

I'm sure you've heard the saying, "To be a great athlete, choose your parents well." That's in part because aerobic capacity largely depends on who your parents are. (Research has shown that identical twins have nearly identical aerobic capacities.) But take heart: While genetics probably sets the upper limit of your VO_2max, proper training can take you very close to the upper limit. Also bear in mind that there are two other physiological factors that contribute to endurance performance: anaerobic threshold and economy.

Anaerobic Threshold

We first looked at anaerobic threshold in Chapter 4. My point there was to explain that it is one of two intensity markers (aerobic threshold is the other) around which your training heart rate, power, and pace should be distributed. In that chapter, I also showed you how to set your training zones by using your anaerobic threshold as the reference point. Now we will complete that discussion of anaerobic threshold by showing you how it explains your fitness.

While aerobic capacity gets a lot of ink in triathlon magazines, high-performance triathletes should focus the bulk of their hard training on anaerobic threshold. Your aerobic capacity isn't going to change much if you've been training and racing with high intensity for 3 years or more. But you may be able to bump up your anaerobic threshold quite a bit.

So what is anaerobic threshold? In Chapter 4, you saw how it sits at a fairly high intensity: about 7 on the scale of 1 to 10 for rating of perceived exertion (RPE). It's the point at which you begin to "redline" as the intensity of a workout increases. Most well-conditioned triathletes can sustain this level of intensity for about an hour. But it is an hour of suffering. This high RPE and redline sensation occur because chemical changes are taking place in the working muscles as they approach their upper limits. For a fit athlete, the anaerobic threshold is typically in the neighborhood of 80 to 85 percent of aerobic capacity. Your sedentary neighbor's anaerobic

High-performance triathletes should focus the bulk of their hard training on anaerobic threshold.

For a fit athlete, anaerobic threshold is typically 80 to 85 percent of aerobic capacity.

threshold is considerably lower, probably in the range of 60 to 70 percent of his or her also-low aerobic capacity.

The higher you can get your anaerobic threshold as a percentage of your aerobic capacity, the faster you will swim, bike, and run. That's why, in this chapter and many of the others, you will see a great deal of emphasis on certain types of workouts that boost anaerobic threshold. Anaerobic threshold is highly trainable if you do the right workouts regularly and frequently.

You will most likely find that you have a different anaerobic threshold for each of the three sports in triathlon. That's why in Chapter 4 I had you field-test each one to set your heart rate zones. It's also one of the reasons why the principle of specificity was explained in Chapter 3. If you want to raise your running anaerobic threshold, you must do run workouts. Hard swim workouts won't raise it. That's because the anaerobic threshold occurs mostly in the muscles, and because you use different muscles when swimming, biking, or running, there is little or no crossover.

Economy

The last of the big three determiners of physiological fitness is economy. Sports science understands less about this one than the other two, but it may be the most important. It has to do with how efficiently you use oxygen while exercising. Measuring oxygen used is just another way of measuring energy used. In the human body, oxygen consumed is directly related to energy expended when you're exercising aerobically. Your exercising economy is much like the economy rating for a car. For a car, it's how many miles per gallon of gas. For your exercising body, it's how many milliliters of oxygen per mile.

The importance of aerobic capacity diminishes with race length, while the importance of economy grows as the race gets longer. This is because at the longer distances, such as an Ironman triathlon, you race at a low percentage of your aerobic capacity. So having a big VO_2max won't be of great benefit. But wasting even a little energy per stroke or stride (by using excessive oxygen) because of poor economy will add up to a lot of wasted energy—and a slow performance—in a long race.

Do you recall how aerobic capacity is increased? It's boosted by doing high-volume training and mixing in high-intensity intervals. Economy is a bit different. There are some things you have control over, but also many you can do nothing about. Some are even contradictory. For example, being tall with long arms and big feet improves economy for swimming. Unfortunately, you can't change those. A cyclist with long thighbones relative to total leg length will likely be economical. For running, though, a long thighbone is a detriment. A runner needs long shinbones for good economy. It also helps to be short and small for running. As a triathlete, your economy is improved by having a high percentage of slow-twitch muscle fibers. These are good for endurance, while fast-twitch muscle fibers are better for sprinters. But your specific mix is largely determined by genetics. There are other changes to our physiology we would also make if we had control over them, such as increasing the number of mitochondria we have (the little powerhouses in the muscle cells that produce energy). But these are all things we have little or no control over.

So what things *can* you control to improve your economy and so use less oxygen as you swim, bike, and run? The most common skill

---

The higher your anaerobic threshold as a percentage of your aerobic capacity, the faster you swim, bike, and run.

Economy is a measure of how efficiently you use oxygen while exercising.

you can alter is technique, which is a judgment of how good you are at making the movements of a sport. If your technique is poor, it can be changed. You must realize, however, that as you work on improvement, there will be a period of time during which you become less economical. This will show up as a higher-than-normal heart rate and a higher RPE at any given pace or power. And it may take weeks, if not months, to make the new technique your normal one. At that point, though, you should be faster at the same heart rates as before, and you should also use less oxygen than before the change. Those are highly positive improvements and well worth pursuing.

Other changes that are beneficial for bike and run economy include reducing excess body weight and using lighter equipment. You can also improve efficiency by installing aerobars on your bike along with other aerodynamic equipment, such as wheels, helmet, and bike frame. As a swimmer, you can improve economy by increasing the flexibility of your shoulders and ankles, especially the ability to point your toes. Interestingly, the research shows that less flexibility in the ankle joint makes for more economical running; it appears to improve the release of energy stored in your calf muscle with each footstrike. This is yet again one of the many conflicting challenges of triathlon: Making improvements in one sport can decrease performance in another.

To improve economy, you need to focus your training with intensity and frequency. Training at a high speed or power has been shown to make athletes more economical at all speeds and power outputs, including the lower range. Long-duration workouts when you are trying to change technique to improve economy are usually just the opposite of what you should do.

One of the best ways to improve your technique and therefore your economy is to do a sport frequently, especially if each session is very brief. For example, to become a more economical swimmer with only 2 hours a week to devote to the sport, swim 4 times a week for 30 minutes each time. That will improve your economy more rapidly than swimming 2 times a week for 1 hour each time.

Plyometric exercises—explosive jumping, bounding, and hopping drills—have also been shown to improve economy for running and cycling. Powerful hill repeats for cycling and running are similar and also beneficial for economy. That's why you will see these types of workouts included in the training discussions that follow.

There is still a great deal of debate about whether or not traditional strength training with weights improves economy. I believe it does, as I have seen so many of the athletes I've coached over the years improve their performances remarkably after a winter of lifting weights—provided they did exercises that closely mimicked the movements of the sport. Doing curls is unlikely to make you a better runner. But doing step-ups may help a lot.

ABILITIES

Now it's time to take all of this scientific mumbo jumbo about the three markers of fitness and begin shaping them into common, triathlon-specific workouts. To do this, I organize all workouts into six categories, called *abilities*. Each of the abilities is related to aerobic capacity, anaerobic threshold, and economy in some way. Here they are:

> To improve economy, you must focus your training with intensity and frequency.

- Aerobic endurance
- Muscular force
- Speed skills
- Muscular endurance
- Anaerobic endurance
- Sprint power

The first three are the most basic and must be well established before you can move on to the last three, all of which are advanced abilities. Let's take a brief look at each of them. I will frequently refer to these abilities throughout the rest of this book when discussing training, so having a working knowledge of them is important.

The Basic Abilities

The basic abilities—aerobic endurance, muscular force, and speed skills—are the most important because they are the platform upon which race fitness is built. The more developed these abilities are, the greater your eventual race fitness.

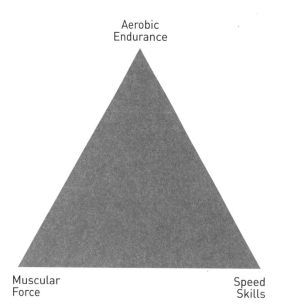

Aerobic
Endurance

Muscular
Force

Speed
Skills

FIGURE 6.1 The basic abilities of training

Aerobic endurance, muscular force, and speed skills are the platform for race fitness.

If your basic abilities are weak, your advanced ability training will be quite limited, and you will never reach your potential.

The basic abilities (Figure 6.1) are generally the ones a triathlete should focus on early in the season (the base period) and return to again for further development after long pre-race tapers and lengthy post-race recoveries. During such low-volume training periods, the basic abilities gradually fade and need to be refreshed.

Aerobic endurance. Aerobic endurance is the ability to keep going for a very long time at a low intensity. It is improved by doing long, relatively easy, steady workouts in heart rate, power, or pace zone 2. Such workouts have a lot to do with building aerobic capacity because they contribute significantly to the volume of your training (recall that high volume boosts VO_2max). Aerobic endurance training does this by making several positive changes to your physiology. For example, by doing lots of aerobic endurance training, some of your fast-twitch muscles begin to take on the endurance characteristics of slow-twitch muscles. Your blood also becomes better at carrying oxygen to the working muscles. Your body builds more capillaries to deliver the oxygen-rich blood to your muscles. The muscle cells make more enzymes to produce energy by using the delivered oxygen. The list of aerobic benefits from training this ability is lengthy. Aerobic endurance training is without a doubt the single most important of the six abilities for a triathlete. As an endurance athlete, you must be aerobically fit.

Later, you will see how it's possible to measure aerobic endurance throughout the season to gauge your progress with a simple test called the *efficiency factor.* This test will tell you on a weekly basis how your aerobic endurance is progressing.

Muscular force. This is the ability to overcome resistance. In swimming, water produces resistance because it is such a thick medium to move through. When you are biking and running, air causes resistance to forward movement. If there is a head wind, the resistance is greater still. When you are riding and running uphill, gravity causes resistance. The better you are at overcoming such resistance, the faster you swim, bike, and run.

In terms of physiology, the key to this ability is your muscular system, especially the primary mover muscles for each sport. If they are well developed (but not bulky), you will excel when resistance is high. If your muscles are weak, though, it doesn't matter how aerobically fit you are; you will always be slow. Muscular force is closely associated with economy. If you can easily overcome resistance, then you are economical.

Muscular force is improved by training against resistance—overcoming gravity with weight lifting, riding and running into the wind when going up hills, and swimming with drag devices and in rough water. By training this ability, you will come to see how such workouts boost your performance. The training is simple—but not easy. Muscular force workouts are typically short repetitions done at a very high intensity with one of the above types of resistance. In the very early stages of your annual training, you can hit the weight room. After that, though, you need to transfer your workouts to the pool and the road, where they become specific to each sport.

Speed skills. Speed skills are the ability to make the movements of the sport in an efficient and

effective manner. As explained above, skill development is one of the best ways to improve economy and therefore boost fitness. The movements of some sports are quite complex and challenging to learn, but all sports involve skill development, whether simple or difficult. In triathlon, the most complex skills are found in swimming. Although biking and running demand less complex movements, they are not devoid of skill. Master the skills of swimming, biking, and running, and your fitness and race performance will improve.

I call this ability *speed skills* because the purpose is to be able to make the movements, no matter how complex, at a speed that is called upon during racing. Here, I'm not referring to body speed—as in how fast you are going—but rather to arm and leg speed. The high cadences at which you swim, bike, and run in a race must be done skillfully. It's easy to master a skill if you do it slowly enough. In fact, that's the way new skills are typically introduced—at a slow cadence. When the demands of the workout or race require a high cadence, your skills must remain efficient. If you become sloppy at high cadences, you will waste energy and your fitness will be poor.

Speed skills are taught and improved with drills, fast repeats of a few seconds' duration, and sport-specific exercises such as plyometrics. As mentioned in the economy discussion above, short-duration, high-frequency training is the best way to master a new skill. In Chapter 12, we will get into the many details of swimming, biking, and running skills.

The Advanced Abilities

Once you have established your basic abilities early in the season, you need to shift your training toward the advanced abilities of muscular

Speed skills are the ability to make athletic movements efficiently and effectively.

endurance, anaerobic endurance, and sprint power (Figure 6.2). These are the keys to high-performance racing for the experienced and competitive triathlete. They have a lot to do with how fast you are and how long you can sustain a high output.

Muscular endurance. This is the ability that ultimately determines how fast you are in a triathlon. Not surprisingly, the training plans later on include a considerable amount of muscular endurance workouts in the final few weeks of training before an important race.

Muscular endurance is the ability to continue swimming, biking, and running for a *moderately* long time at a *moderately* high effort. The duration is "moderate" because it's shorter than what you do for aerobic endurance workouts. The intensity is greater than that of aerobic endurance training, but not as intense as that of anaerobic endurance training. When training this ability, you will be at or just below anaerobic threshold. So it's "moderately" intense.

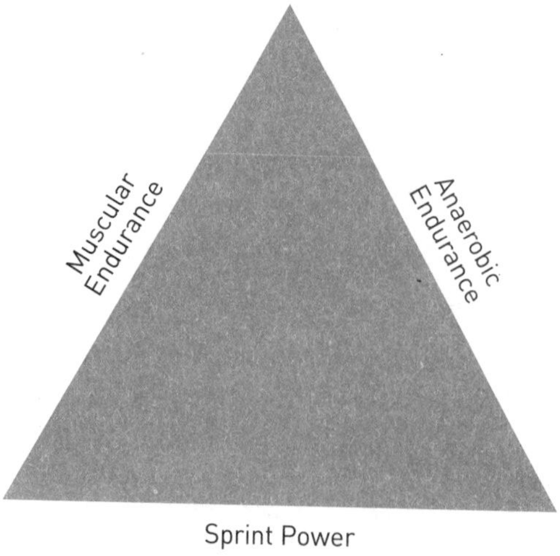

Muscular
endurance
involves
moderately high
effort for
a moderately
long time.

FIGURE 6.2 The advanced abilities of training

Your muscular endurance is improved by doing long (6–12 minutes) intervals with short recoveries, or long (20–60 minutes) steady efforts in heart rate, power, or pace zones 3 and 4. These are hard workouts, but they pay off with greatly improved fitness. Bear in mind that just like anaerobic threshold, muscular endurance workouts must be specific for each sport. To improve running muscular endurance, you must do running workouts. Swim intervals won't boost your run muscular endurance. By following the training guidelines in later chapters, you will do a considerable amount of this type of training in all three sports.

Anaerobic endurance. This is the ability to exercise for a few minutes at a very high effort—well above your anaerobic threshold. Anaerobic endurance training is the single best workout for improving your aerobic capacity. I know the terms *anaerobic endurance* and *aerobic capacity* sound contradictory. I'll try to explain what is something of a scientific misnomer that dates back to the 1960s in exercise physiology.

Whenever you are exercising above the anaerobic threshold, you are, by definition, *anaerobic*. In other words, as described in the discussion of anaerobic threshold above, acidic hydrogen ions are accumulating in the muscles. This process is accompanied by other cellular changes that ultimately contribute to short-term fatigue. But whenever you are using oxygen to produce energy, you are by definition *aerobic*. And you are still burning oxygen when you are at your aerobic capacity, even though the term *anaerobic* means without oxygen. So when doing anaerobic endurance workouts, you are building muscle fatigue very rapidly, but you are still, to some extent, using oxygen to produce energy. *Anaerobic* is therefore an inaccurate term, but after 50 years of use, I'm afraid it's here to stay.

Anaerobic endurance workouts call for short—a few seconds to a handful of minutes—and highly intense intervals done in zone 5 with equal to somewhat shorter recovery breaks between them. You should take on your anaerobic endurance training sparingly and with great caution. It is very strong medicine. It's not candy. In the training guidelines later in this book, you will see how I emphasize these workouts at only a few selected times throughout the season. You need to do them, but be prudent.

Sprint power. As the name implies, sprint power is the ability to sprint at very high power outputs for a few seconds. It's improved by very short (less than 20 seconds), maximum-effort intervals with long recoveries (several minutes). It's an ability that is critical to bicycle road races, such as the flat stages of the Tour de France, but is of little consequence for triathlon. The outcome of a multisport race seldom comes down to a sprint to the finish line. So this is the one ability of the six you probably don't need to worry about.

DETERMINING ABILITY LIMITERS

Chapter 5 introduced you to the concept of limiters. A limiter is a goal-specific weakness that stands between you and the successful accomplishment of a goal. Why do I call it a "goal-specific" weakness? It's because not all of your weaknesses are limiters for your race performance. Let's look at an example. An athlete may not be very good at climbing hills on a bike.

That's definitely a weakness. But if the most important race of that athlete's season doesn't have any hills, then this weakness is not a limiter. It's not standing in the way of success. That's why limiters are goal-specific. You can think of your limiters as a mismatch between your weaknesses and the demands of the event for which you are training. All athletes have limiters, even the pros. It's just that the limiters are more obvious for some athletes than for others. This is certainly true of the three sports of triathlon. One or two of them are limiters for you, meaning that you are weaker in one than in another. For example, you may be an excellent cyclist and runner but only moderately accomplished as a swimmer. In this case, swimming is a limiter because it's a weakness that is certainly challenged during a triathlon. And then within swimming, the specific ability that may be holding you back the most could be speed skills. You may also determine that rough, open-water swimming is a weakness. But if your most important races are always done in calm water, then it's not a limiter.

In the same way, we could assess your strengths and weaknesses in all three of the sports to determine your ability limiters. Once we figure these out, we have a good idea of how to focus your training going forward.

How do we determine your ability limiters by sport? You may already have a good sense of your strengths and weaknesses. You undoubtedly know which of the three sports is your strongest and which is your weakest. You may even have a sense of why that is so, from an abilities perspective. A quick guide for determining your weaknesses is provided in Sidebar 6.1. This set of simple and straightforward questions should help you assess your abilities. Follow the

A limiter is a specific weakness that stands between you and your goal.

SIDEBAR 6.1 **Assessment of Your Basic Abilities by Sport**

Read each statement below and decide if you agree or disagree as it applies to you. Check the appropriate answer. If unsure, go with your initial feeling. Do this three times—once each for your swimming, biking, and running.

A→ AGREE   D→ DISAGREE

_____ 1. I swim/bike/run with a slow stroke rate/cadence.

_____ 2. I prefer races with relatively short swim/bike/run portions.

_____ 3. As the swim/bike/run intervals get shorter and quicker, I do better than most of my training partners.

_____ 4. I'm stronger than my training partners at the end of very long swim/bike/run workouts.

_____ 5. I'm stronger in the weight room than most other athletes my size.

_____ 6. I prefer long swim/bike/run workouts to short ones.

_____ 7. I swim in rough water/bike uphill/ run uphill better than most in my age group.

_____ 8. I really enjoy high-volume swim/bike/run-training weeks.

_____ 9. I consider my swim stroke/bike cadence/run stride to be short and quick.

_____ 10. I have always been better at short but fast swim/bike/run workouts than at long endurance workouts.

_____ 11. I finish long swim/bike/run workouts stronger than most of my training partners.

_____ 12. I'm more muscular than most swimmers/ cyclists/runners of my age and sex.

_____ 13. My upper body (swim) and leg (bike/run) strength is quite good.

_____ 14. I consider my swim/bike/run technique to be very good.

_____ 15. I'm confident of my swim/bike/run endurance at the start of long workouts.

SCORING: For each of the following sets of statements, count and record in the space provided the number of "Agree" answers you checked each of the three times you responded to the above statements. Do this once each for swim, bike, and run.

STATEMENTS   1, 5, 7, 12, 13: Number of "Agrees" _____ Muscular force

2, 3, 9, 10, 14: Number of "Agrees" _____ Speed skills

4, 6, 8, 11, 15: Number of "Agrees" _____ Aerobic endurance

SCORES BY SPORT: Record your score below for each of the three basic abilities by sport. The lower the score, the more likely that ability is a weakness, and possibly a limiter, for you. A score of 0 or 1 certainly indicates a weakness, while a score of 4 or 5 is a good indicator of a strength.

SWIM		BIKE		RUN	
Muscular force score	_____	Muscular force score	_____	Muscular force score	_____
Speed skills score	_____	Speed skills score	_____	Speed skills score	_____
Aerobic endurance score	_____	Aerobic endurance score	_____	Aerobic endurance score	_____

instructions for this sidebar and then return to reading about how to use the results.

This strength-and-weakness assessment tool is by no means perfect, but it may help you to confirm your suspected weaknesses in the three basic abilities. Determining ability weaknesses can be quite difficult, especially if you are an accomplished triathlete. As you've seen from having completed the sidebar, assessing abilities goes well beyond simply knowing your weakness among the three sports. The key to purposeful training is knowing which of the nine total basic abilities are in need of repair.

So what about your advanced ability weaknesses? They result from poor basic abilities that you should now know. Figure 6.3 can help determine yours. Note that each of the advanced abilities is on a side of the triangle, with the basic abilities at the corners. Each advanced ability is based on the two basic abilities at the two ends of its side. For example, the advanced ability *muscular endurance* is the product of the two basic abilities *aerobic endurance* and *muscular force*. If either of these two basic abilities is weak, the resulting advanced ability is also likely to be weak.

If either your *aerobic endurance* or *muscular force* is weak, then your *muscular endurance* is also likely inadequate.

If both *aerobic endurance* and *muscular force* are weaknesses, then there's little doubt that *muscular endurance* is a weakness.

By comparing your results from Sidebar 6.1 with Figure 6.3, you can get a pretty good idea of what your weaknesses are. Again, of course, this doesn't mean they are limiters. We'll return to this matter of weaknesses versus limiters shortly.

For novice triathletes, the basic abilities are the typical limiters. This is where novices should

focus their training time. There is no need for them to work on the advanced abilities until the basic ones are well established, which may take 1 to 3 years of basic training. For experienced athletes who have devoted several years to improving aerobic endurance, muscular force, and speed skills, the common limiters are the advanced abilities of muscular endurance and anaerobic endurance. But, as you will see when we get to the topic of planning your season in Chapter 7, the experienced athlete should still re-establish the basic abilities each season before progressing to training in advanced abilities.

There are many other possible weaknesses beyond the six abilities in Figure 6.3 that may be limiting your performance. The others have mostly to do with lifestyle-related matters and include such behaviors as training inconsistency, limited time available for training, lack of confidence, limited support from family and friends, poor nutritional choices, insufficient

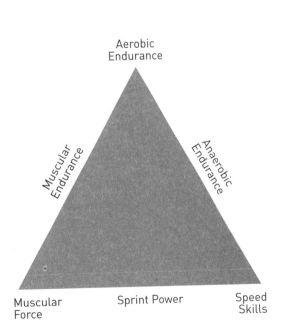

FIGURE 6.3 The complete training triad

athletic equipment, an inadequate training environment, a propensity to overtrain, frequent illness or injury, inappropriate body composition, insufficient sleep, unusual psychological stress, a physically demanding job, and many more. These must also be addressed if you are to perform anywhere near your potential as a triathlete. I suspect you know which apply to you and that you already know what to do about them. This book touches on a few of them, but the primary focus here is upon your basic and advanced performance limiters.

ABILITIES AND TRAINING

Let's review. An ability strength or weakness is something you have determined, either from experience or from Sidebar 6.1, that you are either good or inadequate at doing in a race. In terms of the basic abilities, that means you have either strong or weak aerobic endurance, muscular force, and speed skills for each of the three sports. For the experienced triathlete, being strong or weak in the advanced abilities means that muscular endurance and anaerobic endurance are also either well developed or lacking.

A limiter is a weak ability that is holding you back when it comes to your most important races of the season because being good at that ability is necessary for success in the event. Your limiters can be either basic or advanced abilities. But typically, if you have a weak basic ability, it also affects one of your advanced abilities.

When it comes to the abilities, races have unique demands. For example, if you're doing a very long race, such as an Ironman, which demands aerobic endurance, and aerobic endurance happens to be your weakness in one of the

three sports, then that is also a limiter. For sprint-distance races, aerobic endurance is unlikely to be a limiter. If the race has challenging hills on the bike course and muscular force for cycling is your weakness, then that's a limiter. But for flat courses, muscular force is less likely to be a limiter, even though it's a weakness. For experienced athletes doing a short-course race, a high level of anaerobic endurance is required. If anaerobic endurance is a weakness, then it's also a limiter. On the other hand, a muscular endurance weakness in a sport is highly likely to be a limiter in any type of triathlon, simply because of the unique demands of the sport. That's why you'll see suggestions for so much muscular endurance training when we get to the later chapters.

You will never realize your potential as a triathlete until you improve your limiters. By now, you should have an understanding of what yours are. Identifying your limiters is not a negative exercise, by the way; it's a positive one because you can then train in such a way as to improve your limiters in order to achieve your goals. It's that simple.

As you attack the process of identifying your limiters, the key question to keep in mind is this: Which limiters are holding me back from high performance? Answering this question is critical in achieving your goals. Most athletes never ask it. They train without purpose, haphazardly doing whatever feels right at the time. For too many, the emphasis is generally only on what they are already good at doing—their strengths. If they are strong in the hills, they do lots of climbing. If long, slow endurance is their favorite way to train, then that's what they mostly do. It never dawns on them that there will never be a breakthrough until they improve whatever it is that is holding them back. Continuing to focus solely on strengths while ignoring limiters means there will be little or no change in performance.

Here's the short take-away: In order to train purposefully, you must know both your weaknesses and the demands of the race for which you are training. That's limiter-based training.

What about your strengths? What are you already good at doing in each of the three sports? How do these fit into your training plan? You certainly don't want to compromise or lose your strong abilities, do you? That's correct, and there are two considerations when it comes to your strengths. The first has to do with training. Some workouts need to emphasize your strengths so that they are maintained. If aerobic endurance is a strong ability, you need to do occasional aerobic endurance training throughout the season. But you don't need to do as much of it as the athlete for whom aerobic endurance is a weakness. It's easier to maintain a strength than to improve a limiter, so you must balance your training appropriately.

The other consideration when it comes to your strong abilities is race selection. If you have a choice when it comes to scheduling your races for the season, you are likely to have better performances in those races that closely match your strengths. If aerobic endurance is a strength, you are likely to do well in long-course races. If your anaerobic endurance is good, then you will excel at short-course races. If you're strong in the hills, hilly races are for you. Race selection has a lot to do with success.

Of course, you don't always have the option to select races that match up well with your abilities. The most important races are often one of a kind. Take it or leave it. A national, regional, or world championship happens only once in

a season, and the course may not match your strengths. Or your favorite race of the season may not match what you are good at doing. In these cases, your only options are to either skip the mismatched race or strengthen your limiters. Given this problem, you will probably choose to race and train to become better with regard to your limiters.

Choosing to do a race that is a mismatch for your abilities also requires building a strategy around your strengths. You will need to get the most possible time savings from your sport-specific strengths while minimizing your losses in the portions of the race where you are weak. That can be a real challenge, but it makes the sport interesting and fun. A good performance in such a situation is all the more rewarding.

SUMMARY: BUILDING FITNESS

This chapter introduced what are generally considered by sports scientists to be the physiological determiners of endurance performance—aerobic capacity (VO_2max), anaerobic threshold, and economy. In summarizing these, recall that aerobic capacity is largely the result of your genetics as optimized by consistent training over many years. The longer your race, the less significant aerobic capacity is in performance, even though it's never a bad thing to have a high VO_2max.

Anaerobic threshold is highly trainable. You should see a steady improvement in your race performance as training raises your threshold to a higher percentage of your aerobic capacity.

Economy may be the best determiner of performance of the three, but sports science is still studying it. Much of what is now known to be

Choose races that closely match your strengths.

important is out of your control, simply because of genetics. Those variables you can control often take a long time to accomplish (e.g., changing your technique), are difficult to achieve (e.g., reducing your body weight), or are expensive (e.g., purchasing a lighter bike).

We also looked at your abilities in this chapter. Abilities are your physiological strengths and weaknesses that are specific to race performance. There are basic abilities—aerobic endurance, muscular force, and speed skills—and advanced abilities—muscular endurance, anaerobic endurance, and sprint power. Each

defines a specific type of workout and is related in some way to the three fitness determiners. Understanding the abilities will help you determine how to train for races.

This brought us to the concept of limiters. If a race requires mastery of one of the six abilities but you have a weakness in that ability, then it is limiting your performance potential. One of the primary purposes of training is to strengthen your limiters. It's also important that you maintain your strong abilities. In the coming chapters, we will delve into how all of this is done in quite a bit of detail.

PART IV

PLANNING
TO RACE

I consider this part to be the heart of the book. Why? Because planning is the single most important thing you can do to improve performance outside actual training.

It's remarkable how having a written plan will help you stay focused on attaining high goals. Too many athletes never experience this because they see no reason to plan ahead. They train one workout at a time, with little thought as to how the series of workouts they have been doing will affect their current level of fitness, or how the workouts they're doing today will blend with future workouts to produce readiness to race at a high level. They're myopic, seeing only today. That may be OK if your only goal for training is to have fun, but if you also want to achieve high-performance goals, then a plan for getting there is essential. So in this section, you'll learn the many intricacies of how to create an annual training plan and a weekly training schedule.

Chapters 7 and 8 will take you step by step through building your annual training plan and laying out a standard training week. These two chapters also provide a great deal of detail about the factors to consider as you prepare your plan. Chapter 9 will offer alternative ways of planning your season and your typical week.

I'd like to suggest that you read all three chapters in this part before you sit down to sketch out your plan. As you read the first two chapters, you'll probably start to see your training from a new perspective, differently from the way you've viewed it in the past. But then Chapter 9 will throw a curveball at you and lay out other ways to plan your training. Once you have read Chapter 9, you can decide which training system may be best, given everything you now know. At that point, you can return to the previous chapters to start planning your season.

By the time you have completed your annual training plan (Appendix A), you will have a working tool that is quite similar to what I use when preparing athletes to achieve high-performance goals. You will learn to rely on your annual training plan throughout the season to guide you to goals that will now be much more achievable. And in the seasons that follow, you will return to this plan to consider how you might tweak it in order to achieve even higher goals.

Your high-performance race results start here.

PLANNING A SEASON

PLANNING IS WHAT got me started down the path to coaching and eventually to writing books about training. As a young athlete in the 1970s, I figured that if I could lay out a season-long training schedule that balanced the frequency, length, and intensity of the workouts, I would gradually build my fitness to a high level and achieve my race goals (I was a runner at the time). So I set about planning my seasons.

My original plans were very basic. I used a calendar to schedule how hard each of the weeks would be for the entire buildup to my most important race. Then, I went back to each week and decided what the key workouts would be. I included intervals, tempo, hills, long runs, strength training, and recovery days. Over time, these basic calendar plans became more sophisticated as I slowly learned the best ways to arrange the hard and easy weeks and the individual sessions.

Somewhat later, I became aware of a new planning method called *periodization*. Soviet bloc countries had been using it for 50 years, but it wasn't introduced to Western countries until the 1970s. At the time, it was revolutionary. Now it's common for athletes around the world to plan and train with this system. Periodization is simply a way of planning the season based on well-defined training periods over a course of days, weeks, months, and even years. Each period has a purpose, I learned, and if the periods are structured in certain ways, they can lead to peak performance for a few select races.

In practical application, I soon discovered that periodization would not have me race-ready all the time. But that was OK; I picked out just a few races every year in which I wanted to do well. Approaching my race season this way meant that I would not be in top race shape year-round, and so I had to accept doing some low-priority races while not in peak form. But on those days when I had an important race, my performance would border on astonishing.

Over the years, as I read books on the topic, talked with other athletes and coaches who used it, and experimented with me as the guinea pig, I improved my periodization model and eventually used it with the athletes I coached. Refining how I periodize training has turned out to be a lifetime activity as new inroads into training for peak performance appear every few years. Learning about the application of sports science to planning and training is a never-ending process. In the time since I wrote the first version of *The Triathlete's Training Bible* back in the late 1990s, a lot of new periodization concepts have been introduced. While this chapter and the next one are similar to those in the original *Training Bible*, many subtle changes have been made. There are also some new periodization concepts that we will look into.

For example, a new method of periodization that was under development in the 1990s became widely used by elite endurance athletes starting in the early 2000s. It's called *block periodization*. In traditional periodization, several abilities (see Chapter 6) are developed concurrently. That method works just fine for nearly all age-group athletes. But for elite athletes whose fitness in the various abilities is close to their upper limits, the low density of traditional periodization—how closely the unique ability workouts are spaced— is a major concern. In order for an elite athlete to make progress with individual abilities, those workouts must be very closely spaced. That isn't possible when several abilities are being trained in each training week.

Because of this concern, coaches began to focus on only one or at most two abilities in each

multiweek block of training. Once that ability was well established, the athlete progressed to the next ability in a new block while doing just enough training of the previously established ability to maintain it. This proved to be an effective periodization method for elites—but not for the vast majority of age groupers.

Many other periodization methods have been developed and refined over the years. The method I will teach you in this chapter is called *classic* or *linear periodization*. It's easy to understand and apply. It's been around for a long time, and it is still the method most commonly used by athletes at all levels. It's the method I described in the first *Training Bible* a few years ago. But there have been some refinements since then that will be introduced in this and the next chapter. In Chapter 9, I will use case studies to show you examples of other periodization methods, including block periodization.

PERIODIZATION OF TRAINING

The starting place for your planning is adopting the belief that training must be a steady and gradual building process. Peak race performance doesn't happen suddenly or mysteriously. Your body must undergo a lot of changes to become race-ready. Each of these physiological changes takes time. They cannot be rushed. You can't force your body to become fit on some sort of artificial schedule. It must be gently coaxed to a higher level of fitness by allowing it to progress naturally.

To honor the body's natural progression, you *must* be willing to make changes to it from time to time. A rigid plan that doesn't allow for days when you are overly tired and doesn't consider

Peak race performance doesn't happen suddenly or mysteriously.

the many other lifestyle demands on your time is worse than no plan at all. Your plan needs to be dynamic to be effective. Every day, you have to take into account how you are feeling. Planning flexibility is critical to your racing success. You must be willing to make changes. That almost always means resting when rest is needed. Chapter 11 will get into the topic of rest and recovery, including "recovery on demand," in detail.

The second periodization concept you need to understand and adopt has to do with a gradually changing training progression. As the season moves forward, your workouts must become increasingly like the race. In other words, as you get closer to the day of your most important race, your workouts must gradually take on the characteristics of that race based on your goals for the race. For example, if your goal is to run in the race at a pace of 7 minutes per mile (4 minutes, 20 seconds per kilometer), then some of your runs off the bike need to be at that pace—and you need to do more of these runs as you get closer to the race. If the bike course will be hilly, then your training should increasingly include hills as you move into the last several weeks of training. If the swim will be in open water, then you need to do some lake or ocean swimming at race intensity, preferably with other triathletes. If race day is expected to be hot, then you need to train in the heat frequently in the last several weeks before the race. Your goal in the last few weeks of training is to make your most important workouts as much like the race as you can.

Planning Details

This latter point on workout progression brings us to a critical principle of periodization—the timing of workouts by ability. Chapter 6 intro-duced the concept of abilities and divided them into two categories—basic and advanced. Figure 7.1 combines these two categories into one diagram. The basic abilities are at the corners of the ability triangle—aerobic endurance, muscular force, and speed skills. At the sides are the advanced abilities—muscular endurance, anaerobic endurance, and sprint power. The critical message from Chapter 6 is that the advanced abilities are the product of the basic abilities. If you want to have good muscular endurance for your race, then you must first fully develop your aerobic endurance and muscular force. In the same way, strong anaerobic endurance results from well-developed aerobic endurance and speed skills. (As mentioned in Chapter 6, triathletes need not train for sprint power.)

For this reason, in linear periodization we begin the season by focusing on the basic abilities, and as training progresses we shift the emphasis to the advanced abilities. It's not a sud-

As the season moves forward, your workouts must become increasingly like the race.

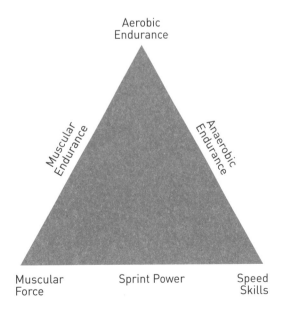

FIGURE 7.1 The basic and advanced abilities

TABLE 7.1 **The Common Periods in a Linear Periodization Model**

PERIOD	LENGTH	PURPOSE	PRIMARY ABILITY FOCUS
Prep	1–4 weeks	Preparing to train	Basic abilities
Base	9–12 weeks	Training to train	Basic abilities
Build	6–8 weeks	Training to race	Advanced abilities
Peak	1–2 weeks	Tapering for race	Advanced abilities
Race	1–3 weeks	Removing fatigue Sharpening fitness	Advanced abilities
Transition	1–4 weeks	Resting and recovering	Basic abilities

den shift from basic to advanced, but rather a gradual change involving a considerable overlap of the two categories.

Sports scientists call the early part of the season, when the basic abilities are emphasized, the *general preparation period*. Most athletes call it the base period. But the general preparation title is actually more descriptive of the purpose of the base period—to prepare in a general way for the latter part of the season. Essentially, when in the general preparation (base) period, you are training to train. Sports scientists call the subsequent period *specific preparation*. Most athletes call it the *build* period. Again, specific preparation is a good name because it implies that the emphasis of training is on workouts that are specific, or similar, to the race for which you are training. In deference to common usage, I will continue to use the terms *base* and *build*, but you should keep the general and specific definitions in mind when you read them here.

Besides the base and build periods, a few other periods must be understood to fully grasp the concept of planning with periodization. In common athlete language, the others are the *prep, peak, race,* and *transition* periods. Table 7.1 lists each of the periods in the order in which

> Base period is for general preparation. Build period is for specific preparation.

they generally occur, along with a description of each.

Overview of Your Plan

By now, you should have an understanding of what the focus of your training should be: You want to minimize your limitations and maximize your already well-established ability strengths. And you should also have a general understanding of the training periods you will use in your annual training plan (ATP). With these in mind, we will develop a plan to fully prepare you for your race by developing both ability categories throughout the current or coming season. This will be a big picture, an overview, of where you are going and what you should work on in preparation for your race. We'll pull together many of the concepts discussed in the previous chapters in order to provide structure and purpose for your training.

If you are coming to this chapter at the start of a brand-new season, your timing is perfect. If, on the other hand, you are already well into the season, incorporating what is discussed here will require some adjusting on your part to blend what you have been doing so far with a new and possibly more highly structured training method. In either case, by the end of this chapter, you will

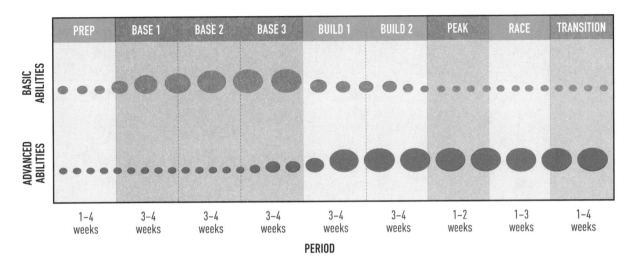

FIGURE 7.2 Overview of linear periodization showing preparation for the first important race of the season

have developed most of your ATP for your next important race. This method may be used over and over in the following seasons, allowing you to easily devise a training plan that provides a purposeful focus for your season and sound fitness on race day. As you finish each season, save the plans you have come up with so that you have a record of what you did in the past along with end-of-season notes on how you will make adjustments in the future based on what you have learned.

Before we start designing your season, it's important to understand how the training of abilities fits into a linear periodization plan. Figure 7.2 lists all of the periods and divides them into subperiods. It shows how the basic and advanced abilities are blended into a training plan as you prepare for the *first* important race of the season.

Note that Figure 7.2 shows how to train only for your season's first race. For the subsequent most important races in your season, you don't have to go through the entire periodization process shown in Figure 7.1 all over again to get ready because you have gradually accumulated

fitness through the course of the season. But there is also a slight loss of fitness associated with the periods around the race period. When you taper for a race during the peak period and recover after the race in the transition period, even if the taper lasts just a few days, your fitness is somewhat compromised, especially the basic abilities. Your fitness built before the initial race won't be entirely lost when you back off from hard training at these times, but you'll need to rebuild some basic fitness before the upcoming second and third races.

Planning to prepare for subsequent races is a much trickier process than planning to prepare for the first race of the year. It all comes down to how much time you have between the first and second races. The more time you have, the easier it is to get ready. In a perfect season, you'd have 12 to 16 weeks between important races. That means that after a short break from training in the few days after the first race (the transition period), you would to return to a bit of base training (base 3) before advancing through the build, peak, and

Planning for subsequent races is trickier than planning for the first race of the year.

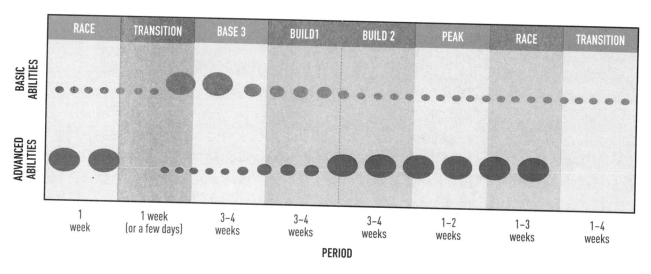

FIGURE 7.3 A suggested preparation plan for the second and third most important races of the season when there are 12 to 16 weeks to train following the previous race

race periods. In this case, your periodization plan would look something like Figure 7.3.

There are likely to be seasons when there are far fewer than 12 weeks separating your second or third most important race from the previous race. The less time you have to prepare, the greater the challenge when it comes to planning.

Figure 7.4 suggests a plan for when there are only 7 to 11 weeks between races.

With fewer than 7 weeks between important races, which often is the case, you must make difficult decisions about what you will do to prepare for the next event. You will still need a transition period following the previous race. This period

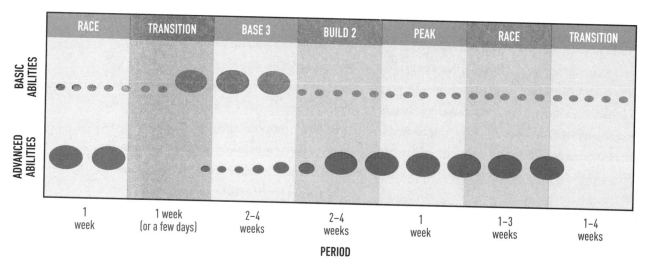

FIGURE 7.4 A suggested preparation plan for the second or third most important race of the season when there are only 7 to 11 weeks to train following the previous race

may last only a few days, depending on how stressful the race was. Long-course races typically require more transition time than short-course events.

Following the transition period's break from serious training, you are ready to return to focused training again. What you must do is decide what you need most at this time—basic or advanced fitness. With only a handful of weeks until your next race, both are important. Unfortunately, I cannot supply a simple plan that will fit all athletes' needs in this situation. Even coaches with an excellent understanding of periodization and physiology will find this a difficult decision. I can, however, give you some excellent guidance: Follow your gut, and then test yourself to see whether the test results and your gut agree.

Regarding your gut feelings, ask yourself how you think your aerobic fitness is at this time. Remember, it's your aerobic fitness that is critical for both muscular endurance and anaerobic endurance.

In terms of objective tests, you can undertake some aerobic threshold workouts (see Appendixes B, C, and D) and compare the results with the results of the same workouts when you did them before the previous race. Study the test results to decide what is most in need of development. If your aerobic endurance is still solid, then go straight to the build period with the focus on either muscular endurance or anaerobic endurance, depending on the type of race you're doing next. You may decide to include both aerobic endurance and either muscular endurance or anaerobic endurance in a sort of blended base-build period with an emphasis on the one most in need.

Of course, the type of race next on your schedule also plays a role in the decision. If it is a short-course race, you may decide to devote most of your limited training time to one ability, such as muscular endurance. In fact, if in doubt, work on this ability regardless of race type, with a special emphasis on your limiting sport. Pay close attention to how you feel in the upcoming race and make notes in your training diary (see Chapter 14) as to how you *should* have trained if it were possible to go back and make changes. That will prove valuable the next time such a scheduling situation comes up.

YOUR ANNUAL TRAINING PLAN

Let's start planning your season. As mentioned earlier, the best time to do this is at the start of a new training year. But you may be coming to this task well into your race season. That's OK. Simply design your plan for the remainder of the year.

There are many formats you can use to do this. You can use a paper calendar on which you write in all of the details that will be described below. Or you can use an electronic calendar on your computer that allows you to make changes quickly and easily. An electronic variation would be to use the ATP feature at TrainingPeaks (www.trainingpeaks.com), which is available to subscribers and follows the procedures I explain in this chapter. Perhaps the easiest way, and certainly the least expensive, is to use a paper-based plan such as the one provided in Appendix A. Normally, you shouldn't make copies of a book because of copyright laws, but you have my permission (and the publisher's) to make copies of the ATP you will find there. If you create a paper plan, be sure to use a pencil because there are certain to be many changes throughout the year.

Don't avoid making a plan just because your race season has started.

In 30 years of coaching, I've never had an athlete's plan go unaltered for an entire season.

Before we get started on the details of your plan, let's briefly review why you are doing this. It isn't to impress anyone or simply to feel organized (although there's a lot to be said for the confidence that comes with such a feeling), but rather to create a dynamic guide to lead you through the coming season. It's easier to lay out a plan at the start of the season, when you can do it from a long-range perspective, than when you are in the heat of the battle. Planning is usually best when emotions don't get in the way.

In the remainder of this chapter, I'm going to take you step by step through the process of laying out an ATP. Now is a good time to make a copy of the ATP in Appendix A and follow along as you read what is coming next. If at any time you get confused, skip ahead to the end of this chapter, where you will find Figure 7.5, which is an example of a completed plan.

We will follow six steps to produce your ATP:

- Establish your season goals.
- Determine your training objectives.
- Set your annual training volume.
- Prioritize your races.
- Divide the season into periods.
- Estimate your weekly volume.

By the end of this chapter, you will have most of your ATP done. All that will remain to complete it is scheduling weekly workouts. We'll do that in Chapter 8.

Step 1: Establish Season Goals

At the top of the ATP in Appendix A, there is a space to write in your season goals. In Chapter 5, you read about how to set your goals for a race season. Short of rereading that chapter, here is a quick summary of the key points.

Set no more than three goals for the season. With more than three, you run the risk of being overwhelmed, and something may be overlooked with all of the details. Having too many goals makes it hard to stay focused on what is truly most important. Having fewer than three is also a good option and will give you an even greater focus, so don't feel that you need to have three to succeed.

State your goals as seasonal outcomes. What is it you will look back on with satisfaction and a feeling of great accomplishment in the coming years? Bear in mind that these are not the subgoals you must accomplish in order to achieve your overarching goals. Those are objectives that we will get to in the next step. An outcome goal for a triathlete is something higher, usually a race result. It can also be something along the lines of "qualify for the national team" (although that usually requires a race outcome to accomplish). Your goals should be measurable. In triathlon, the most common measurement is your race finishing time, so it is the most likely measurement to include when you are defining your goals. Goals based on race placement in your age group, such as "podium at XYZ race," depend too much on who shows up on race day in your age group. While making the podium is a worthy accomplishment, you have no control over who the other competitors are or how fit they may be. You have control only over your performance. Your goals should reflect that.

So now it's time to write your goals at the top of the ATP. Go ahead and pencil them in, and be sure to make them measurable.

Planning is usually best when emotions don't get in the way.

Step 2: Determine Training Objectives

There is a space near the top of your ATP for four training objectives, which address your ability limiters. Chapter 5 provided an in-depth explanation of training objectives, and Chapter 6 addressed limiters. Let's refresh your memory on both of these.

Training objectives are subgoals for your season. If you achieve them, then you can expect to achieve your season goals. Typically, training objectives will be accomplished during workouts. But they may also be achieved in less important races that you do before your season goal events.

The purpose of the training objectives is to "fix," or correct, the goal-specific weaknesses—your limiters—that are preventing you from achieving your season goals. In Chapter 6, you determined your race-specific weaknesses (your ability limiters) and you assessed your basic abilities (aerobic endurance, muscular force, and speed skills) as well as your advanced abilities (muscular endurance and anaerobic endurance). Now it's time to establish subgoals for improving those limiters.

A training objective is simply a statement about one of your ability limiters and how you will know when it is corrected. Let's take a look at some basic abilities limiters as training objectives. For example, if your basic swim limiter is speed skills, which is common for triathletes, then a training objective might be, Improve average pace when doing form 25s at a comfortable effort before starting the build period. (This workout will be addressed in Chapter 12.) Another example, this time for aerobic endurance during running, might be, Increase my run efficiency factor by 10 percent by March 1. (The run efficiency factor workout is described in

Appendix D.) A muscular force objective might be, Leg press 2.5 times my body weight by the end of base 1. (See Chapter 13 for details.)

Here are some examples of training objectives for the advanced ability of muscular endurance: Swim 1,000 meters in less than 15 minutes by the end of build 2. Bike 20 minutes with a normalized power of 250 watts by April 15. Run a local 10-km race in less than 42 minutes by 4 weeks prior to my Olympic-distance triathlon. For the advanced ability of anaerobic endurance, training objectives might be something like these: Swim 100 meters in less than 80 seconds by March 30. Run 1,200 meters in under 4 minutes, 30 seconds by the end of build 1. Climb Maniac Hill on my bike in less than 3 minutes by April 15.

Now is a good time for you to contemplate your ability limiters as determined in Chapter 6 and record training objectives that address them at the top of your ATP. Again, note that you may not have a limiter for every ability in every sport. Narrow it down to the four or fewer limiters that are most likely to affect your race performances for your most important races. If you improve these, you are highly likely to achieve your season goals.

Step 3: Set Annual Training Volume

At the top of the ATP, there is a space to indicate your annual volume. This is how many cumulative hours you will train over the course of the season, including all of your sport-specific workouts, strength training, and cross-training time. Athletes who train with Dr. Andy Coggan's training stress score (TSS) system, as supported by TrainingPeaks.com, should indicate anticipated TSS volume for the year in the annual volume

Training objectives are subgoals for your season.

space. The nice thing about TSS is that it includes training intensity along with time. With annual training hours, of course, only training time is considered. And as explained in Chapter 4, of the two factors—time and intensity—that contribute to a workout's fitness benefits, intensity is the more critical one for the high-performance athlete. Even if you are already well into your race season, you should still indicate how many hours or at what TSS you anticipate training for the remainder of this season.

How do you determine annual training hours or TSS? One way is to look back at how much total volume you trained in the previous year. Again, this should include all swim, bike, run, strength, and cross-training workouts. If you successfully managed the amount you did last year, consider increasing the volume 10 percent or so for the new season. This is generally a good idea for athletes in the first 5 years of triathlon training because they probably still have room for growth. If you are beyond 5 years in the sport, you may want to keep annual hours the same as last year but do more intensity in training in the new season. This will, of course, increase TSS by perhaps 10 percent, but not hours.

Another way to estimate annual volume is to determine your typical average training hours or TSS for a week and multiply that by 45. Using 45 as a multiplier allows for weeks or cumulative days when you don't train during the year, as when you are sick or injured, taking recovery days, experiencing business and career interruptions, taking a family vacation, or taking transition period training breaks. Of course we hope that the first two on the list won't happen, but they have a way of showing up from time to time. A third option is to base annual volume on

your longest race and general goal for that event (Table 7.2).

The annual training volume for many athletes is determined not by what they are capable of doing but rather by lifestyle: career, family, and other commitments. For these athletes, weekly volume is set according to the maximum weekly time usually available to train. Athletes in a time crunch may be able to manage a greater training volume physically, but their other commitments cut that volume to a lesser amount. If this describes your situation, multiply the common weekly hours available to you by 45 and record this in your ATP.

This annual volume number will actually have little meaning for the time-constrained athlete because the weekly volume will be much the same from week to week, with the possible exception of rest-and-recovery weeks and during the peak and race periods. There may also be weeks or days when you can increase your training volume if temporary lifestyle changes free up some time. Otherwise, because weekly time is restricted, this athlete will need to vary intensity significantly throughout the season to produce race readiness. In that case, note that TSS is of much greater value than training hours as a marker of annual volume because it also takes intensity into consideration. Increasing or decreasing training intensity, even if weekly hours stay the same, is reflected by a changing TSS. Whereas a low-intensity week may produce 45 TSS points per hour, a high-intensity week can result in 55 per hour. A long-term hourly TSS of 50 is a common average. The time-crunched triathlete can estimate weekly TSS throughout the season by using the standard number of weekly hours available to set training volume.

Training stress score includes training intensity with time.

TSS will reflect increasing or decreasing training intensity, even if weekly hours stay the same.

TABLE 7.2 **A Rough Guide for Determining Annual Training Volume**

LONGEST RACE DURATION	FINISH THE RACE		HIGH PERFORMANCE	
	ANNUAL HOURS*	TSS*	ANNUAL HOURS*	TSS*
Up to 3 hours	300–400	(15,000–17,500)	400–800	(20,000–40,000)
3–8 hours	400–500	(17,500–22,500)	600–1,000	(30,000–50,000)
More than 8 hours	500–700	(22,500–30,000)	800–1,200	(40,000–60,000)

* Suggested goal range.

This guide is based on the expected duration of your longest race in the season and your general goal for that event; volume is listed in both annual hours and TSS.

Step 4: Prioritize Races

Your season may start whenever you feel the time is right, so long as you have enough time to prepare for your first race of the season. First, you will need to recover from the last season, of course. That can take a month or so. Then allow about 24 weeks to become race-ready for the new season. For most athletes in the Northern Hemisphere, training typically starts sometime in the period of October through January. What we'll do next is set up your ATP to indicate this start-up and the weeks that follow.

In the "Week" column on your ATP, row 01 is the first week of the new season. Next to that column is the "Mon." column. Here, you will write in the date of your season's first Monday. Next, record all of the dates for the Mondays of the coming season in the column labeled "Mon." For example, the first Monday of October may be the second day of that month. So under "Mon.," write in 10/2, meaning October 2. The next row down would then be October 9 and is recorded as 10/9. This is done for the rest of the season so that every weekly row starts with Monday's date.

After recording all of the Mondays for the season, write in the races you intend to do in the coming season in the column labeled "Races."

Place them on the ATP in the appropriate weeks based on their dates. It's quite likely that your planned races for the new season have not yet announced their exact dates, but you probably know roughly when they will occur, so use those expected dates. For example, let's say that you have an event scheduled for Saturday, May 5, in the coming season. It would be listed in the row that starts with Monday, May 1, and is marked as 5/1 because that row includes all the dates from May 1 through May 7. If you have two races the same weekend, list them both in that row.

Once you have listed all of your planned events in the "Races" column, assign a priority to each by writing in A, B, or C in the "Pri." column next to the race name. Table 7.3 will help you determine priorities.

You are going to create your season's plan around the A-priority races, so I'd strongly suggest having no more than three. Because you will taper—meaning that you will reduce—your training during a 2- to 3-week stretch before the race and then recover for at least a few days during the post-race transition period—again with reduced training—you will lose fitness, especially from your basic abilities. Because you're giving up a bit of fitness to gain race form (see Chapter 3 for details on form), there is a downside to these

Start your season whenever the time is right, so long as you have time to prepare for your first race.

TABLE 7.3 Race Prioritization

RACE PRIORITY	MAXIMUM NUMBER PER SEASON	RACE IMPORTANCE	SPECIAL RACE-DAY PREPARATION
A	3	Most important. Your season's success is determined by these.	Include a 1- to 2-week peak period before race week.
B	8	Of secondary importance. You want to do well, however.	Reduce training stress for 2 to 5 days before race day.
C	Unlimited	Least important. Use as race tune-ups, tests, hard workouts, social events, or for experience.	No special preparation. Treat these as workouts.

You can never have enough base fitness.

most important races. That means you must be conservative in choosing how many to do in a season. Three is about the most that can be managed with time still left to rebuild fitness and come to peak form before the next A-priority race. The more spread out on the calendar the A-priority races are, the better you are likely to do in each of them, as described above in the section "Overview of Your Plan."

With regard to race performance, there are two basic ways to design your season. One is to do no more than three A-priority races, as suggested above, with a taper for 2 to 3 weeks before each. This is highly likely to result in your best possible race performances. You can still do several B-priority races, for which you back off of training for 2 to 5 days prior, as shown in Table 7.3. Think of it as a mini-taper with a resulting small peak in race form. The second way is not to do any A races and instead do lots of B races without a true peak for any of them. Your performances aren't likely to be the best possible, but doing this may well make your race season more enjoyable. I've known many good athletes who enjoy racing frequently. You can do that if you don't schedule any A races that have to be preceded by a long taper.

Another possibility is that you may have only one A-priority race scheduled for the entire sea-

son. That presents a different kind of problem. It takes about 6 months to progress through the standard periodization process before the first race of the year. With as long as 12 months until your race, what do you do with the "extra" 6 months? There are two common solutions. The first, and probably the best, is to designate a second A race that is about 12 to 16 weeks before your most important A race. Go ahead and train for that first race, including a taper prior and a short transition period after. This will give you a chance to see how well you can perform while testing your training for high-priority races. What you learn from that will undoubtedly add to your performance at the more important race. The second way of solving this dilemma is to start your base-period training as described in this chapter, but when you complete base 3, do not continue into the build period. Instead, repeat base 3 as many times as is needed to leave you about 12 weeks until your most important A-priority race. Then start the build period of training. You can never have enough base fitness, so this second method will do a lot to prepare you quite well for the specific, racelike training that precedes the "true" A race.

Note in Table 7.3 that the C-priority races are treated as workouts, meaning you rest before them about the same as you would rest before a hard workout. These events are done strictly as "throwaway" results—meaning you don't expect to be in top form or even race-ready. They are typically done as tune-ups before A or B races to get back into the mind-set and routine of racing if it's been some time since the last one. They may also serve as tests of fitness, hard workouts, or social events done with friends. For the novice triathlete, they are also done for experience. When you are new to the sport, one of the fastest ways to learn what triathlon is all about is to go to races—lots of them. The first year as a triathlete should be a learning experience. Participating in C races is one of the best things you can do to learn.

The longer your A-priority races are, the fewer C races you should do. Ironman and half-Ironman races require doing lots of long training sessions, especially on the bike. Because these are usually done on the weekends when you have available time, and because races also are on the weekends, you're likely to have a time conflict. Something has to go. I'd strongly suggest making that something the C races. You're probably going to train better if you do only a couple of B races in addition to your long-course, A-priority race. For Ironman triathletes, I'd suggest only one B race, preferably a half-Ironman, in the last 12 weeks before your A race. That B race is probably best done around 3 to 7 weeks prior.

Step 5: Divide Season into Periods

The next task in completing your ATP is to periodize the season. Table 7.4 will guide you through that process. It expands on Table 7.1 by dividing the seasonal periods into subperiods and by basing period duration on age. We'll come back to that latter point shortly.

The purpose of each subperiod, as described in the table, is generally the way it is done during training for most events. But there may well be differences in the way you train during any given period in the season. For example, when training elite Ironman triathletes, I may have them train their anaerobic endurance ability in base 3 to boost their aerobic capacities before they start the build period, during which there is a heavy emphasis on muscular endurance. In traditional linear periodization, anaerobic endurance workouts are not done in the base period at all. But there are times when this is appropriate for certain athletes. Feel free to experiment with the model suggested in Table 7.4. You may discover something that works well for you but isn't commonly done. The only hard-and-fast rule in periodization that I would strongly suggest you adhere to is this: The closer in time that you get to your A-priority race, the more like the race your training must become. Otherwise, training periodization can be quite flexible.

Before we continue, I want to explain something about the age and subperiod durations shown in Table 7.4. Subperiod duration actually has more to do with recovery than with age. The age delineation in Table 7.4 is merely a way to simplify this planning, even though age is not always an accurate marker of recovery. Let me elaborate. Regardless of age, breaks from focused and serious training are needed every few weeks in order to shed some of the accumulating fatigue of training. Some athletes need these recovery breaks more frequently than others. How often has to do with several physiological variables, with hormone production perhaps the most important. It's hormones such as growth hormone, testosterone, estrogen, insulin-like

The longer your A-priority races are, the fewer C races you should do.

TABLE 7.4 **Purposes and Durations of Subperiods Relative to Age and Durations of Planned Recovery**

SUBPERIOD	PURPOSE	DURATION (UNDER AGE 50)	DURATION (OVER AGE 50)	PLANNED RECOVERY DURATION
Prep	Preparation for training: cross-training, weights, functional strength, general athleticism	1–4 weeks	1–4 weeks	Recovery not needed
Base 1	General training: aerobic endurance, muscular force, speed skills	4 weeks	3 weeks	Last 4–7 days of base 1
Base 2	General training: aerobic endurance, muscular force, speed skills, limited muscular endurance	4 weeks	3 weeks	Last 4–7 days of base 2
Base 3	General training: aerobic endurance, muscular force, speed skills, more muscular endurance	4 weeks	3 weeks (repeat base 3)	Last 4–7 days of base 3
Build 1	Specific training: muscular and/or anaerobic endurance; maintaining aerobic endurance, muscular force, speed skills	4 weeks	3 weeks	Last 4–7 days of build 1
Build 2	Specific training: muscular and/or anaerobic endurance; maintaining aerobic endurance, muscular force, speed skills	4 weeks	3 weeks (repeat build 2)	Last 4–7 days of build 2
Peak	Specific training: simulating a portion of the race every 72–96 hours; otherwise, recovery workouts	1–2 weeks	1–2 weeks	Recovery not needed
Race	Specific training: short intervals at race intensity or greater and decreasing in number daily; rest	1 week	1 week	Recovery not needed
Transition	Rest and active recovery	1–4 weeks	1–4 weeks	Recovery not needed

Planned recovery breaks from training are included at the end of each subperiod.

growth factor, and others that have a lot to do with how well and how quickly an athlete recovers from hard training sessions, and these hormones decrease with age. The less we produce, the more slowly we recover and therefore the more frequently we need recovery breaks from training. Sometime around age 50, the low production of hormones is evident. That's why recovery typically has to be included more frequently for older athletes than younger ones, and why Table 7.4 shows more frequent recovery for

over-50 athletes at several times throughout the season. But I've known many over-50 athletes who recovered quite quickly. I've also known under-50 athletes who recovered slowly. So even though this table uses age to suggest period duration, you may not fit into these two categories neatly based simply on your age. In other words, use the columns for under 50 and over 50 after giving considerable thought to your usual rate of recovery. That decision is best based on your past experience with accumulating fatigue.

In the "Planned Recovery Duration" column, the "Last 4–7 days" during the base and build periods is a rather broad range. Again, some athletes recover slowly and may need an entire week of reduced training before returning to serious training, while others recover quite quickly and need only 4 days—or something between these extremes. Your recovery in one of these short breaks may also vary from one subperiod to the next. So consider this an "on-demand" decision. If you are still tired after 4 days, take another day—or more—to recover. We'll explore this topic more thoroughly in Chapter 11.

OK, that was a lot of details. Now let's move on to the central focus of this section—periodizing your season.

Periodizing means assigning training periods to each week of the year in the "Period" column of your ATP. You'll fill in this column by working backward. Start with the first A-priority race of the season. At the intersection of the "Period" column and the row, or week, of your first A-priority race, write in "Race" in the "Period" column. Then go up one more row and write in "Peak." Go up another row and again write in "Peak." This will give you a 3-week taper before your race—two peak weeks and a race week. Some athletes in some situations come into better race-day form with only 2 weeks of tapering. Again, this is a part of the individualization you need to consider when designing your plan for the season. There is nothing I can tell you that determines which way to go other than to say it's based entirely on your experience. It's OK to experiment with this to determine which is better for you. But for now, if in doubt, make it two peak weeks.

In the row above your first "Peak" week, write in "Build 2." Now you must decide if you will plan

3- or 4-week subperiods based on the discussion above about recovery and age. If you are using 4-week subperiods, write in "Build 2" three more times so that you have 4 weeks of "Build 2" above your first "Peak" week. If you are using 3-week subperiods, write in "Build 2" in only three rows. Now do the same thing—3 or 4 weeks each—for build 1, base 3, base 2, and base 1. Note that you may use different subperiod durations—3 or 4 weeks—for the base and build periods. Some athletes recover quite quickly when focused primarily on the basic abilities, as in the base period, but somewhat more slowly when training the advanced abilities. So these athletes may opt to use 3-week subperiods in build and 4 weeks for each of the base subperiods. Again, this is a personal decision based on experience. If unsure, keep your base and build subperiod durations the same.

In the row above your first week in the season of base 1, write in "Prep." This can vary from only 1 week to as many as 4 weeks. I should add that there have been times when I've completely omitted it for some athletes when they had a limited amount of training weeks before the first race. I've also extended it beyond 4 weeks when athletes had excessive time until an A-priority event and we decided to hold off on base training for whatever reason. The most common point of determination here is the number of training weeks available before the first A-priority race. If everything works out just right, your first prep or first base 1 week on the ATP will coincide with when you intend to start training for the coming season.

Now go back down to the row immediately below your first "Race" week. It's possible that you will have one or two more races in the fol-

Work backward to fill in the Period column of your ATP.

lowing 1 or 2 weeks. If so, write in "Race" for each such week so that you have two or three consecutive rows labeled "Race." It's rare in triathlon to have multiple A-priority races in consecutive weeks, but it does happen. Now write in "Tran" (for *transition*) in the first week after your single A race or the last of your back-to-back A races. As noted in Table 7.4, this week may last a few days or can be as long as 4 weeks. I've even had athletes take up to 6 weeks if their season was exceptionally stressful. If this first transition period comes early in your season, which is common, then I'd suggest taking just a few days off from focused training. This may be only 3 or 4 days but could be 7 days depending on lingering mental and physical fatigue from the race or muscle soreness. (After your last A race of the season, you will probably need a much longer break, more on the order of 4 weeks.) The idea of transition is to give not only your body but also your mind some rest. It's all right to "exercise" in the transition period, but "training" is forbidden. The purpose is to rest and rejuvenate by not having a workout routine that must be followed.

The novice athlete—someone in the first year of triathlon training—will focus on the basic abilities for an entire season and will not do any build periods. In this case, base 3 is repeated and replaces all of the build subperiods.

Planning up to the first A-priority race schedule of the season is now complete. It was actually pretty easy; we just followed a formula. For your subsequent A races, though, you have decisions to make and some periods to leave out. For example, when scheduling beyond the first A race, you will not repeat the prep period and probably not base 1 or base 2 either. However,

you may want to return to base 3 after the first transition period if your basic abilities, especially aerobic endurance, have obviously declined in the last few weeks surrounding the first A race. Repeating base 3 is common when the first A race was a short event and the next is long. You may even want to do base 3 twice if there are enough weeks remaining until the second A race. If your basic abilities are lacking, that weakness will greatly detract from training and racing for the rest of the season. But if your basic abilities are still strong after the first A race, then you may want to start back into training with a build 1 or build 2 period.

A note of caution: Don't shortchange the base abilities in order to do more high-intensity training. For the details of how to schedule these subsequent weeks, see Figures 7.3 and 7.4 above along with the accompanying discussion.

Of course, at this point you are guessing about what sort of fitness you'll have several months from now. That's another reason why the ATP is likely to change throughout the season. But for now, if you have enough weeks between races, include base 3 as the starting point for training after the first transition period of the season.

Finish filling in the "Period" column on the ATP through the end of the season by assigning subperiods that lead to each A-priority race. And remember that for the B-priority races on your schedule, you will include a few days of reduced training to help you be ready for them. A B race that comes at the end of a rest-and-recovery week is perfect, but not always possible. Later on, should you decide that the plan you have isn't right for the subsequent races, you can always make changes.

Don't shortchange the base abilities in order to do more high-intensity training.

Step 6: Estimate Weekly Volume

You now have most of your ATP complete and should also have a general idea of what you will do in training at various times during the upcoming season. What remains to be done is setting the number of hours or TSS you will train weekly—your volume. Once weekly volume is determined, you're ready to take care of the final details—the actual workouts. We'll get to that in the next chapter.

Tables 7.5 and 7.6 will help you complete the "Volume" column. In the top row of the table you use, find your "Annual Hours" or "Annual TSS" that matches what you recorded at the top of the ATP. Then read down that column to see how much volume to train in each week by subperiod. Write these numbers in the appropriate weekly rows of the "Volume" column on your ATP. Your weekly volume is not a rigid number that must be accomplished. It's meant only to be ballpark

Weekly volume includes all three sports plus strength training and crosstraining.

TABLE 7.5 Weekly Training Hours

PERIOD	WEEK	ANNUAL HOURS																		
		300	350	400	450	500	550	600	650	700	750	800	850	900	950	1,000	1,050	1,100	1,150	1,200
Prep	All	5.0	6.0	7.0	7.5	8.5	9.0	10.0	11.0	12.0	12.5	13.5	14.5	15.0	16.0	17.0	17.5	18.5	19.5	20.0
Base 1	1	6.0	7.0	8.0	9.0	10.0	11.0	12.0	12.5	14.0	14.5	15.5	16.5	17.5	18.5	19.5	20.5	21.5	22.5	23.5
	2	7.0	8.5	9.5	10.5	12.0	13.0	14.5	15.5	16.5	18.0	19.0	20.0	21.5	22.5	24.0	25.0	26.0	27.5	28.5
	3	8.0	9.5	10.5	12.0	13.5	14.5	16.0	17.5	18.5	20.0	21.5	22.5	24.0	25.5	26.5	28.0	29.5	30.5	32.0
	4	4.0	5.0	5.5	6.5	7.0	8.0	8.5	9.0	10.0	10.5	11.5	12.0	12.5	13.5	14.0	14.5	15.5	16.0	17.0
Base 2	1	6.5	7.5	8.5	9.5	10.5	12.5	12.5	13.0	14.5	16.0	17.0	18.0	19.0	20.0	21.0	22.0	23.0	24.0	25.0
	2	7.5	9.0	10.0	11.5	12.5	14.0	15.0	16.5	17.5	19.0	20.0	21.5	22.5	24.0	25.0	26.5	27.5	29.0	30.0
	3	8.5	10.0	11.0	12.5	14.0	15.5	17.0	18.0	19.5	21.0	22.5	24.0	25.0	26.5	28.0	29.5	31.0	32.0	33.5
	4	4.5	5.0	5.5	6.5	7.0	8.0	8.5	9.0	10.0	10.5	11.5	12.0	12.5	13.5	14.0	15.0	15.5	16.0	17.0
Base 3	1	7.0	8.0	9.0	10.0	11.0	12.5	13.5	14.5	15.5	17.0	18.0	19.0	20.0	21.0	22.5	23.5	25.0	25.5	27.0
	2	8.0	9.5	10.5	12.0	13.5	14.5	16.0	17.0	18.5	20.0	21.5	23.0	24.0	25.0	26.5	28.0	29.5	30.5	32.0
	3	9.0	10.5	11.5	13.0	15.0	16.5	18.0	19.0	20.5	22.0	23.5	25.0	26.5	28.0	29.5	31.0	32.5	33.5	35.0
	4	4.5	5.0	5.5	6.5	7.0	8.0	8.5	9.0	10.0	10.5	11.5	12.0	12.5	13.5	14.0	15.0	15.5	16.0	17.0
Build 1	1	8.0	9.0	10.0	11.5	12.5	14.0	15.5	16.0	17.5	19.0	20.5	21.5	22.5	24.0	25.0	26.5	28.0	29.0	30.0
	2	8.0	9.0	10.0	11.5	12.5	14.0	15.5	16.0	17.5	19.0	20.5	21.5	22.5	24.0	25.0	26.5	28.0	29.0	30.0
	3	8.0	9.0	10.0	11.5	12.5	14.0	15.5	16.0	17.5	19.0	20.5	21.5	22.5	24.0	25.0	26.5	28.0	29.0	30.0
	4	4.5	5.0	5.5	6.5	7.0	8.0	8.5	9.0	10.0	10.5	11.5	12.0	12.5	13.5	14.0	15.0	15.5	16.0	17.0
Build 2	1	7.0	8.5	9.5	10.5	12.0	13.0	14.5	15.5	16.5	18.0	19.0	20.5	21.5	22.5	24.0	25.0	26.5	27.0	28.5
	2	7.0	8.5	9.5	10.5	12.0	13.0	14.5	15.5	16.5	18.0	19.0	20.5	21.5	22.5	24.0	25.0	26.5	27.0	28.5
	3	7.0	8.5	9.5	10.5	12.0	13.0	14.5	15.5	16.5	18.0	19.0	20.5	21.5	22.5	24.0	25.0	26.5	27.0	28.5
	4	4.5	5.0	5.5	6.5	7.0	8.0	8.5	9.0	10.0	10.5	11.5	12.0	12.5	13.5	14.0	15.0	15.5	16.0	17.0
Peak	1	6.5	7.5	8.5	9.5	10.5	11.5	13.0	13.5	14.5	16.0	17.0	18.0	19.0	20.0	21.0	22.0	23.5	24.0	25.0
	2	5.0	6.0	6.5	7.5	8.5	9.5	10.0	11.0	11.5	12.5	13.5	14.5	15.0	16.0	17.0	17.5	18.5	19.0	20.0
Race	All	4.5	5.0	5.5	6.5	7.0	8.0	8.5	9.0	10.0	10.5	11.5	12.0	12.5	13.5	14.0	15.0	15.5	16.0	17.0

If you are using hours instead of TSS, find your annual hours in the top row. Then scan down that column to find your weekly hours for each subperiod in your season.

TABLE 7.6 **Weekly TSS**

PERIOD	WEEK	ANNUAL TSS																		
		15K	17.5K	20K	22.5K	25K	27.5K	30K	32.5K	35K	37.5K	40K	42.5K	45K	47.5K	50K	52.5K	55K	57.5K	60K
Prep	All	240	280	320	360	400	440	480	520	560	600	640	700	720	760	800	840	880	920	960
Base 1	1	280	330	380	430	480	520	570	620	670	710	760	810	850	900	950	1,000	1,040	1,090	1,140
	2	310	370	420	470	530	580	630	680	730	780	840	890	950	1,000	1,050	1,100	1,150	1,210	1,260
	3	350	400	460	520	580	630	690	750	810	860	920	980	1,030	1,090	1,150	1,210	1,260	1,320	1,380
	4	240	280	320	360	400	440	480	520	560	600	640	700	720	760	800	840	880	920	960
Base 2	1	290	335	380	430	480	520	570	620	670	710	760	810	850	900	950	1,000	1,040	1,090	1,140
	2	330	385	440	500	550	600	660	720	770	820	880	940	990	1,040	1,100	1,150	1,210	1,260	1,320
	3	370	440	500	560	630	690	750	810	880	940	1,000	1,060	1,120	1,190	1,250	1,310	1,370	1,440	1,500
	4	240	280	320	360	400	440	480	520	560	600	640	700	720	760	800	840	880	920	960
Base 3	1	330	385	440	500	550	600	660	720	780	820	880	940	990	1,040	1,100	1,150	1,210	1,260	1,320
	2	370	440	500	560	630	690	750	810	880	940	1,000	1,060	1,120	1,190	1,250	1,310	1,370	1,440	1,370
	3	410	475	540	610	680	740	810	880	950	1,010	1,080	1,150	1,210	1,280	1,350	1,420	1,480	1,550	1,620
	4	240	280	320	360	400	440	480	520	560	600	640	700	720	760	800	840	880	920	960
Build 1	1	370	440	500	560	630	690	750	810	880	940	1,000	1,060	1,120	1,190	1,250	1,310	1,370	1,440	1,370
	2	370	440	500	560	630	690	750	810	880	940	1,000	1,060	1,120	1,190	1,250	1,310	1,370	1,440	1,370
	3	370	440	500	560	630	690	750	810	880	940	1,000	1,060	1,120	1,190	1,250	1,310	1,370	1,440	1,370
	4	240	280	320	360	400	440	480	520	560	600	640	700	720	760	800	840	880	920	960
Build 2	1	410	475	540	610	680	740	810	880	950	1,010	1,080	1,150	1,210	1,280	1,350	1,420	1,480	1,550	1,620
	2	410	475	540	610	680	740	810	880	950	1,010	1,080	1,150	1,210	1,280	1,350	1,420	1,480	1,550	1,620
	3	410	475	540	10.5	680	740	810	880	950	1,010	1,080	1,150	1,210	1,280	1,350	1,420	1,480	1,550	1,620
	4	240	280	320	360	400	440	480	520	560	600	640	700	720	760	800	840	880	920	960
Peak	1	290	335	380	430	480	520	570	620	670	710	760	810	850	900	950	1,000	1,040	1,090	1,140
	2	240	280	320	360	400	440	480	520	560	600	640	700	720	760	800	840	880	920	960
Race	All	240	280	320	360	400	440	480	520	560	600	640	700	720	760	800	840	880	920	960

If you are using TSS instead of hours, find your annual TSS in the top row. Then scan down that column to find your weekly TSS for each subperiod in your season.

guide to how much training you do in a given week. This number can and should be changed to suit your situation when you come to that particular week, or any given day, in your season. We'll get to setting daily durations and making timely decisions about weekly volume in Chapter 8.

Your weekly volume includes all three sports plus strength training and any other crosstraining you may do. Again, in the next chapter we'll examine how these hours or TSS are distributed.

SUMMARY: PLANNING A SEASON

Having read this chapter—a big and complex one—you can probably understand why I said at the start that I see this as the most important section of the book. Many of the details from previous chapters have been brought together here. And while building your ATP may have seemed a bit tedious, I am certain you'll find that it will pay

ANNUAL TRAINING PLAN

Athlete _Jane Doe_

Annual Volume _500 hours_

Year _2017_

							SWIM							BIKE							RUN						
WEEK	MON.	RACES	PRI.	PERIOD	VOLUME	WEIGHTS	AEROBIC ENDURANCE	MUSCULAR FORCE	SPEED SKILLS	MUSCULAR ENDURANCE	ANAEROBIC ENDURANCE	SPRINT POWER	TESTING	AEROBIC ENDURANCE	MUSCULAR FORCE	SPEED SKILLS	MUSCULAR ENDURANCE	ANAEROBIC ENDURANCE	SPRINT POWER	TESTING	AEROBIC ENDURANCE	MUSCULAR FORCE	SPEED SKILLS	MUSCULAR ENDURANCE	ANAEROBIC ENDURANCE	SPRINT POWER	TESTING
01	11 / 21			Prep	8.5																						
02	11 / 28			↓	8.5																						
03	12 / 5			Base	10.0																						
04	12 / 12				12.0																						
05	12 / 19				13.5																						
06	12 / 26			↓	7.0																						
07	1 / 2			Base 2	10.5																						
08	1 / 9				12.5																						
09	1 / 16				19.0																						
10	1 / 23			↓	7.0																						
11	1 / 30			Base 3	11.0																						
12	2 / 6				13.5																						
13	2 / 13	(Tri camp)			15.0																						
14	2 / 20	Sprint Tri Race	C	↓	7.0																						
15	2 / 27			Build 1	12.5																						
16	3 / 6				12.5																						
17	3 / 13				12.5																						
18	3 / 20	Olympic Tri Race	B	↓	7.0																						
19	3 / 27			Build 2	13.0																						
20	4 / 3				12.0																						
21	4 / 10				12.0																						
22	4 / 17	10K Run Race	B	↓	7.0																						
23	4 / 24			Peak	10.5																						
24	5 / 1			↓	8.5																						
25	5 / 8	Gulf Coast HIM	A	Race	7.0																						
26	5 / 15			Tran	—																						

FIGURE 7.5 Example of an Annual Training Plan (continued on next page) →

Season Goals

1. _Sub–5:00 at Gulf Coast HIM_
2. _Break 5:10 at IM 70.3 Silverman_
3. _____

Training Objectives

1. _Leg Press 320 lbs. 3 times by Jan 1_
2. _Increase bike FTP to 230w by Mar 26_
3. _Swim 1000m in 515 by Apr 23_
4. _Run half marathon in <1:45 by July 23_

							SWIM							BIKE							RUN						
WEEK	MON.	RACES	PRI.	PERIOD	VOLUME	WEIGHTS	AEROBIC ENDURANCE	MUSCULAR FORCE	SPEED SKILLS	MUSCULAR ENDURANCE	ANAEROBIC ENDURANCE	SPRINT POWER	TESTING	AEROBIC ENDURANCE	MUSCULAR FORCE	SPEED SKILLS	MUSCULAR ENDURANCE	ANAEROBIC ENDURANCE	SPRINT POWER	TESTING	AEROBIC ENDURANCE	MUSCULAR FORCE	SPEED SKILLS	MUSCULAR ENDURANCE	ANAEROBIC ENDURANCE	SPRINT POWER	TESTING
27	5/22			Base 3	11.0																						
28	5/29			↓	13.5																						
29	6/5			↓	7.0																						
30	6/12			Base 3	13.5																						
31	6/19			↓	15.0																						
32	6/26			↓	7.0																						
33	7/3			Base 3	13.5																						
34	7/10			↓	15.0																						
35	7/17	Half Marathon	B	↓	7.0																						
36	7/24			Build 1	12.5																						
37	7/31			↓	12.5																						
38	8/7	Olympic Tri Race	C	↓	12.5																						
39	8/14			↓	7.0																						
40	8/21			Build 2	12.0																						
41	8/28			↓	12.0																						
42	9/4			↓	12.0																						
43	9/11	Olympic Tri Race	B	↓	7.0																						
44	9/18			Peak	10.5																						
45	9/25			↓	8.5																						
46	10/2	Silverman 70.3	A	Race	7.0																						
47	10/9			Tran	—																						
48	10/16				—																							
49	10/23				—																							
50	10/30				—																							
51	11/6																											
52	11/13																											

FIGURE 7.5 (continued)

off with better training and racing in the coming season. Yours should look similar to Figure 7.5—an example of an ATP for a triathlete whose A-priority races are at the half-Ironman distance. Note that there are some parts of your ATP that aren't complete yet—the "Weights," "Swim," "Bike," and "Run" portions. Those all have to do with workout details and will be completed in the next chapter.

You may find it hard to adjust to using such a detailed plan if you have never trained with one before. New ways of thinking are difficult to adopt, especially if you've trained by the seat of your pants for several years. Having a plan is almost like having a coach. It fosters confidence and direction for your training. Once you get used to it, I think you will find that your workouts and race performances improve significantly.

To make your plan work, you must resolve to view it as a work in progress, not an inflexible mandate. I'd strongly suggest reviewing and modifying your ATP at the end of every week as you plan for the coming week's training. Chapter 8 will explain how to do that. When you find yourself running out of enthusiasm for getting organized, as everyone does from time to time, remind yourself of the reason you should do this—to achieve your goals and be the best triathlete possible. The time spent planning will pay off. I've seen it help many athletes achieve high goals in 30-plus years of coaching.

Now let's bring all of the pieces together as we walk through the final step—how to determine the details of the training weeks for your season. That's the subject of Chapter 8.

PLANNING A WEEK

BEFORE WE GET into the details of weekly training, let's review a key point from Chapter 7. As we pointed out earlier, your training must become progressively more like the race as you approach race day. But this does not mean that only the workouts close to the race are critical, and that workouts early in the season are unimportant. Those early workouts establish the fitness platform on which you build your race-specific workouts later, so of course they are important. If your base period goes well, you should be able to manage a great deal of racelike training in the build period. In the build period, you develop fitness by doing workouts that are race-specific in terms of intensity and duration. That's the key to high performance, and that's why you are creating a periodization plan.

Many athletes think of periodization as rigid guidelines that must be followed without deviation: aerobic before anaerobic training, volume before intensity, specific workouts at specific times, little concern for day-to-day recovery, and so on. Periodization is often considered an inflexible, demanding way of viewing the world of training. But it isn't that way at all. When done correctly, periodization is actually free-flowing and creative. You can do anything with it you can imagine—so long as it works.

In fact, you should always be seeking better ways to train by experimenting. Would you race faster if you made a few small changes to your ATP or to your weekly routine? Well, your ATP is not carved in stone. Feel free to make adjustments to what was presented in Chapter 7 and to what you will read here. As long as you maintain the fundamental principles of periodization that have been found to work well, then you can definitely make small tweaks here and there to fit your particular needs. You'll see that Chapter 9 offers some alternatives to the classic, linear model I've described so far for your plan.

For some athletes, all of this may seem like overkill—much too serious. How serious you are, which I take to mean how focused you are on training to improve your race performance, depends on a couple of things. The first is how challenging your race goal is. It's OK to take a long break and have a low-key season occasionally in which you race just to have fun. If some races are only social outings and you aren't concerned about the outcomes, then there is no reason for serious training. In fact, it may not be "training" at all because that usually implies having goals and a plan. Instead, all you need is an unstructured exercise program and a goal of having a good time while staying fit. Do what you want, when you want. It's OK to have nonserious seasons when race results are unimportant.

For seasons in which you are focused on achieving high goals, your changing levels of seriousness are reflected in your periodization plan. For example, the transition period at the very end of the season should not be serious at all. You're recovering from the previous season. You don't need a weekly routine now. In fact, you shouldn't have one. Have fun. Relax. Do what you feel like doing when you feel like doing it. Or take the day off. There's no structure at all. The only thing that matters is to arrive fully rested when it's time to start training again. That's when the preparation period begins.

The prep period is the next step in your season and not all that serious either. You're just beginning to introduce some structure. In fact, the only structured workouts are done in the weight room,

as you will soon see. Otherwise, it's play, not training. The other workouts should be open-ended, allowing you to have fun with an exercise program by doing whatever you find enjoyable, such as hiking with your family, cross-country skiing with friends, and generally having a good time through exercise. While having fun, you will gain some general fitness.

Things get more serious in the base period. Now you begin more challenging swim, bike, and run workouts, along with serious strength training. But the workouts are not difficult at first. This gradually changes over the course of about 3 months. By the start of the build period, your training should become much more focused as the sessions take on the characteristics of your A-priority race. The peak and race periods lift your seriousness to the highest level of the season, with workouts laser-focused on preparing for the race.

Once the A race is done, it's time to rest your body and mind again with another transition period. And it can well be that your mind is what needs the most recovery. Serious training is mentally demanding. This transition period lasts a few days to a few weeks depending on whether it happens midseason or at the end of the season.

My point here is that planning does not mean that you are always serious and focused on challenging workouts and high-performance race results. Training ebbs and flows throughout the year. Creating a detailed plan, while it may seem tedious now, will greatly improve your chances of having a successful, high-performance season when the time is right. So hang in there with me as we finish your ATP for the coming season.

SCHEDULE WEEKLY WORKOUTS

In Chapter 7, you completed the first six steps of creating your ATP for the season. All that remains now is to add the weekly details about training. Your ATP thus far should be complete for "Annual Volume," "Season Goals," "Training Objectives," a calendar of the season by Monday dates for every week ("Mon."), your "Races" and their priorities ("Pri."), a breakdown of the season by "Period," and your "Volume." Now it's time to do the final step of scheduling weekly workouts. This involves adding a "Weights" column for your weight training routine and each week's ability-focused workouts in the columns under the headings "Swim," "Bike," and "Run." Should you need an example along the way, see Figure 8.1, which is a continuation of what you saw in Figure 7.5.

Weights

In Chapter 13, I will present the case for why you should *probably* be doing strength training—lifting weights. You may decide not to do so for any number of reasons that will be explained there. For now, though, let's assume you will be following a periodized strength program in which your weight lifting routine will change throughout the season, just as your swim, bike, and run workouts do. The major task here is to match up the two periodization schemes by recording each strength phase in the "Period" column on your ATP. For now, we will just do a general overview for each strength period; Chapter 13 will cover the details.

Start at the top of the ATP in the "Weights" column. Record the abbreviation, as described in what follows, for each strength period, and work your way down through each week of the season.

Preparation period. In this period, write in *AA* ("anatomical adaptation") in the "Period" column. This is the strength period in which you become accustomed to the various exercises you will do in the weight room (again, the exercises will be explained in detail in Chapter 13). You will probably need 2 weeks of AA, with two or three sessions per week. If you have more than 2 weeks in your prep period, then also write in *MT* ("muscular transition") for the remaining weeks. This is the time when you gradually increase the loads while reducing the repetitions. Again, this usually requires 2 weeks, with four to six total sessions. If you don't have 2 weeks remaining in your prep period, put *MT* into the first part of base 1.

Base 1 period. Write in 4 weeks of *MS* ("maximum strength")—the most challenging strength workouts of the season. If you don't have 4 weeks remaining open in base 1, roll the remaining weeks of MS over into base 2. You should complete MS before starting the hard swim, bike, and run training of the base 3 period. The exception might occur when you have multiple base 3 periods back to back. This may be the case if you need to include "extra" training weeks for the periodization plan to match the timing of an A-priority race in your schedule.

Base 2, base 3, build 1, build 2, and peak periods. Strength training for all of the remainder of the periods in the buildup to your first A-priority race is recorded as *SM* ("strength maintenance").

You will probably need 2 weeks of anatomical adaptation (AA), two or three sessions per week.

You should complete muscular strength (MS) before the hard training of the base 3 period.

ANNUAL TRAINING PLAN

Athlete **Jane Doe**
Annual Volume **500 hours**
Year **2017**

WEEK	MON.	RACES	PRI.	PERIOD	VOLUME	WEIGHTS	SWIM: AEROBIC ENDURANCE	MUSCULAR FORCE	SPEED SKILLS	MUSCULAR ENDURANCE	ANAEROBIC ENDURANCE	SPRINT POWER	TESTING	BIKE: AEROBIC ENDURANCE	MUSCULAR FORCE	SPEED SKILLS	MUSCULAR ENDURANCE	ANAEROBIC ENDURANCE	SPRINT POWER	TESTING	RUN: AEROBIC ENDURANCE	MUSCULAR FORCE	SPEED SKILLS	MUSCULAR ENDURANCE	ANAEROBIC ENDURANCE	SPRINT POWER	TESTING
01	11 / 21			Prep	8.5	AA	X		X					X	X						X		X				
02	11 / 28			↓	8.5	AA	X		X				X	X	X						X		X				X
03	12 / 5			Base 1	10.0	MT	X		X					X	X						X		X				
04	12 / 12			↓	12.0	MT	X		X					X	X						X		X				
05	12 / 19				13.5	MS	X		X					X	X						X		X				
06	12 / 26			↓	7.0	MS	X		X				X	X	X						X		X				X
07	1 / 2			Base 2	10.5	MS	X		X	X				X	X						X		X	X			
08	1 / 9			↓	12.5	MS	X		X	X				X	X						X		X	X			
09	1 / 16				14.0	SM	X	X	X	X				X	X	X	X				X	X	X	X			
10	1 / 23			↓	7.0	SM	X		X				X	X	X						X		X				X
11	1 / 30			Base 3	11.0	SM	X	X	X	X	X			X	X	X	X	X			X	X	X	X	X		
12	2 / 6			↓	13.5	SM	X	X	X	X	X			X	X	X	X	X			X	X	X	X	X		
13	2 / 13	(Tri camp)		↓	15.0	SM	X	X	X	X	X			X	X	X	X	X			X	X	X	X	X		
14	2 / 20	Sprint Tri Race	C	↓	7.0	SM	X		X				X	X	X						X		X				X
15	2 / 27			Build 1	12.5	SM	X	X	X	X	X			X	X	X	X	X			X	X	X	X	X		
16	3 / 6				12.5	SM	X	X	X	X	X			X	X	X	X	X			X	X	X	X	X		
17	3 / 13				12.5	SM	X	X	X	X	X			X	X	X	X	X			X	X	X	X	X		
18	3 / 20	Olympic Tri Race	B	↓	7.0	SM	X		X				X	X	X						X		X				X
19	3 / 27			Build 2	12.0	SM	X	X	X	X	X			X	X	X	X	X			X	X	X	X	X		
20	4 / 3				12.0	SM	X	X	X	X	X			X	X	X	X	X			X	X	X	X	X		
21	4 / 10				12.0	SM	X	X	X	X	X			X	X	X	X	X			X	X	X	X	X		
22	4 / 17	10K Run Race	B	↓	7.0	SM	X		X				X	X	X						X		X				X
23	4 / 24			Peak	10.5	SM				X							X							X			
24	5 / 1			↓	8.5	SM				X							X							X			
25	5 / 8	Gulf Coast HIM	A	Race	7.0	SM				X							X							X			
26	5 / 15			Tran	—																						

FIGURE 8.1 Continued example of an Annual Training Plan   →

Season Goals

1. Sub-5:00 at Gulf Coast HIM
2. Break 5:10 at IM 70.3 Silverman
3. _____

Training Objectives

1. Leg Press 320 lbs. 3 times by Jan 1
2. Increase bike FTP to 230w by Mar 26
3. Swim 1000m in 515 by Apr 23
4. Run half marathon in <1:45 by July 23

							SWIM							BIKE							RUN						
WEEK	MON.	RACES	PRI.	PERIOD	VOLUME	WEIGHTS	Aerobic Endurance	Muscular Force	Speed Skills	Muscular Endurance	Anaerobic Endurance	Sprint Power	Testing	Aerobic Endurance	Muscular Force	Speed Skills	Muscular Endurance	Anaerobic Endurance	Sprint Power	Testing	Aerobic Endurance	Muscular Force	Speed Skills	Muscular Endurance	Anaerobic Endurance	Sprint Power	Testing
27	5/22			Base 3	11.0	MS	X	X	X	X				X	X	X	X				X	X	X	X			
28	5/29			↓	13.5	MS	X	X	X	X				X	X	X					X	X	X				
29	6/5			↓	7.0	MS	X		X					X	X		X				X	X		X			X
30	6/12			Base 3	13.5	SM	X	X	X	X	X			X	X	X	X				X	X	X	X	X		
31	6/19			↓	15.0	SM	X	X	X	X	X			X	X	X	X				X	X	X	X	X		
32	6/26			↓	7.0	SM	X		X					X	X		X				X	X		X			X
33	7/3			Base 3	13.5	SM	X	X	X	X	X			X	X	X	X	X			X	X	X	X	X		
34	7/10			↓	15.0	SM	X	X	X	X	X			X	X	X	X	X			X	X	X	X	X		
35	7/17	Half Marathon	B	↓	7.0	SM	X		X					X	X		X				X	X		X			X
36	7/24			Build 1	12.5	SM	X	X	X	X	X			X	X	X	X	X			X	X	X	X	X		
37	7/31			↓	12.5	SM	X	X	X	X	X			X	X	X	X	X			X	X	X	X	X		
38	8/7	Olympic Tri Race	C	↓	12.5	SM	X	X	X	X	X			X	X	X	X	X			X	X	X	X	X		
39	8/14			↓	7.0	SM	X		X					X	X		X				X	X		X			X
40	8/21			Build 2	12.0	SM	X	X	X	X	X			X	X	X	X	X			X	X	X	X	X		
41	8/28			↓	12.0	SM	X	X	X	X	X			X	X	X	X	X			X	X	X	X	X		
42	9/4			↓	12.0	SM	X	X	X	X	X			X	X	X	X	X			X	X	X	X	X		
43	9/11	Olympic Tri Race	B	↓	7.0	SM	X		X					X	X		X				X	X		X			X
44	9/18			Peak	10.5	SM				X							X							X			
45	9/25			↓	8.5	SM				X							X							X			
46	10/2	Silverman 70.3	A	Race	7.0					X							X							X			
47	10/9			Tran	—																						
48	10/16				—																						
49	10/23				—																						
50	10/30				—																						
51	11/6																										
52	11/13																										

As the name implies, at these times you are simply maintaining the strength gains made in MS. Whereas you were doing gym workouts two or even three times each week in previous weeks, now you are lifting weights only once per week. So the strength workouts are now not only less frequent but also much easier, allowing you to train hard in the pool and on the road. What you must avoid is having a few weeks when both strength training and triathlon-specific training are at high workloads.

Race period. During this period, if it lasts only 1 week, leave the "Weights" column blank. There is no strength training during this week. But if you have two or three races in consecutive weeks, then add SM for the second week only.

Transition period. Leave the "Weights" column blank here. There is no need to lift weights during this period because the focus is on rest and recovery.

You have now created a periodized strength training program in preparation for your first important race of the season. In subsequent periods, as you prepare for your second and third important races of the season, it's generally a good idea to include a few sessions of MS. Of course, there may not be enough time if your A races are separated by only a few weeks. In that case, something has to give, and the logical candidate is strength training. So either record SM or leave the column blank. At this point, it comes down to your time available and limiters. If your limiters are muscular force and muscular endurance, then some MS may be beneficial. And of course you don't have to make this decision now. It can wait until after the first A race. This is one of those times when self-coaching relies heavily on the art of training because there is no science to tell us exactly what must be done.

Again, if you become confused while trying to periodize your strength training program, refer to Figure 8.1 for assistance.

Swim, Bike, and Run Abilities

I'm going to show you how to assign workouts by sport and by ability, as is typically done in a linear periodization model. But realize that there are many ways to periodize and plan workout scheduling besides the linear model. These often involve customization and creativity. In Chapter 9, I'll show you some of these other methods.

Assigning workouts by sport is done on your ATP by marking the type of workouts you will do each week in the appropriate ability columns under the "Swim," "Bike," and "Run" headings. The abilities were described in Chapter 6—aerobic endurance, muscular force, speed skills, muscular endurance, and anaerobic endurance. Notice on the ATP that sprint power is also listed as an ability under each sport, but we won't use it because it has little value for nondrafting races.

In addition to the standard six abilities, a column titled "Testing" is included for each sport. At various times throughout the year, you should check your training zones for accuracy and test your progress as described in Chapter 4 and Appendixes B, C, and D. You would typically do this near the end of a rest-and-recovery week, and the following discussion will show you how it's done.

The process for assigning ability-based workouts and testing for the entire season is simple but tedious. You're going to place an X in the ability column for each type of workout you'll do

---

Avoid having weeks when both strength training and tri-specific training workloads are high.

Schedule regular checks of your training zones for accuracy and tests of your progress.

by sport in the appropriate row for each week of the season. This will help you to make decisions when it's time to determine the specifics of your workouts. We'll get into these details shortly. Again, if you are creating an ATP on paper, use a pencil because there will undoubtedly be changes as you get into the season.

Preparation period abilities. As you've seen so far, the preparation period is quite low-key with the purpose of moving toward structured training, once again following an extended rest-and-recovery break in the transition period. The only serious training now is in the weight room. Your focus should be only on becoming accustomed to the strength exercises and, after a few such sessions, gradually moving to heavier loads for each exercise (as described in Chapter 13). The only sport-specific abilities to be included now are "Aerobic Endurance" and "Speed Skills." Place an X in these two columns for each sport—swim, bike, and run—for every week in your prep period. Also put an X in the "Testing" column for the last prep period week.

Base 1 period abilities. In this period, the emphasis is definitely on strength training because you are now using heavy loads and low reps. These make for very challenging workouts two or three times each week, so the sport-specific workouts are quite easy. As with the prep period, place an X in the "Aerobic Endurance" and "Speed Skills" columns for each week in this period. And also put an X under "Testing" for the last week of this period.

Base 2 period abilities. In base 2, you will begin to cut back on strength training by following a maintenance program with reduced training stress and only one session per week. This allows more time and energy for workouts intended to improve your swim, bike, and run abilities. The workouts for all three sports will now include "Muscular Force" and "Muscular Endurance" in addition to the continuation of "Aerobic Endurance" and "Speed Skills" workouts. Mark each of these columns with an X for every week of base 2 except for muscular force sessions, which may be omitted as long as you are still doing MS sessions in the gym. That may be the situation if your prep period was short. This is illustrated in Figure 8.1.

The muscular force workouts at this time are intended to take the strength built in the gym by lifting weights and convert it to swim, bike, and run strength by doing workouts that emphasize this ability. This will eventually morph into swim, bike, and run power development with the potential for making you faster. More on that later. While muscular force has become the primary focus of training at this point, muscular endurance is only being introduced. These muscular endurance workouts are not very long or difficult now, but over the next several weeks they will become the primary focus of your training. In the last week of base 2, put an X in the "Aerobic Endurance," "Speed Skills," and "Testing" columns.

Base 3 period abilities. This is the period when training becomes somewhat more specific to the type of race for which you are training and your level of competition. It is a transitional period. Up until now, it really did not matter all that much if you were training for a sprint-distance race or an Ironman. The types of workouts were much the same. But now there is a shift in emphasis.

Muscular force workouts at this time convert gym strength to swim, bike, and run strength.

In build 1 and build 2, training becomes specific to your A race.

Regardless of your race type, start by marking the ability columns for each sport exactly as you did in base 2: aerobic endurance, muscular force, speed skills, and muscular endurance. And as before, the last week of base 3 is aerobic endurance, speed skills, and testing.

The major concerns of training in this period are your race distance and your level of competition. For the athlete who is doing half- and full-Ironman-distance races and also has a goal of racing at a very high level of competition, it can be quite effective now to include some anaerobic endurance–ability workouts. If long course and highly competitive apply to you, then mark an *X* in the "Anaerobic Endurance" columns in all three sports for each week except the last week of the period, as shown in Figure 8.1. I'll explain the rationale behind this below in the sections on training routines, which may help you decide whether or not to include these sessions in your base 3.

Build 1 and build 2 period abilities. By the time you get to this point in the season, your general, or base, fitness should be very well developed. You should be muscularly strong and able to swim, bike, and run skillfully for relatively long durations. But you aren't yet race-ready. In the build 1 and build 2 periods, the training becomes specific to your A race. For the next several weeks, you will build fitness to match the exact demands of your race. While the abilities selected will remain largely the same as in the base periods, the individual workouts will become much more racelike.

Put an *X* under every ability column for each of the three sports for both build 1 and build 2 for all but the last weeks of each period. This, of

course, implies a lot of workouts, but now there are a couple of changes taking place that help you manage your training time. The first is that workouts for aerobic endurance, muscular force, and speed skills generally become maintenance-only sessions, depending on the event for which you are training, much as is the case with your SM weight sessions. So these brief, base-period-like swim, bike, and run sessions for aerobic endurance and speed skills can be merged with the advanced sessions as part of the warm-up, or even included in recovery workouts. The other change now occurring that keeps your total training time manageable is that multiple abilities are combined into single sessions. We do that to make these workouts more racelike. The typical race doesn't demand only one ability for each leg of the race. Races nearly always place multiple demands on you, with flat sections, hills, descents, head winds, cornering, rough water, fast starts, surges, fatigue, and finishing kicks. You need to prepare for all of these that are expected in your race.

For the long-course athlete, anaerobic endurance training is quite limited in the build periods. That's why I suggested starting that type of training in base 3 for competitive athletes racing this distance. Sprint- and Olympic-distance athletes will place a greater emphasis on anaerobic endurance training in the build periods. So while all athletes, regardless of race distance, will do anaerobic endurance training at this time, the amount of such training will vary considerably.

As with the base period, the last week of each build period is marked with an *X* in the columns for "Aerobic Endurance," "Speed Skills," and "Testing."

Peak period abilities. Now your training shifts to workouts that closely match the demands of your race that is only 2 or 3 weeks away. This means an increased emphasis on the expected intensity of the race while workout duration is decreased. Also eliminated from the training routine are workouts that emphasize the basic abilities of aerobic endurance and muscular force. Speed skills sessions may continue as a variation on recovery workouts. Aerobic endurance and muscular force should be quite well developed by now. The long-course triathlete will not do anaerobic endurance training at this time, but it continues for short-course racers. So if you are racing a half-Ironman-distance or an Ironman-distance race, mark your ATP for the peak-period weeks with an *X* in the "Muscular Endurance" column only. Sprint- and Olympic-distance athletes should mark both the "Muscular Endurance" and "Anaerobic Endurance" columns. There is no testing in the peak period.

Race period abilities. The emphasis in your race week is on rest, with workouts that are quite brief but still focused on intensity. Mark your race week just as you did for the peak period. Later in this chapter, I will introduce the details of how the peak and race weeks are organized.

Transition period abilities. You've just completed an A-priority race, so this is the time in the season when you kick back and take a break, with no structured training, no key workouts, and no scheduled volume. The purpose of this period, which may last a few days to a few weeks, depending on where you are in the season, is mental and physical rest. Do not mark any abilities in this period. Leave the spaces blank. You can still exercise, but any training or exercise you do should be an unplanned, spur-of-the-moment decision and should be short and easy. There is more on this in Chapter 11.

Planning for later-season races. You have the easy part of your ATP completed for the season—preparing for the first A race. The hard part is assigning workouts for the remaining A-priority races later in the season. An overview of how to do this is found in Chapter 7 in the section "Overview of Your Plan." In summary, the biggest decision you need to make after the first A race of the season is how well maintained your aerobic endurance is. Given your emphasis on muscular endurance and anaerobic endurance in the build, peak, and race periods, there is a strong possibility that you have lost some aerobic endurance fitness. One way to determine this is to do an aerobic threshold workout (see Appendixes B, C, and D) to see how your efficiency factor compares with what it was back in your last base 3 period (the aerobic threshold workout and efficiency factor are explained in those appendixes). If it is at much the same level as earlier, then you can go straight into a build period in preparation for your next A race. If your efficiency factor for cycling or running is lower than the previous base 3 best workout result by 10 percent or more, I'd suggest starting back into base 3 training after the transition period following the first A race of the season and continuing in that period until your efficiency factor is less than 5 percent lower. The emphasis should be on aerobic endurance.

In the example in Figure 8.1, you can see that the athlete returned to base 3 for 9 weeks to re-establish not only aerobic endurance but also muscular force (note the MS weight sessions) and

After your first A race of the season, you need to test aerobic endurance.

speed skills. Her last base 3 period culminates with a B-priority race and then goes straight into two back-to-back build periods, two peak weeks, and a race week. This is a nearly perfect plan when there are ample weeks between races. That's highly likely when there are only two A races in a season. But when there are three, the timing is considerably tighter, so planning becomes more challenging. Again, all of this was discussed in more detail in Chapter 7. Figures 7.3 and 7.4 will help you decide how to plan when you have fewer than 16 weeks between races.

For subsequent races following the first A race of the season, after you've written in the periods necessary to best prepare you, mark the swim, bike, and run abilities as described above as determined by your race distance and your level of competitiveness. Figure 8.1 will help you see how to do this.

Period Progression by Sport

Notice that in assigning workout types by ability category, I assumed that the progression of each sport was synchronized. In other words, as you started base 3, you were ready to move on to doing muscular endurance workouts in all three sports. That may not be the case for various reasons. The most likely reason why the progression won't be the same for all three sports is that you have more natural ability or experience in one and another is a limiter. What this means is that you must pay close attention to your progression for each sport and be willing to modify your periodization planning by changing the length of a period in order to make sure that your sport limiter is allowed ample time to develop. This is most likely to happen when you are doing base-type training.

I've found, however, that for most athletes, the 12 or so combined weeks of the base 1, 2, and 3 periods is usually ample time to develop all of the assigned abilities in each of the sports. Of course, your fitness and performance in the three sports will never be exactly the same. One will always be your strongest while another will always be a limiter. But as previously explained, a major purpose of training is to improve your limiting sport so that the difference between it and your other sports is reduced.

The bottom line here is that it may be necessary to do basic-ability training, especially for aerobic threshold, in one of the sports while advanced-ability training is being done for the other two. The written plan may not reflect this. It may show that you are in a build period even though one of the sports has not caught up. If two of your sports need to return to the basic abilities, then it's best to return to the base 3 period for all three of them. Of course, you can't plan for this when you are creating your ATP. It is something you come to realize during the training process and make the adjustments as you go along.

WEEKLY AND DAILY TRAINING

Here, you will design a training routine for each week in each period, with the exception of rest-and-recovery weeks and the transition and preparation periods. The latter two don't need weekly routines because they are meant to be unstructured. We'll get into the details of the routines for rest-and-recovery weeks in Chapter 11. Tables 8.1, 8.2, and 8.3 near the end of this section show my suggested weekly routines. These may or may not work for you given

> The 12 weeks of base 1, 2, and 3 are usually enough to develop all of the abilities in all three sports.

> If two of your sports need to return to the basic abilities, it's best to return to base 3 for all three.

your particular lifestyle. As you will see, there are several factors to consider when you design your own personalized routine.

Base and Build Week Routines

Once a weekly training platform is laid out, it can usually be repeated for a few weeks so long as everything else in your daily schedule, such as work, family, and other commitments, remain stable. Continuity in training is beneficial both physically and mentally. Your body and mind like it when the routine stays much the same week after week. When a new period begins, however, there may be a need to change the weekly routine. Going from the base period to the build period means a shift of intensity and duration that may necessitate change. But I'd suggest keeping the periods as similar as possible because doing so usually makes for consistent and effective training.

Let's start working on your personalized weekly routine. On a sheet of paper or on your computer, write down the days of the week in a column at the left side of the page:

- Monday
- Tuesday
- Wednesday
- Thursday
- Friday
- Saturday
- Sunday

Next, you need to decide the days you will swim, bike, run, and do strength workouts in the gym. Make sure your plan is realistic. Does it fit your lifestyle and your capacity for training? The most common mistake is to make the training week overly hard by scheduling too many workouts. I'll help you make decisions about this, but only you can know if the finished product is truly realistic.

A good starting point is to look at what you've done in the past. You might simply sketch in what your swim, bike, run, and gym routine has been like recently. On which days have you typically done each type of workout? If you are uncertain about what the best days may be, bear with me as I take you through the many considerations.

Anchor Workouts

"Anchors" are workouts that are tied to specific days and times. Write these into your weekly plan first, and build all the other sessions around them.

By necessity, anchors are usually the same every week. A common one for triathletes is lap swimming when it is available. Another swim anchor may be done when your masters swim team sessions are held. Group workouts such as track sessions or group rides may be bike anchors. If you have any such anchor workouts that must be done on given days of the week at certain times, pencil them in on the weekly calendar you started above so that you have the beginnings of a weekly routine. If they are always at a given time, note that, too.

Pay attention to the common stress levels of these sessions, especially those that are group workouts. How hard are they typically? Once you have planned the entire week, you may see there are days when you need to move to a slower lane, "sit in" on the ride, or run with a slower group. This may be because there was a very hard workout shortly before the anchor workout. Or it may be a time in the season when several challenging sessions are needed in a week. Each week, you need

Anchor workouts are tied to specific days and times.

to decide ahead of time what it is you need from a group workout—or any workout—and then stick with your decision. Be cautious about getting caught up in "racing" when your goal was skill refinement or aerobic endurance. My experience is that athletes who frequently train with groups and fail to control their competitiveness burn out earlier in the race season than those who mostly train alone. To stay enthusiastic until your last race of the year, you must control the desire always to push the limits when training with a group. Later in this chapter, we'll return to the matter of previewing and refining the coming week.

Breakthrough Workouts

Once you have noted the anchor workouts on your weekly routine, it's time to decide when to schedule the breakthrough training sessions for the week. These are the sessions that are stressful enough to produce greater fitness—you *break through* to a new level of fitness. The primary concerns here are arriving at them rested and ready, and recovering for a day or so afterward. Your weekly schedule should reflect this.

For some, the anchor workouts are the breakthroughs, or at least make up a portion of them. These key weekly workouts are usually high-intensity or long-duration sessions, and they are your most important workouts relative to seasonal goals and the training objectives on your ATP. You should schedule these so that your recovery time after the hardest anchor sessions (which are also high-intensity or long-duration sessions) is adequate for you to recover before the next breakthrough workout. Of course, breakthrough workouts encompass each of the three sports and, in the base 1 and possibly the early base 2 periods, the most challenging weight

workouts (Chapter 13 will go into the details of strength building in the gym).

The types of breakthrough workouts you do in a given week depend on the time in the season and your race goals. For example, it's common in the base period to have breakthrough workouts for the basic abilities, such as aerobic endurance and muscular force. The stress of the aerobic endurance sessions comes from their long duration and moderate intensity (see Appendixes B, C, and D for details). The muscular force workouts are stressful because of the heavy loads placed on the muscles. The build period is usually focused on the advanced abilities—muscular endurance and anaerobic endurance. These are stressful because of the high intensity. But such generalizations about when these workouts are done in the season don't always hold true. For example, I previously explained that it's not unusual for advanced long-course triathletes to do anaerobic endurance training in the base 3 period in order to boost aerobic capacity. Later in the build period, they will limit such training to infrequent maintenance sessions. Some refer to this intensity-before-duration method as *reverse periodization*, but it really isn't. Periodization, by my definition at least, is marked by a gradual shift in training regimens from non-specific training to increasingly race-specific training. For long-course triathletes, anaerobic endurance training is very much *unlike* the race, so it's not a reversal at all when done in the base period. Doing such workouts in the build period would indeed be reverse periodization—and of questionable value to the half- or full-Ironman athlete who must primarily do racelike workouts such as muscular endurance at that time.

Back to planning. At this point, you should have anchor and breakthrough workouts for

Breakthrough workouts must be stressful enough to produce greater fitness.

each of the three sports written onto your weekly routine on the appropriate days. Weight training in the gym at this point requires a bit more information to plan. As mentioned, in the early part of the base period—base 1 and perhaps early base 2—you may be lifting 2 days each week. On your weekly routine, separate them by at least 2 days so they are scheduled for Monday and Thursday, Tuesday and Friday, or some similar pairing that works for your lifestyle. Treat these as breakthrough workouts, meaning that a day of recovery is typically needed afterward. After the early base period, you will lift only once each week until the next race, and you should reduce the gym workouts to a moderate intensity so they are no longer breakthroughs.

The general weekly routine you have now designed should work for your base and build periods with the few exceptions for weight lifting, as noted. What remains to be scheduled are recovery sessions and speed skills workouts that are not very strenuous. Both are still critical to your race-day performance. If you are doing two or more sessions in a day, they will often be done on the same day as a breakthrough workout (more on this below), and they'll also take place on the days between breakthrough workouts.

Recovery Between Workouts

Chapter 11 will get into the details of short-term recovery during hard training weeks. For now, you need to give consideration only to how you schedule weekly workouts in order to allow adequate time to refresh before the next breakthrough session. Going into these sessions tired is counterproductive. You are unlikely to experience a "breakthrough" when fatigued. You will more than likely experience just the opposite—a setback. Recovery

is just as critical to your fitness gains and your success on race day as the breakthrough workouts. Do not overlook the value of recovery days.

The more experienced you are, the more stressful the breakthrough workouts can be. That's because you recover faster after several years of training. Conversely, those who are new to serious training need to limit the number of breakthrough sessions in a week. They recover more slowly. Age also plays a role, as both junior and senior athletes need longer recovery breaks from training before breakthrough sessions (see my book *Fast After 50* for more details on age and training). The bottom line here is that young athletes, especially those in their 20s and early 30s who have been in the sport for a few years, can typically schedule several breakthrough workouts in a week—perhaps one or two in each sport. Be conservative in making this decision. A common mistake athletes make in planning is not allowing enough recovery time between breakthrough workouts. As a result, they go into these sessions overly tired and show little progress throughout the season. It's far better to be overly recovered.

Two-a-Days

It's common for experienced age-group triathletes to do two workouts a day. Most pros frequently do three-a-days. The demands of a sport such as triathlon make multiple daily sessions a necessity for performance at the highest level. But if you are a novice and your goal is to cross the finish line of a race, then multiple daily workouts are likely not necessary. A single workout each day, with a day off from all training once each week, will give you six total sessions weekly with two sessions in each sport. The two sport-specific workouts should be separated by 2 days,

After the early base period, reduce the gym workouts to a moderate intensity.

Recovery is as critical to fitness and success on race day as breakthrough workouts.

such as run on Monday and Thursday, swim on Tuesday and Friday, and bike on Wednesday and Saturday, with Sunday a day off.

For the intermediate or advanced triathlete with 2 years or more in the sport, some of the two-a-day triathlon workouts may be "bricks," which are workouts combining two or more sports, such as bike-run, swim-bike, or swim-bike-run sessions. Such workouts may be done year-round, but they are quite beneficial in the build period when breakthrough workouts become racelike. While the brick workout is one continuous session, I consider it as two or three workouts because multiple sports are involved.

The obvious advantage of doing two-a-day workouts is that you can fit in more training in each sport weekly than if you do only one each day. That's important to high-level performance when you are training for three sports. With only one session each day, you can manage only two or three workouts per sport in a week.

Of course, as with everything in life, there is also a downside to working out twice in a single day. Doing two or three workouts in a single day means increased fatigue. Some athletes seem to handle that quite well and bounce back quickly. Others, especially novices, juniors, and seniors, recover more slowly. So several stressful, back-to-back, double-workout days can lower the quality of your training and therefore your fitness and performance. You'll get worse, not better. More stress also raises the specter of overtraining from trying to do too much in too short a period of time. Raising the workload significantly by doing two-a-days can cause you to become overtrained in just a few weeks, depending on how well you cope with training stress (see Chapter 10 for more on overtraining).

In addition, two-a-day workouts raise the possibility of injury, which is especially common in running. I've coached many triathletes over the years who have "glass legs." They're fragile. It doesn't take much stress to cause a soft-tissue injury that leaves them hobbled for days, if not weeks. Running on tired legs as the second workout of a two-a-day, especially after cycling or lifting weights, is very risky for some. If this is a concern of yours, it's better to do the run earlier in the day when your legs are likely to be fresher, then ride or go to the gym later.

While cycling isn't nearly as orthopedically stressful as running, there is still an increased risk for a bike-related injury from two-a-days. For the cyclist, the knees are where overuse injuries are likely to occur. This may be related to poor pedaling skills, unusual biomechanics, too much climbing in a gear that is too high, or, most commonly, a poor bike setup (we'll cover these matters in later chapters).

Sports Distribution

How many workouts should you do in each sport in a base or build week? The more experienced you are, and the faster you recover, the more training sessions you can do. For the highly experienced triathlete, I'd suggest doing at least three workouts in each sport weekly, with a day or more of separation between those in a single sport. If you can manage more than nine sessions in a week, then the "extra" ones should be on the bike or in your limiting sport. Why the bike? About half of a triathlon is spent cycling, so it's the sport that contributes the most to your race performance. But if you are a strong cyclist and your limiter is swimming or running, then you may devote more of the weekly sessions beyond

Two-a-day workouts squeeze in more training but also produce more fatigue.

nine to that sport. We'll return to this topic later and take it to the next level in the section "Weekly Volume Distribution" (page 127).

Finalizing Your Weekly Base and Build Routine

You should now have all of your workouts recorded on your standard weekly routine for the base and build periods. In doing this, you should have given consideration to anchor and breakthrough workouts, recovery, multiple workout days, sports distribution, and especially your lifestyle. You must realize that it's not possible to create a perfect weekly plan given three sports, nine or so workouts, and only seven days. This makes last-minute adjustments to your standard training week a necessity in order to allow for recovery and optimizing your time. I'll tell you more about that later in this chapter.

Table 8.1 provides my suggestion for what a base and build training week may look like for the experienced triathlete. Of course, I don't know your level of proficiency as a triathlete, your age, how well you handle training stress, or your lifestyle, so what you see here is only an example. Use it to help tweak your weekly plan.

In this table, breakthrough workouts are indicated as *BT*. These vary by period but typically are aerobic endurance, muscular force, muscular endurance, and anaerobic endurance workouts (see Appendixes B, C, D, and E for details). The exact type of breakthrough workout that *you* do depends on your strengths, limiters, and the seasonal period you are currently in. Note in this example that in the early base period, the athlete does only four breakthrough sessions in a week, with weight training accounting for two of these. But after the early base period, when weight

training is reduced, the athlete does six breakthroughs: two for swimming, three on the bike, and one for running. These more challenging sessions may be introduced gradually throughout the base period and be common in the build period. Nonbreakthrough workouts are intended for recovery, skill improvement, or the maintenance of previously well-established abilities, especially aerobic endurance.

Peak and Race-Week Routines

While the base and build periods make up by far the greatest portions of your training year, there are other periods, as you learned in Chapter 7, that also need structure. These are the peak and race periods that are scheduled in the last weeks before your A-priority races. These two periods combined may last 2 to 3 weeks, depending on the type of race you're training for, how previous training has gone, and how your body responds to reduced training volume.

The other periods discussed in Chapter 7 and included on your ATP, the preparation and transition periods, don't have planned weekly routines. There are no fixed schedules because they are meant to be unstructured. Their objectives are the gradual return to training (the prep period) and a break for the body and mind following the highly structured training that led to your most recent A race (the transition period).

Let's take a closer look at the peak and race periods to see how they may be structured to produce the best possible performance on race day.

Peak Week Routine

One of the most important but least understood times in the season is the peak period, which usually starts 2 to 3 weeks before an A-priority

Peak period usually starts 2 to 3 weeks before an A-priority race.

TABLE 8.1 Example of a Standard Training Week for Base and Build Periods

Monday	Weights BT* (BT in early base period only; otherwise SM)	Rest and recovery
Tuesday	Swim BT (BT following early base only)	Bike BT (BT following early base only)
Wednesday	Run	Bike (optional after early base period)
Thursday	Swim BT (BT following early base only)	Weights BT (in early base period only; omitted in later periods) or Bike BT (included after early base period)
Friday	Run	Rest and recovery
Saturday	Swim	Run BT
Sunday	Bike BT	Run (optional; done as a brick with a very short run or can be a race in build, but if B-priority then no BTs on Thursday or Saturday)

* BT indicates a breakthrough workout, and SM indicates strength maintenance. Nonbreakthrough workouts are active recovery or skill enhancement.

race. If training goes well in this period, you can come into great form on race day. If it goes poorly, much of the work done in the base and build periods can be wasted. It's a critical time in the season when things must go right if you are to race well.

Athletes often make two mistakes in the peak period. The first is training too hard. What's needed is some mix of rest and hard training—with the emphasis on rest. Self-coached athletes often don't trust that what they've done so far is enough, so they tend to do too much hard work in the last few weeks. On the other hand, a few rest too much and don't train hard enough because they've heard that rest produces greater fitness. They're not exactly right. Rest actually produces greater form (see Chapter 3), which can be called freshness. Resting also results in an insignificant loss of fitness. Whenever you reduce the training load, fitness begins to diminish slowly, but that's OK; you become more race-ready as fatigue is rapidly lost. That's the purpose of the peak period in a nutshell.

> Resting results in a loss of fitness, but you become race-ready as you shed fatigue.

The trick is to lower fatigue gradually, maintain fitness at a relatively high level, and steadily increase form. Then you are peaked and ready to race. So how do you do that? Here's how.

Starting 2 to 3 weeks before your A-priority race, do a race-intensity workout every third day that simulates the conditions of the race. Then make these workouts gradually shorter as you progress through the peak period. With the workouts becoming shorter, your weekly volume is also dropping. That's good. It should drop rather rapidly. Something such as a 30 to 50 percent drop each week is about right.

The intensity for these racelike workouts should be similar to what you're expecting in the race, but the intensity must reach at least zone 3 for heart rate, pace, or power—"moderately hard." Such an intensity is the key to maintaining fitness while reducing the volume of your training. The two recovery days between these race simulations are key to reducing fatigue while elevating form. They should be low-intensity, low-duration workouts that also become shorter as the peak

TABLE 8.2 **Example of a 2-Week Peak Period Routine**

Monday	Weights (SM*) or day off from training	Rest and recovery
Tuesday	Swim BT	Bike BT (may be a swim-bike brick)
Wednesday	Run	
Thursday	Swim	Bike
Friday	Bike BT	Run BT (best done as a brick)
Saturday	Swim	
Sunday	Bike	Run (done as a brick to rehearse transition)
Monday	Swim BT	Bike BT (may be a swim-bike brick)
Tuesday	Bike or day off from training or weights (SM)	
Wednesday	Swim	Run
Thursday	Bike BT	Run BT (best done as a brick)
Friday	Swim	
Saturday	Run	
Sunday	Bike BT	Run BT (best done as a brick)

* BT indicates a breakthrough workout, and SM indicates strength maintenance. Nonbreakthrough workouts are active recovery or skill enhancement.

This example is for an experienced triathlete doing several two-a-day workouts per week during base and build periods.

period progresses. So what you are doing when peaking is mixing the two key elements—intensity and rest—to eventually produce race readiness on race day.

This is a simple process for single-sport athletes such as cyclists and runners. For the triathlete, the peaking process described here is a bit more complex. For example, the tapering procedure described above may be modified by sport. For example, running, which is more orthopedically stressful, typically requires a longer taper than does cycling, and the cycling taper is usually longer than that for swimming. There are other elements to consider, such as the length of the race (long-course races mean long tapers), how fit you are (high fitness means long tapers), how easily injured you are (injury-prone athletes should taper longer), and how

old you are (older athletes often need longer tapers).

With all of this in mind, Table 8.2 provides an example of how a 2-week peak period may be designed. In this example, the breakthrough workouts are done as muscular endurance intervals (see Appendixes B, C, D, and E) when race intensity is expected to be in zone 2, 3, or low 4 for heart rate, pace, or power, and as anaerobic endurance intervals when race intensity will be in zones 4 and 5. Nonbreakthrough workouts are for rest, recovery, and skill maintenance. These sessions are done in zones 1 and 2. All workouts gradually get shorter as this period progresses. As in the base and build periods, this routine may not work for you without modification, but it will help you get started in designing your own routine.

Peaking mixes the key elements of intensity and rest to produce race readiness.

Race-Week Routine

The week of the race is unique compared with how you've been training throughout the season and even in the peak period. You should emphasize rest even more than previously, yet you still need to do a bit of intensity work to maintain fitness. The one thing you can leave out is long workouts. Your aerobic endurance will do fine with only a few days remaining before your race. Let's get into the details of this last critical week of training.

In race week, do three or four workouts in which you include several 90-second intervals with 3-minute recoveries following a warm-up. Cool down afterward. For short-course races, the intensity is "hard" to "very hard" perceived exertion, or zone 4 or 5 for power or pace (see Chapter 4 for details on intensity). For long-course races, the intensity is zone 3 power or pace, or a perceived exertion of "somewhat hard." Do not use heart rate to gauge intensity for these intervals; they are too brief. Your heart would not have enough time to respond and achieve the targeted zone in only 90 seconds.

Over the course of the week, you need to decrease the number of intervals, which means the individual workout times will also gradually decrease. Table 8.3 provides the suggested details of how many intervals to do by sport for each day of the week, depending on whether your race day is Saturday or Sunday.

For most athletes, I've found that the easiest day of race week should be 2 days before the race. This is usually a day off or, at most, a very short and low-intensity session. It's often a day of travel to the race venue, especially when the race is a short-course one. The longer the race (and also the greater the heat or altitude relative to where you train), the earlier in the week you should arrive at the venue. Note that the day before the race also includes some racelike intensity with a very brief session. I'd suggest doing the three sports in their race order the day before the race.

It's also a good idea to do the final training swim of the week at the same time that the race starts so that you can see how things look in the water at that time of day. This has to do with where the sun is and how landmarks appear.

After the swim, if it is very early, have a light breakfast. Allow a break for digestion, and then do a bike-run brick on the course with one 90-second effort in each sport at race intensity, as you've done throughout the week. The bike ride may last only 20 minutes including warm-up, and that high-intensity effort should be followed by a transition to a short run of about 10 minutes with one 90-second effort. Follow that with a short cooldown jog. Stay off of your legs as much as possible the remainder of the day.

You must realize that many factors influence your readiness on race day besides workouts. Diet, sleep, and lifestyle are important. Things should remain similar to your normal, *restful* routine in this regard. Regardless of how well we manage things, sometimes the taper works and sometimes it doesn't. We're biological organisms, not robots. That's simply the way the real world is for humans. What you should do before every race is keep a record in your training diary (see Chapter 14) of what you did in the last few days to prepare for an important race. If things go well, repeat this process as closely as possible for subsequent races. If things don't go well, study what you did and make appropriate adjustments the next time.

Race week is unique compared with season training, even in the peak period.

The easiest day of race week should be 2 days before the race.

TABLE 8.3 Examples of Race-Period Routine for a Saturday or Sunday Race

	SATURDAY RACE	SUNDAY RACE
Monday	Swim or day off from training	Swim or day off from training
Tuesday	Swim BT* (5) + bike BT (3)	Swim BT (5) + bike BT (3)
Wednesday	Brick: bike BT (4) + run BT (2)	Brick: bike BT (4) + run BT (2)
Thursday	Day off from training or very easy and short bike ride; possible travel day	Swim BT (3) + run BT (1)
Friday	Swim BT (1) + bike BT (1) + run BT (1)	Day off from training or very easy and short bike ride; possible travel day
Saturday	Race	Swim BT (1) + bike BT (1) + run BT (1)
Sunday	Day off from training	Race

* BT indicates a breakthrough workout. These are 90-second intervals with 3-minute recoveries done at race intensity, but at least at a perceived exertion of "somewhat hard" or zone 3 for pace or power. The nonbreakthrough workouts here are for rest, recovery, or skill maintenance. Nonbreakthrough workouts are done in zones 1 and 2. All breakthrough workouts gradually decrease the number of intervals as the week progresses. The suggested number of 90-second intervals per sport on each day is shown in parentheses.

These examples are for an experienced triathlete doing several two-a-day workouts in the base and build periods.

Weekly Volume Distribution

Let's take a step back and review an important training concept discussed in Chapters 3 and 4. There, I explained the relative importance of workout frequency, duration, and intensity.

You may recall that for the novice athlete, the frequency of workouts should be the primary focus. At this level, the athlete is making a rather significant lifestyle change, so too little motivation simply to exercise regularly is the greatest obstacle to race fitness. This athlete simply needs to get out the door frequently.

For the intermediate athlete, who may be in the second or third year of the sport and for whom training frequency is no longer an issue, the most important of the three variables is workout duration. These intermediates need to increase the distance or time of certain workouts in order to develop general endurance.

For the advanced athlete who has been training for 3 years or more, however, intensity is the key. This doesn't mean going all out or extremely hard. It means doing certain workouts at an intensity that is specific to the goal event. If you want to run a 7-minute pace off the bike, you need to do a lot of training at a 7-minute pace. There may also be sessions that are somewhat more intense and some that are very slow. Even though the advanced athlete is best advised to focus on intensity, this doesn't mean that frequency and duration are of no consequence. They are still important, but they typically are not performance limiters at this level.

You may also recall from Chapter 3 that the combination of frequency and duration is called *volume*. It has to do with the number of miles, hours, kilometers, or TSS points in a period of time such as a day, week, month, or year. All too often, this is the number that advanced athletes become obsessed with maximizing. That's a mistake that can lead to poor performance and even overtraining. Again, this doesn't mean that weekly volume is unimportant; it means only

For the advanced athlete who has been training for 3 years or more, intensity is key.

that it is less important than intensity. Advanced athletes still need to get their weekly volume right. Too much and you're always tired, with poor performance in the planned breakthrough workouts. Too little and you're undertrained. Given a choice, you should take the latter. It would be better, however, if we got your volume right. That's where we're headed next.

Daily Duration and TSS Distribution

How do you get the volume of your training right every day and every week? The starting point for answering the first part of this question was discussed in Chapter 7 and detailed in Tables 7.2, 7.5, and 7.6. Using these tables, you recorded your projected "Annual Volume" at the top of your ATP and then broke that number down into "Volume" in the column with that header. Now we need to break down weekly volume further into daily volume and then into individual workout duration. This is a big task, but by the time you've completed it, your weekly plan will be complete. Let's get started.

Tables 8.4 and 8.5 provide a suggested breakdown of the "Volume" column on your ATP into suggested hours or TSS for each day of the week. This daily distribution may certainly be changed to better fit your unique lifestyle needs. The tables are tied to the days of the week in Tables 8.1, 8.2, and 8.3. So if you change the daily routines for these figures, then the days of the week for the following tables also need to be changed so that they match.

Tables 8.4 and 8.5 break down your weekly volume into daily hours and daily TSS. Start by finding in the left column of the appropriate table the weekly hours or TSS for any given week on your ATP. They may not match exactly for TSS,

so find the closest one. To the right is a suggested division of the weekly volume into daily hours or TSS for each day of the week. On any given day, the hours or TSS are then subdivided among the sports in which you are doing workouts. Besides swim, bike, and run, weight lifting sessions are also included in the weekly volume.

There's no need to use these tables right now because the time to determine daily volume and workout durations is during planning for the upcoming week. Return to this section when you are doing the final planning for a training week to find your planned weekly volume distribution. How you divide those hours or TSS by sport is then the next step in your weekly planning.

Workout Duration and TSS Distribution

Further dividing your daily volume into workout hours or TSS for swimming, biking, running, and weight lifting starts by determining your expected time by sport in your A-priority races. For most athletes, the race time distribution is roughly 10 percent swimming, 50 percent biking, and 40 percent running. Of course, this may not be exactly what you expect to do in your race. If you are a very good runner, you may expect to spend less than 40 percent of your total race time running. But your swimming may not be nearly as good, so more than 10 percent of your race time is in that portion of the race. This same calculation may be done with TSS. Your common time or TSS distribution by sport gives you a good idea of how much volume you should devote to each sport, on average, in a standard training week.

Determine what you think your time splits will be for each leg of your next A-priority race and then use that to decide what percentage of time or TSS will be devoted to swimming,

TSS distribution by sport tells you how much volume you should devote to each in a standard training week.

TABLE 8.4 **Daily Training Hours**

WEEKLY HOURS	MONDAY	TUESDAY	WEDNESDAY	THURSDAY	FRIDAY	SATURDAY	SUNDAY
4:00	0:00	1:00	0:00	1:00	0:00	1:30	0:30
4:30	0:00	1:00	0:00	0:45	0:30	1:30	0:45
5:00	0:00	1:00	0:00	1:00	0:30	1:30	1:00
5:30	0:00	1:00	0:30	1:00	0:30	1:30	1:00
6:00	0:00	1:15	0:30	1:00	0:45	1:30	1:00
6:30	0:00	1:15	0:45	1:00	1:00	1:30	1:00
7:00	0:00	1:30	0:45	1:15	1:00	1:30	1:00
7:30	0:00	1:30	0:45	1:15	1:00	2:00	1:00
8:00	0:00	1:30	1:00	1:15	1:00	2:00	1:15
8:30	0:30	1:30	1:00	1:15	1:00	2:00	1:15
9:00	0:45	1:30	1:00	1:30	1:00	2:00	1:15
9:30	0:45	1:30	1:00	1:30	1:00	2:30	1:15
10:00	0:45	2:00	1:00	1:30	1:00	2:30	1:15
10:30	1:00	2:00	1:00	1:30	1:00	2:30	1:30
11:00	1:00	2:00	1:00	1:30	1:30	2:30	1:30
11:30	1:00	2:00	1:00	1:30	1:30	3:00	1:30
12:00	1:00	2:00	1:00	2:00	1:30	3:00	1:30
12:30	1:00	2:00	1:00	2:00	1:30	3:30	1:30
13:00	1:00	2:30	1:00	2:00	1:30	3:30	1:30
13:30	1:00	2:30	1:00	2:00	1:30	3:30	2:00
14:00	1:00	2:30	1:00	2:00	1:30	4:00	2:00
14:30	1:00	2:30	1:30	2:00	1:30	4:00	2:00
15:00	1:00	2:30	1:30	2:30	1:30	4:00	2:00
15:30	1:00	2:30	1:30	2:30	2:00	4:00	2:00
16:00	1:00	3:00	1:30	2:30	2:00	4:00	2:00
16:30	1:00	3:00	1:30	2:30	2:00	4:00	2:30
17:00	1:00	3:00	2:00	2:30	2:00	4:00	2:30
17:30	1:00	3:00	2:00	2:30	2:00	4:30	2:30
18:00	1:00	3:00	2:00	3:00	2:00	4:30	2:30
18:30	1:00	3:30	2:00	3:00	2:00	4:30	2:30
19:00	1:00	3:30	2:00	3:00	2:30	4:30	2:30
19:30	1:00	3:30	2:00	3:00	2:30	4:30	3:00
20:00	1:00	3:30	2:30	3:00	2:30	4:30	3:00
20:30	1:00	3:30	2:30	3:00	2:30	5:00	3:00
21:00	1:00	3:30	2:30	3:30	2:30	5:00	3:00
21:30	1:00	3:30	2:30	3:30	3:00	5:00	3:00
22:00	1:00	4:00	2:30	3:30	3:00	5:00	3:00
22:30	1:00	4:00	2:30	3:30	3:00	5:00	3:30
23:00	1:30	4:00	2:30	3:30	3:00	5:00	3:30

→

TABLE 8.4 (continued)

WEEKLY HOURS	MONDAY	TUESDAY	WEDNESDAY	THURSDAY	FRIDAY	SATURDAY	SUNDAY
23:30	1:30	4:00	2:30	3:30	3:00	5:30	3:30
24:00	1:30	4:00	2:30	4:00	3:00	5:30	3:30
24:30	1:30	4:00	2:30	4:00	3:30	5:30	3:30
25:00	1:30	4:30	2:30	4:00	3:30	5:30	3:30
25:30	1:30	4:30	2:30	4:00	3:30	5:30	4:00
26:00	1:30	4:30	2:30	4:00	3:30	6:00	4:00
26:30	1:30	4:30	3:00	4:00	3:30	6:00	4:00
27:00	1:30	4:30	3:00	4:30	3:30	6:00	4:00
27:30	1:30	4:30	3:00	4:30	4:00	6:00	4:00
28:00	1:30	5:00	3:00	4:30	4:00	6:00	4:00
28:30	1:30	5:00	3:00	4:30	4:00	6:00	4:30
29:00	1:30	5:00	3:30	4:30	4:00	6:00	4:30
29:30	2:00	5:00	3:30	4:30	4:00	6:00	4:30
30:00	2:00	5:00	3:30	5:00	4:00	6:00	4:30
30:30	2:00	5:00	3:30	5:00	4:30	6:00	4:30
31:00	2:00	5:30	3:30	5:00	4:30	6:00	4:30
31:30	2:00	5:30	3:30	5:00	4:30	6:00	5:00
32:00	2:00	5:30	4:00	5:00	4:30	6:00	5:00
32:30	2:00	5:30	4:00	5:30	4:30	6:00	5:00
33:00	2:00	5:30	4:00	5:30	5:00	6:00	5:00
33:30	2:00	6:00	4:00	5:30	5:00	6:00	5:00
34:00	2:00	6:00	4:30	5:30	5:00	6:00	5:00
34:30	2:00	6:00	4:30	5:30	5:00	6:00	5:30
35:00	2:00	6:00	5:00	5:30	5:00	6:00	5:30

Find your weekly volume for a given week on your ATP in the "Weekly Hours" column. To the right is the distribution of those hours into daily volume.

biking, and running in a week. For example, if you expect to finish the race with 13 percent of your total time as swimming, then it may be a good idea to devote around 13 percent of your weekly training time or TSS to the swim. Of course, you may feel that greater gains will result from shifting even more volume from your strongest to your weakest sport. That's generally a good idea. Just don't move so much training away from your strongest sport that it becomes a weakness.

Planning the Training Week

How do you lay out your training plan for the coming week? This is something you should do near the end of the preceding week. Now that you have a good idea of how to distribute the weekly volume by sport, it's merely a matter of how much time to train each day in each sport (including strength training).

Start by subtracting the anticipated time or TSS for weight lifting from the week's total in

TABLE 8.5 **Daily TSS**

WEEKLY TSS	MONDAY	TUESDAY	WEDNESDAY	THURSDAY	FRIDAY	SATURDAY	SUNDAY
240	0	50	0	50	20	80	40
260	0	50	0	60	20	80	50
280	0	50	20	60	20	80	50
300	0	50	30	60	30	80	50
320	0	60	30	60	40	80	50
340	0	60	30	60	50	90	50
360	0	70	40	60	50	90	50
380	0	70	40	60	50	100	60
400	10	70	50	60	50	100	60
420	30	70	50	60	50	100	60
440	40	70	50	70	50	100	60
460	40	70	50	70	50	120	60
480	40	90	50	70	50	120	60
500	50	90	50	70	50	120	70
520	50	90	50	70	70	120	70
540	50	90	50	70	70	140	70
560	50	90	50	90	70	140	70
580	50	90	50	90	70	160	70
600	50	110	50	90	70	160	70
620	50	110	50	90	70	160	90
640	50	110	50	90	70	180	90
660	50	110	70	90	70	180	90
680	50	110	70	110	70	180	90
700	50	110	70	110	90	180	90
720	50	130	70	110	90	180	90
740	50	130	70	110	90	180	110
760	50	130	90	110	90	180	110
780	50	130	90	110	90	200	110
800	50	130	90	130	90	200	110
820	50	150	90	130	90	200	110
840	50	150	90	130	110	200	110
860	50	150	90	130	110	200	130
880	50	150	110	130	110	200	130
900	50	150	110	130	110	220	130
920	50	150	110	150	110	220	130
940	50	150	110	150	130	220	130
960	50	170	110	150	130	220	130
980	50	170	110	150	130	220	150
1,000	70	170	110	150	130	220	150

$\rightarrow$

TABLE 8.5 (continued)

WEEKLY TSS	MONDAY	TUESDAY	WEDNESDAY	THURSDAY	FRIDAY	SATURDAY	SUNDAY
1,020	70	170	110	150	130	240	150
1,040	70	170	110	170	130	240	150
1,060	70	170	110	170	150	240	150
1,080	70	190	110	170	150	240	150
1,100	70	190	110	170	150	240	170
1,120	70	190	110	170	150	260	170
1,140	70	190	130	170	150	260	170
1,160	70	190	130	190	150	260	170
1,180	70	190	130	190	170	260	170
1,200	70	210	130	190	170	260	170
1,220	70	210	130	190	170	260	190
1,240	70	210	150	190	170	260	190
1,260	90	210	150	190	170	260	190
1,280	90	210	150	210	170	260	190
1,300	90	210	150	210	190	260	190
1,320	90	230	150	210	190	260	190
1,340	90	230	150	210	190	260	210
1,360	90	230	170	210	190	260	210
1,380	90	230	170	230	190	260	210
1,400	90	230	170	230	210	260	210
1,420	90	250	170	230	210	260	210
1,440	90	250	190	230	210	260	210
1,460	90	250	190	230	210	260	230
1,480	90	250	210	230	210	260	230
1,500	90	250	210	230	210	280	230
1,520	90	270	210	230	210	280	230
1,540	90	270	210	250	210	280	230
1,560	90	270	210	250	210	280	250
1,580	90	270	210	250	210	300	250
1,600	90	290	210	250	210	300	250
1,620	90	290	210	270	210	300	250

Find your weekly volume for a given week on your ATP in the "Weekly TSS" column. To the right is the distribution of the TSS into daily volume.

Table 8.4 or 8.5. That's sometimes overlooked in weekly planning. What remains is then divided among the three sports as described in the preceding section by giving consideration to your race distribution by sport. Be sure to make adjustments to this distribution by moving some portion of the remaining weekly volume from your strongest sport to your weakest. How much is your call. I'd suggest no more than about 10 percent. Combined workouts, or bricks, often raise issues during planning. For the purposes of weekly planning, the multiple sports in a brick are considered as separate workouts even though they are done as a single nonstop session.

Next to be considered for planning your weekly workout schedule are the anchor workouts. Record each of them on the days and at the times they will be done. These typically happen on predetermined days and at standard times. And they usually have fixed, or at least predictable, durations or TSS. Write the anchor workouts into your training diary and subtract their total duration or TSS, by sport, from the weekly volume planned for each sport.

Next, write down your breakthrough workouts for each sport on the days you will do them. You must be realistic in deciding how many you will do. Too many is far worse than too few. You may, for example, do one breakthrough in each sport during the week. That's fairly common for advanced triathletes. Or you may decide to do an additional breakthrough workout in your weakest sport. Or perhaps you race at an elite level and can manage two or more breakthroughs in each sport each week. Each of these workouts has a fairly common duration or TSS, so record them along with the times each day when you will do these hardest sessions. Of course, some of your anchor workouts may also be breakthroughs.

By adding up your weekly time or TSS for gym workouts, anchor sessions, and breakthroughs, then subtracting that total from your planned weekly volume on your ATP, you have the time or TSS that will be divided among the remaining workouts. These are usually low-intensity and low-volume active recovery and speed skills sessions. Decide how that remaining time or TSS will be distributed for these workouts.

You now have a detailed weekly plan. While this procedure probably seems quite time-consuming, after a few weeks of doing it I'm certain you'll find you can do it quickly. In fact, you'll find, I'm sure, that there is a common pattern you follow most weeks of the season, which makes the process quite simple once you get on to it. It will also improve your training and ultimately your racing.

The only weekly routine and volume distribution we haven't covered so far is for the rest-and-recovery weeks, which are critical to the quality of your training and for avoiding overtraining. Chapter 11 will cover how to distribute weekly volume at these times.

WORKOUT SPECIFICS

Now that you have a weekly plan, let's move on to the specifics of individual workouts. This is where the rubber meets the road. The specific workout details described here have to do with the topics of workout timing, brick sessions, anaerobic endurance workouts for long-course athletes, and missed workouts.

Workout Timing

Preparing for three sports is complicated and difficult; among multisport events, only heptathlon and decathlon are as demanding as triathlon. For the serious triathlete who has a family, a career, and many other commitments, the challenge can be overwhelming. That's why weekly planning is so beneficial. It allows you to make the most of your limited time and energy.

Multiple sports in a brick are considered as separate workouts even though they are done nonstop.

Doing the right workouts at the right times can be a real conundrum. This is apparent every day when the training plan calls for two (or even three) workouts. The way you wedge them into your day goes well beyond the range of this book because it involves your own daily lifestyle and how you manage time. For most athletes, the solution is based on piecing together a patchwork of sessions—early in the morning, during the lunchtime break at work, late in the day, and on weekends. Hard-charging triathletes commonly have a busy daily routine aside from sport, which makes managing time an extremely important aspect of high performance.

One scheduling matter we can tackle right off the bat has to do with the optimal order of workouts in a day. When should you do your swim, bike, and run workouts, relative to one another? On some days, your anchor workouts will decide this for you. For example, if you swim with a masters group that meets early in the morning on certain days, then the order of workouts that day is settled. You may encounter the same story for your other anchor workouts, such a club track session or group ride after work. But what do you do about the order of workouts when there are no anchors? Sometimes, even these are decided for you. Runs are typically shorter workouts than bike rides—or even swims when you include travel time to the pool—so your available time may make the decision for you.

Let's address two scheduling concerns I always take into consideration when planning a week for an athlete. The first has to do with workout intensity and duration relative to training purpose and recovery when two-a-days are being done. The other involves planning long

runs and rides on the weekend, which is the time when most triathletes schedule these.

Stepping back a bit, in Chapter 6 I told you about the importance of identifying and improving your limiters. The most basic of these is your sport limiter. Which is your weakest sport—swim, bike, or run? Which one will have the greatest impact on your performance if it's improved? If you are equally strong in all the sports, the order of impact is bike, run, and then swim, simply because of race time in all three sports. We discussed this earlier in the chapter, but now we're looking at it in a slightly different way. If you are even a little weak as a cyclist, that slight weakness will be magnified because of race time on the bike. The same is true to a lesser extent for running. Swimming has the least relative impact on overall race performance simply because it makes up such a short portion of the race. That doesn't mean it's unimportant; if you can't make the swim cutoff time, then nothing else is important about your ability as a cyclist and runner. So you must address your sport limiter regardless of its relative importance to race performance.

What does this have to do with the order of training per sport on a given day? Quite a bit, actually. Doing two-a-day sessions increases the importance of your limiting sport when it comes to scheduling. If you need to improve in one sport far more than the other one planned for that same day, you should take into consideration the order in which they will be done. It's undoubtedly better to tackle the workout for your limiting sport first, especially if your energy and motivation after the first workout are diminished; it's seldom effective to work on improving your limiting sport when you are tired. That's especially true when the limiting-sport workout is planned to be a breakthrough. You don't want to go into breakthroughs tired. Hence, the breakthrough session for the limiting sport is best done before the other session.

What about when both workouts are breakthroughs? If the first session is only for active recovery—meaning short and with low intensity—then the order of scheduling is of little concern. If you are not a morning person, though, and tend to have higher-quality workouts later in the day, then you should schedule the breakthrough workout for your limiting sport later in the day. In this situation, it's critical that you make the first workout easy enough that it doesn't hurt the breakthrough workout for your limiter.

The other common issue that must be addressed for triathletes is the order of their long ride and run workouts, which are typically done on the weekends. The common way of scheduling these is for the long bike ride to be done on Saturday and the long run on Sunday. The thinking is usually along this line: *I will be tired when I start the run in a race; therefore, I need to do my long run on Sunday when I'm tired from the long ride on Saturday.* But that's wrongheaded thinking. The fatigue you experience while running the day after a long ride is not the same as the fatigue you feel as soon as you exit T2 in a race. Instead, a long run on Sunday following a Saturday long ride increases your risk for an injury while lowering the quality of your run. Running injuries are common among triathletes. And running on tired legs is a common cause of injury. If running is a limiter, then doing that workout when leg-weary on Sunday will have little benefit.

The best solution is to do one of the long workouts—probably the run because it's a bit shorter than a long ride—on Tuesday, Wednesday, or Thursday. That way, with the long ride scheduled for the weekend, you will probably be fresh for both of them. Of course, this depends on what other workouts you may have on weekdays and whether they can be positioned not to affect your long weekday session.

If you must do both long workouts on the same weekend, I'd suggest doing the long run on Saturday and the long ride on Sunday. Another common solution is to do the long bike workout on one weekend and the long run the following weekend. You will need to decide which solution best fits your schedule.

Brick Workouts

When should you do brick workouts and how should they be done? Here, we're going to examine only continuous, bike-run bricks because they are the most common and the ones that have the greatest potential for affecting your race performance. The most challenging aspect of the swim-bike brick is the transition, especially the quick stripping of your wet suit. (You should rehearse your T1 transition several times during the peak and race periods.) Apart from the issue of the wet suit, though, the swim-to-bike brick is not nearly as difficult as the bike-to-run brick.

You can do the bike-run brick year-round, but it's best done in the build period when workouts are becoming increasingly racelike. In this regard, the brick is nearly the perfect race-preparation session. During the build period, it can be beneficial to do frequent short runs after most bike rides, if not all of them. They'll go a long way in preparing you for what is one of the most challenging parts of the race—the first 2 to 3 miles (3–5 km) of the run.

> If you must do long workouts on the same weekend, do the long run on Saturday and the long ride on Sunday.

It takes only 15 to 20 minutes of running off the bike to reap the benefits of a brick workout. Going longer may be mentally beneficial, but there is little to be gained physiologically. That's why I seldom have triathletes run longer than a few minutes after a bike ride, although I do have them do the runs frequently. The exception is when they need to overcome the anxiety of running for a long duration after a hard ride. But even then, I keep the preceding ride short, although it's usually intense with the inclusion of muscular endurance intervals (see Appendix C). Keeping the ride brief improves the quality of the run and reduces the risk for injury. A steady diet of long runs following long rides is a sure way to experience a breakdown of some sort, such as injury, illness, or low motivation. Over the course of the build period, frequent short-run bricks are more valuable than a few long-duration runs.

There are three lessons to be learned from doing frequent, short-run bricks. The first has to do with polishing transition skills. T2 rehearsal starts even before you get off the bike. Near the end of *every* ride in the build period, take your feet out of your shoes while staying clipped in. Get used to pedaling with your feet on top of your shoes instead of in them. Again, that's every ride. That way, your shoes will still be clipped in when you start the next ride so you can practice getting into them while moving. That's a skill many triathletes fumble coming out of T1. As you come into your workout "transition" after dismounting the bike, rehearse getting into your running shoes. Practice this frequently, too, to make it second nature in a race. The build period is the time to hone these skills, not the day before the race.

Short-run bricks are also good for becoming familiar with what it feels like to run when your legs are not yet warmed up for running and are still recovering from the bike ride. This takes some getting used to every season. You can also use short bricks to rehearse pacing early in the run when your legs feel rubbery. In the build period, set the pace at the level you expect to run in the race. Don't overdo it; once you're a few minutes into the run and thoroughly warmed up, the pacing benefits begin to decrease. The rest of the run leg in your race will come down to your aerobic endurance, muscular endurance, and anaerobic endurance, and all of those are best developed in stand-alone run sessions. That's yet another reason why short-run bricks are usually a better option than long-run bricks.

Anaerobic Endurance Workouts

I've mentioned several times in this and previous chapters that advanced, long-course triathletes should consider doing anaerobic endurance workouts in all three sports in the base 3 period. So who are "advanced" athletes, and what is an anaerobic endurance workout? Advanced triathletes are those who have been seriously training in the sport for more than 3 years and are competitive in their age groups. An anaerobic endurance workout is one involving short intervals (usually less than 4 minutes for each interval) done at a very high intensity—well above the anaerobic threshold—with short recoveries (again, 4 minutes or less). The primary benefit of doing such a workout is boosting one's aerobic capacity (see Chapter 4 and the Glossary for details).

So why don't I recommend that short-course triathletes also do anaerobic endurance intervals in the base 3 period? The answer takes us back to my underlying philosophy of periodization: Workouts should become increasingly like the

A-priority race as preparation for the race progresses over time. In the base period, workouts are largely unlike the race. The build period is the time when racelike workouts become the focus of training. For this reason, short-course triathletes don't need to start earlier than the build period because their anaerobic endurance workouts are similar to what they can expect in a race. They will get plenty of such training in the last several weeks before the race. On the other hand, anaerobic endurance workouts are quite dissimilar to what can be expected in long-course triathlons—they aren't racelike—so such workouts are best done before the build periods starts.

Long-course triathletes typically devote most of the high-intensity training time in the build period to muscular endurance workouts. By doing anaerobic endurance workouts in base 3, they can lift their aerobic capacities to a high level before starting the build period, and then maintain it with less frequent anaerobic endurance intervals in the last few weeks before their race.

Missed Workouts

In Chapter 2, I told you how important consistent training is to high-performance racing. There, I mentioned that the biggest mistake most self-coached triathletes make is inconsistent training. It's not that they don't want to train better. It's just that they frequently violate an even more basic tenet of smart training that is at the heart of consistency: moderation. When you moderately increase the training stress—the frequency, duration, and intensity of workouts—in conservatively measured amounts, you wind up training consistently week after week. Over time, that consistency adds up to great fitness. But if you pile on huge doses of training with overly long or hard workouts, or skip a

rest-and-recovery break, you greatly increase your risk for injury, burnout, illness, and overtraining. Any one of these will interrupt your training consistency. Fitness is lost whenever there is a break in training for even a few days and you have to take a step back in training and begin over again. It's common for triathletes to make such a mistake once or twice each season; when that happens, they never realize their full potential.

Unfortunately, some "outside" force is just as likely to interfere with your training, even if you do everything right with regard to training and recovery. For example, you're probably a very busy person with many commitments, such as family, career, and other responsibilities. Something here will interfere with training from time to time. It's a given. You're also likely to catch a bad cold or the flu just from being around other people. This can happen a couple of times in a season. So even if you are smart about your training load, it's still quite likely that you will have to vary your training to accommodate an interruption several times during the season. Most of these interruptions will probably last only a day or so. But a longer break from training is also likely to happen. Let's take a look at how to modify your training plan when workouts are missed, regardless of the reason.

Missing 3 days or fewer. Return to training as if nothing happened. Don't try to make up the missed workouts. Cramming more workouts into a few days creates the potential for a breakdown and more lost training time. It's not a big deal to miss a handful of workouts if it rarely happens.

Missing 4 to 6 days. This may be the hardest scenario to deal with. If the lost time was due to illness,

The build period is the time when racelike workouts become the focus of training.

Long-course triathletes typically devote high-intensity time in the build period to muscular endurance workouts.

as is quite often the case, you probably really won't be ready to return to normal training right away, even if the symptoms are gone. Your body's chemistry has probably changed, which will affect your capacity for exercise. This may show up as a high heart rate and an elevated perceived exertion at what have normally been easy-to-moderate paces and power outputs. In this case, you will need to treat it as more than 7 days missed, even though you are starting back into training again (see "Missing 1 or 2 Weeks" below).

If missing 4 to 6 days of training was not due to illness, but rather to something such as business travel, and you are ready to get started right away, you will need to make some adjustments to the plan. The first change is to consider the lost training time as a rest-and-recovery period. This is the best way to handle it, but it will still throw off the scheduling of training for your A-priority race. Your training periods will no longer be synchronized to bring you to a peak of form on the day of the race. Too much fitness was lost.

There are a couple of ways to resolve this dilemma. The first option, if you are in the base or build periods, is to reduce the length of the current period by 1 week. If you still aren't synchronized, do the same for the following period. The second option is to reduce the peak period from 2 weeks to 1 week. Neither of these choices is perfect. Both are going to result in less race readiness and perhaps a compromised performance. But that's the reality of missing a week of training. You can't miss several workouts and have the same fitness as if no training was missed. Unfortunate, but that's just the way life is.

Once you are ready to train again, you will need to step back and make up probably two or three key workouts that were missed. Decide which were the most important ones given your limiters and reschedule them. This may well mean pushing other workouts farther ahead into the plan. Eventually, something will have to give. You'll either have to miss one of the culminating workouts planned for later on or decide you are progressing well enough to skip or modify one of the workouts remaining in the plan. There are simply too many variables here for me to be able to tell you exactly how to handle your situation. You'll have to decide which of your missed workouts were the most important for your race preparation and go from there.

Missing 1 or 2 weeks. If you missed this time because of illness and you were in the build period, start back into training with the base 3 training block. If you were in the base period, go back to the previous base period or even the preparation period if you were in base 1. Stay with that period for 3 to 4 weeks or until your workouts indicate that you are back to where you left off before the lost training. You will know you've reached that level because your heart rate and perceived exertion will again match pace and power, as they did before you got sick. But if in doubt, give it another day or two before going to the next step.

When your training metrics and vigor return to normal, repeat the last week of hard training you did before the interruption. If that week goes well, then begin moving forward with your original training plan but start from a later time in the season. If it doesn't go well, repeat the test week. At some point, you will need to leave out 1 to 3 weeks (or even more) of planned training. That could mean omitting build 2 and perhaps the first week of the peak period. Make sure you complete the full base period, however.

Missing more than 2 weeks. If you were in the build period when this training pause happened, return to base 3 and start over again from there. If you already were in the base period, back up one period from where you left off and start training again from that point. As with the previous scenarios, you will have to leave out some significant portion of your plan—at least 2 weeks. The priority for omissions, in order, is the first week of peak, build 2, and build 1. Again, complete all three base periods.

If any of your training time was lost in the last week of build 2 or the peak period, continue with your training as if nothing has happened. But as with all of these situations, if the lost time was due to illness, be conservative with both duration and intensity as you start back by opting to train with short- to medium-distance workouts and intensity primarily in zones 1 and 2 until you are back to feeling normal.

SUMMARY: PLANNING A WEEK

What should a training week look like in each of the periods? Table 8.6a–f provides examples of how each may be arranged. Your actual plans may not be the same because of the other demands in your daily life. But these samples should give you a general guide for laying out your training weeks. Workouts in these figures are listed as basic (aerobic endurance, speed skills, muscular force) or advanced (muscular endurance, anaerobic endurance) abilities. (Chapter 6 describes these workout categories, and Appendixes B, C, D, E, and F provide the specific workouts within each category.) Making a choice for which specific type of workout to do on a given

day depends on your limiters, activity availability (such as gym, pool, or masters swim days), and the race distance for which you are training. Note that the preparation and transition periods are not included in these figures because they are highly variable; they depend on how you feel on any given day.

That pretty much wraps it up. You should now have your ATP completed down to the level of daily workout types by ability. You should also have a good understanding of how to assign workouts for the base, build, peak, and race periods. The first time you design an ATP down to this level, it is quite a tedious and time-consuming task. But once you have done it and you understand the how and why, future seasons will be much easier. Most importantly, you now have a plan for the upcoming season that can keep you on track for achieving your high-erformance goals. The key here is to visit your plan weekly and use it as a guide to make daily and weekly decisions about your training.

Let's briefly review the central points made in Chapter 8. To do this, I'd like to draw your attention back to the figures and tables in this chapter because they illustrate some important topics. Figure 8.1 serves as an example of how to design your ATP, and Tables 8.1, 8.2, and 8.3 help with scheduling daily workouts by period. Use these as guidelines to help lay out your plan. Tables 8.4 and 8.5 provide guidance in distributing your total daily training volume by hours or by TSS. That volume may be further divided into workout duration or TSS by following the guidelines in the section of this chapter titled "Daily Duration and TSS Distribution." These tools will help you create a personalized training plan in the same way that top triathlon coaches do it.

If you lost training time in the last week of build 2 or peak, continue as if nothing has happened.

TABLE 8.6A Example of the Base 1 Training Period

ACTIVITY	MONDAY	TUESDAY	WEDNESDAY	THURSDAY	FRIDAY	SATURDAY	SUNDAY
Swim		Basic		Basic		Basic	
Bike	Basic		Basic		Basic		Basic
Run		Basic	Basic			Basic	
Weights	MS phase			MS phase			

TABLE 8.6B Example of the Base 2 Training Period

ACTIVITY	MONDAY	TUESDAY	WEDNESDAY	THURSDAY	FRIDAY	SATURDAY	SUNDAY
Swim		Basic		Basic		Basic	
Bike	Basic		Basic	Basic	Basic		Basic
Run		Basic	Basic			Basic	
Weights	SM phase						

TABLE 8.6C Example of the Base 3 Training Period

ACTIVITY	MONDAY	TUESDAY	WEDNESDAY	THURSDAY	FRIDAY	SATURDAY	SUNDAY
Swim		Advanced		Basic		Basic	
Bike			Basic	Basic	Advanced		Basic
Run		Basic	Advanced			Basic	
Weights	SM phase						

All that remains is putting your plan to work by referring to it every day in the season as you prepare for your races. The critical remaining action is to keep it current. Having a plan is not enough. It must be rethought and revised. I have never coached an athlete who went through an entire season without changes to the plan.

One more thing: I want to reiterate my suggestion in the introduction to Part IV. If you've just read Chapters 7 and 8 for the first time, or are returning to these chapters as you prepare for subsequent seasons, then you should read the following chapter before putting the finishing touches on your annual, weekly, and daily training plans. In Chapter 9, you will learn about alternative ways to schedule your training that may cause you to rethink and refine the plan you're creating.

TABLE 8.6D Example of the Build 1 and Build 2 Training Periods

ACTIVITY	MONDAY	TUESDAY	WEDNESDAY	THURSDAY	FRIDAY	SATURDAY	SUNDAY
Swim		Advanced		Basic		Advanced	
Bike			Basic	Advanced	Basic		Advanced
Run		Basic	Advanced			Basic	Basic
Weights	SM phase						

TABLE 8.6E Example of the Peak Training Period

ACTIVITY	MONDAY	TUESDAY	WEDNESDAY	THURSDAY	FRIDAY	SATURDAY	SUNDAY
Swim		Advanced	Basic	Basic		Basic	
Bike	Basic		Basic	Basic	Advanced	Basic	
Run		Advanced			Advanced		Basic
Weights	SM phase						

TABLE 8.6F Example of a Race Training Period with a Sunday Race

ACTIVITY	MONDAY	TUESDAY	WEDNESDAY	THURSDAY	FRIDAY	SATURDAY	SUNDAY
Swim		Advanced		Advanced	Off	Advanced	Race
Bike	Basic	Advanced	Advanced	Advanced	Off	Advanced	Race
Run	Basic		Advanced		Off	Advanced	Race
Weights							

PLANNING ALTERNATIVES

THE LAST TWO chapters have shown you the way to plan your season that is the most popular one among athletes in all sports around the world. That, however, doesn't mean it's the best way for you to organize your training. There are many other ways of doing it that may be equally good, if not better. Some athletes may respond well to the periodization model described in those chapters, while others may lose performance on the same plan. In this chapter, I'll suggest some alternatives to that periodization model.

How will you know which model is best for you? There's no way of knowing short of simply experimenting. And amazingly, what you discover may not remain the same over time. Next season—or even in a few weeks—you may find that what was working well no longer seems effective. Training experimentation is a never-ending process.

The only things that truly remain constant year after year are the general principles of training described in Chapter 3:

- **Progressive overload:** The training load must gradually become greater over time to improve fitness.
- **Specificity:** The types of workouts you do must be similar to the race for which you are training.
- **Reversibility:** Fitness is lost when the training load decreases, which is sometimes necessary, in small portions, to allow you to be "on form" for a race or to recover from hard training.
- **Individuality:** Your training needs are unique to you in many ways—both physically and mentally—and so your training must reflect your personal characteristics.

Here's another key principle that you must include: As you get closer to race day, your workouts must become increasingly like the A-priority race for which you are training. That's similar to the specificity principle above. If your training is different from the demands of the race, then the reversibility principle kicks in. You will lose race-specific fitness. That might happen if, for example, you stop training at goal race intensity as you get closer to the race and start doing long, slow distance instead. The result will be that you become better at running slowly for a long time, but not at your goal race intensity for the race distance. So no matter which periodization method you decide to use after reading this chapter, you must always be aware of how race-specific your workouts are becoming throughout the season.

As you also learned in Chapter 3, the only training variables that can be changed throughout a season are the frequency, duration, and intensity of your workouts. Other than "mode" (swim, bike, or run), there is nothing else to adjust, regardless of your levels of experience and performance. These are at the heart of planning your season. Periodization is nothing more than the management of these three variables in order to be race-ready at the right time.

This chapter will provide alternatives so that you can decide how to arrange them throughout the season. You may decide to stay with the periodization model described in the previous two chapters. If you've never followed a plan before, that's a good place to start. Or you may have used that system in a previous season and now want to try something different. If so, start with whichever of the approaches described below that seems most appealing. If you dis-cover that it does not meet your needs, make adjustments until you find what does.

LINEAR PERIODIZATION ALTERNATIVES

Chapter 7 took you step by step through the process of developing an ATP based on what sports science calls *linear periodization*. The name implies a straightforward and somewhat simple process of developing aerobic fitness first (the base period), followed by an emphasis on race-specific intensity (the build period) before taper of the duration of workouts (the peak period) and finally rest in order to be on form for the race (the race period).

This linear method is the original periodization model and has been very popular among athletes in a wide range of sports—from body builders to triathletes—since the 1960s. It offers several advantages. For example, it's a proven system that has been used and refined over several decades, unlike some other systems that are relatively new and still not well defined for all sports. It carries a low risk for overtraining because the progression is gradual and rest-and-recovery periods are planned. You don't have to be a sports scientist to understand it. Linear periodization is simple and makes sense even to novices. It's easy to measure progress because there are well-defined ability outcomes that are developed independently in each period. This keeps athletes motivated and on course to achieve their goals.

Throughout the late 20th century, coaches, athletes, and sports scientists introduced several other approaches to periodization to meet unique needs while they addressed what they

As you approach race day, your workouts must become like your A-priority race.

Linear periodization carries a low risk for overtraining.

had identified as flaws in the linear system. The most common concern was that the linear format sets an upper limit on how many A-priority races an athlete can peak for in a season—typically two or three. Related to that was the concern that this peak of fitness can be maintained for only 1 to 3 weeks at most. The linear format also is generally not as effective for highly experienced elite athletes as it is for novices and intermediates. Beyond that, many athletes find linear periodization to be monotonous because training stays largely the same for weeks at a time. And finally, for the triathlete, it can be difficult to manage progress in three sports with a linear system because the sports may not always be in the same days concurrently. That makes for a rather confusing plan.

What can you do about these flaws while still reaching a peak of fitness on race day? Let's start by looking at some small but significant changes made to the linear model to better fit your needs. Then, in the remainder of this chapter, we'll examine some "nonlinear" periodization models. Along the way, consider how each alternative method would work for you given your lifestyle, what's worked for you in the past, and what appeals to you now.

I would be remiss if I didn't point out that a periodization plan is perhaps not even needed at all. The alternative is random training—doing what you want when you feel like it. That may seem rather "loosey-goosey," but it may not be all that bad for some triathletes. Random training actually works well for novices who simply need to exercise frequently and for whom performance is judged based on crossing the finish line with a smile. Some highly advanced athletes may even appear to be training randomly. While they may not have a written plan and seem to make last-minute decisions about workouts, most have a plan in their heads. They know what's needed and the order in which their abilities are best developed. Such a method is best suited to triathletes who have been around the sport for many, many years and have learned what works best for them. Most of us are better advised to have a written plan, even if it's only a rough outline, of how training should progress to avoid the many pitfalls on the way to high-performance racing.

With all of this in mind, let's a take a look at some common ways you can tweak linear periodization so that it better fits your needs.

Time-Limited Periodization

Perhaps the most common challenge for the serious age-group athlete who wants to follow a simple linear periodization plan is having limited time available for training. Tables 8.4 and 8.5 suggest weekly volumes throughout the season based on the annual volume from Tables 7.2, 7.5, and 7.6. It's simple enough, but what do you do if you have the physical capacity for managing high annual and weekly volumes but your lifestyle just doesn't allow it? Perhaps the time constraints set by your career, family, and other responsibilities make it impossible to train at a high volume.

Let's look at an example to see how to resolve this common problem. An athlete may decide she is capable of training 600 hours in a year. She's come close to that in the past, so there's reason to believe it is a good number. Based on an annual volume of 600 hours per year, she should be capable of training, on average, about 13 hours per week, with a big week of around 18 hours in base 3, week 3 (according to Table 7.5). While that will push her to her limit, it seems realistic

Time-limited periodization works around the problem of inadequate time for high volume.

given her capacity for training. But what if she can't do that many hours because of limited time for training? Maybe the most she can do, once all of her weekly responsibilities are accounted for, is 15 hours a week. Table 7.5 suggests there should be 7 weeks with training greater than 15 hours in preparation for her first race of the season. What does she do?

First of all, it would not be a good idea to change to an annual volume of 500 hours, even though the biggest week would then be 15 hours. Why not? Simply because the training plan would then be too easy for her. While the training load would still adhere to the principle of progressive training, it wouldn't be great enough in most weeks to produce an increase in fitness. The weekly volume would be far too low for her throughout much of the season.

Instead, the best option is simply to train to a schedule of 600 annual hours but lop off the weekly volume at 15 hours when she comes to those 7 higher-volume weeks.

Won't that also cause a loss of fitness? She could potentially reach a slightly higher level of fitness by putting in those few bigger weeks. So what does she do about that? There really aren't too many options. She has to start by simply shortening the longest workouts in those highest-volume weeks. She may also consider slightly increasing the intensity of some of the workouts in those weeks when training time is reduced. An easy, zone 1 recovery ride may no longer be necessary given the shortened workouts. It's apparent she could handle more, so she could consider bumping up the intensity to zone 2. The general rule is that as duration goes down, intensity can go up. I can't tell you exactly which workouts she can do that with—or even if she

should do it. It all comes down to the art of self-coaching. When she reaches those high-volume weeks, she'll have to make some decisions based on how she is feeling at the time and how her training has been going. My overarching advice to her is to be conservative when increasing the intensity of workouts in those few modified weeks. One additional zone is plenty, and for only a few workouts.

Another fix that may work for her is to move the "excess" hours from a chopped-off, high-volume week to a lower-volume week. Using the example from above, this would make nearly all of the weeks in the base period into 15-hour weeks. She could do the same in the build period so that volume is also increased across the board; in that case, total training time would remain the same as the unaltered plan called for.

These fixes aren't as good as keeping the volume as it was originally called for in Table 7.5, but they are probably better for most time-crunched athletes than simply training to a lower annual volume. Of course, while I was using hours in this example, the same changes could be made if your training is instead based on TSS, as in Table 7.6.

Crash Periods

Many athletes have discovered that their fitness surges markedly after very hard training for several days, followed by a few days of rest and recovery. In fact, a few studies over the last 30 years have confirmed that training this way is effective for producing a high level of fitness in a short period of time. This is a rather risky way to increase fitness, however. So what I'm going to tell you here is only for triathletes who have been training seriously for a number of years and have reached a high level of performance. Others

As duration goes down, intensity can go up.

should avoid it, especially novices and athletes in the first 3 years or so of triathlon training. Instead of becoming more fit, you may end up overtrained, sick, or injured.

If you become infatuated with this training method and overuse it, those negative outcomes are just as likely as a hoped-for boost in fitness. That's why I call it a *crash period*. I hope I've caught your attention with that title because overdoing it will wreck your season, and maybe even your triathlon career. I've seen that happen. But when the method is used conservatively, it has the potential to be quite an effective periodization method, especially for users of the linear model.

So how do you use it correctly? The answer begins with including only a few continuous days of such training, and also limiting how frequently you train this way. And just as important, being willing to abandon such a training period at the first sign that things aren't going as they should. Let's take a closer look at these restrictions.

A crash period is several consecutive days of increased training load. A few days to a week of such training is common. It seldom should extend beyond 10 days, even for elite athletes who are capable of managing heavy training loads.

The training load can be boosted by increasing training volume or intensity for the crash days. The more common option is to increase volume. An increase of around 50 percent in the number of hours or TSS over what was originally planned in your linear periodization plan (see Tables 7.5 and 7.6 for weekly volume) is common for most athletes. If you decide to increase the intensity of training, keep the volume as it was originally scheduled and do a workout that is higher in intensity for a few consecutive days.

Most of these higher-intensity sessions should be at or just below the anaerobic threshold (see Chapter 4), with only a few as high as your aerobic capacity. I'd suggest doing nearly all of these high-intensity sessions at the lower end of that spectrum. That would make them mostly *muscular endurance* workouts (see Appendixes B, C, D, and E).

Most of the high-volume and high-intensity workouts during a crash period should be done on the bike or in the pool. Running workouts done at a high training load require great caution because this is the sport in which many triathletes are most likely to become injured when pushing their limits.

For most athletes preparing for an A-priority race, the best times to include a crash period are the third week of base 3 and the third week of build 2 (see Tables 7.5 and 7.6). Both are the high points of training during race preparation and are followed by rest-and-recovery periods. The timing is nearly perfect in this regard. One way to plan such training would be to do a high-*volume* crash in the base 3 period and a high-*intensity* crash in build 2. Each crash period may last about 5 to 7 days and be immediately followed by a few days of rest and recovery. The typical rest-and-recovery period following a crash is 3 to 5 days long. Table 9.1 is an example of how a 6-day crash period followed by 4 days of rest and recovery may look. *High* in this figure means either high volume or high intensity, depending on the type of crash period being used. *Low* means an easy or recovery workout in terms of both volume and intensity, or perhaps even a day off from training.

It's common to use a training camp as a crash period. This is a good way to boost motivation for

A crash period is several consecutive days of increased training load.

The most difficult crash period workouts should be done on the bike or in the pool.

TABLE 9.1 Linear Periodization Example of 6-Day Crash Period Followed by 4 Days of Rest and Recovery

	ACTIVITY	MONDAY	TUESDAY	WEDNESDAY	THURSDAY	FRIDAY	SATURDAY	SUNDAY
Week 1	Swim		High*		High		High	
Crash	Bike			High	High	High		High
	Run		High	Low			High	
	Weights	SM phase						
Week 2	Swim		Low			Start next period		
Recovery	Bike			Low				
	Run				Low			
	Weights	SM phase						

* High and low refer to workout duration or intensity.

such demanding training. Just be cautious that you don't allow your motivation to push you over your limits. It's OK to miss a group workout at a camp. I always encourage athletes at my camps to take a day off or greatly reduce the training load on any day when they are feeling especially fatigued. Again, be cautious with such training.

Inverse Weeks

You may have noticed in Tables 7.5 and 7.6 that in the three base periods, volume increases somewhat in each subsequent week within a period. For example, Table 7.5 shows a gradual weekly increase in hours in base 3 for the 500-hour column:

Week 1: 11.0

Week 2: 13.5

Week 3: 15.0

Please understand that these weekly hours (or TSS if you train that way) don't have to be precise. They are intended to be ballpark numbers—albeit a small ballpark. But I've generally found that most athletes come very close to achieving the scheduled weekly volumes when following a plan. Toward the right end of Table 7.5, the weekly increases are much larger, on the order of around 4 to 5 hours per week. In Table 7.6, on the right side, the TSS values also increase by large amounts.

Having coached hundreds of triathletes over three-plus decades, I've run into many who found these weekly increases to be overly taxing. They were often wasted by the time they got to the third week, more because of the accumulation of training volume than because the third week in and of itself was a problem. Workout quality seemed to decline as the weekly training volume increased. For these athletes, I've found it sometimes works better if the weekly increase in hours is reversed, so that the first week in a 4-week period is the biggest and the last is the smallest. The weekly volume is inverted—it declines from the start to the finish of the period. I really don't know if this method has a physical or psychological effect, but having a decreasing weekly volume seems to improve the capacity for hard training for some athletes. For the same 500-hour annual volume in the base 3

A decreasing weekly volume seems to improve the capacity for hard training for some athletes.

example above, the progression of weekly hours is then like this:

Week 1: 15.0

Week 2: 13.5

Week 3: 11.0

That may not seem like a big deal, but it could make a difference in how well your training goes as the period progresses.

Another option for the athlete who still finds the cumulative volume increase over 3 weeks to be a problem is to change the format from 4 weeks to 3 weeks, with the last several days still dedicated to rest and recovery. I'll get into the details of this shortly in the section "Slow-Recovery Athletes."

Reverse Linear Periodization

I mentioned this version of the linear periodization model earlier. Basically, it takes much of the linear model and turns it upside down. Instead of starting the base period by gradually building workout duration and then in the build period focusing on racelike intensity, reverse periodization starts with high-intensity but low-duration workouts and shifts toward an emphasis on low intensity with high volume. This way of training is popular with athletes who live where the winters are cold, the hours of daylight are short, and the weather is not conducive to riding or running outdoors. When the linear periodization model is reversed, the short but intense workouts are done in the winter and the longer, less intense sessions in the summer. Problem solved. Maybe.

As is often the case, solving one problem creates a new one. As I explained in Chapter 3, for the advanced triathlete the key to success

is racelike intensity—not duration. The shorter the A-priority race, the greater the problem for making the workouts similar to the race by reversing duration and intensity. The reason is specificity. Remember that from earlier in this chapter? It's an underlying principle of training and periodization. Training must become increasingly like your A-priority race over time. So if you are an advanced athlete training for a short-course race, you'll get faster by focusing on higher intensity in the build-period weeks—not on workout duration.

If, however, you are doing a long-course race, this approach may prove to be an effective training strategy. Why? Because the intensity in a long-course race is low (well below the anaerobic threshold) and the duration is quite long. In fact, I had already suggested this basic strategy for the long-course triathlete in Chapter 7 when I mentioned doing high-intensity interval training in base 3 to boost aerobic capacity before starting the lower-intensity, longer-duration workouts of the build period. Reverse linear periodization merely takes that small change to a grander level.

Let me repeat that I would not suggest this strategy for the short-course triathlete. Doing long, slow workouts in the last few weeks before such an A-priority race is unlikely to produce high performance. What an athlete needs then is racelike intensity, which is quite high for short-course racing.

Should you decide to follow a reverse linear plan, all you need do is redesign Table 8.6a–d to something similar to what is shown in Table 9.2a–d. These figures are intended only as examples of how training weeks *may* be designed for some athletes. They are not necessarily how you should organize your training weeks. In

For the advanced triathlete, the key to success is racelike intensity—not duration.

Reverse linear periodization can work for long-course races, but not short courses.

TABLE 9.2A Reverse Linear Periodization Example of Workouts in Base 1 Period

ACTIVITY	MONDAY	TUESDAY	WEDNESDAY	THURSDAY	FRIDAY	SATURDAY	SUNDAY
Swim		SS		AE		ME	
Bike	MF		SS		ME		AE
Run		SS	ME			AE	
Weights	MS phase			MS phase			

TABLE 9.2B Reverse Linear Periodization Example of Workouts in Base 2 Period

ACTIVITY	MONDAY	TUESDAY	WEDNESDAY	THURSDAY	FRIDAY	SATURDAY	SUNDAY
Swim		SS		AE		AnE	
Bike	MF		SS	AE	AnE		AE
Run		SS	AnE			AE	
Weights	SM phase						

these figures, the workouts listed for each sport and day are the abbreviations for the basic and advanced abilities described in Chapter 6 and also found in Appendixes B, C, D, and E:

- AE: aerobic endurance
- MF: muscular force
- SS: speed skills
- ME: muscular endurance
- AnE: anaerobic endurance

I suggest leaving the peak and race periods unchanged by continuing to follow the examples in Table 8.6e and f. Note that the AE workouts in the base periods are short low-intensity (zones 1 and 2) recovery sessions, whereas in the build period they are longer low-intensity sessions done mostly in zone 2.

The examples provided in Table 9.2a–d represent only one way of using a reverse linear model to organize training. There are other ways to do it. However you decide to do it, what is most important is emphasizing high intensity early in the season, then high duration as you get closer to the race. Be sure not to make your training become less like the race, especially in terms of intensity, as you get into the build period.

Slow-Recovery Athletes

In Chapter 11, I'll get into the details of the rest-and-recovery periods that come at the end of each base 1, base 2, base 3, build 1, and build 2 period. But for now, I want to address a couple of periodization alternatives related to rest and recovery that can have a big impact on the quality of your training.

One of the critical issues in designing a periodization plan, regardless of which type you may use, has to do with how quickly you recover from hard training, especially in the base and build periods. Some athletes recover quickly. They usually do well with a periodization plan based on 4-week base and build subperiods, as described in Chapter 7 and illustrated in Figures

TABLE 9.2C Reverse Linear Periodization Example of Workouts in Base 3 Period

ACTIVITY	MONDAY	TUESDAY	WEDNESDAY	THURSDAY	FRIDAY	SATURDAY	SUNDAY
Swim		AE		ME		AnE	
Bike			AE	AE	AnE		ME
Run		AE	AnE			ME	
Weights	SM phase						

TABLE 9.2D Reverse Linear Periodization Example of Workouts in Build 1 and 2 Periods

ACTIVITY	MONDAY	TUESDAY	WEDNESDAY	THURSDAY	FRIDAY	SATURDAY	SUNDAY
Swim		AE		ME		AE	
Bike			AE	AE	ME		AE
Run		AE	ME			AE	ME
Weights	SM phase						

7.5 and 8.1. For the first 3 weeks or so (it can be a few more than 21 days—to be explained in Chapter 11) of each 4-week subperiod, quick-recovery athletes train with a high training load—either high in duration or high in intensity, depending on the period. Then they go into a rest-and-recovery break that typically lasts 3 to 5 days.

For the athletes who recover more slowly, training needs to be organized differently. These athletes need more frequent rest-and-recovery periods. They can't wait 3 weeks or so before taking a break. They need a break after 2 weeks or so (again, this may be a bit more than 14 days, as will be explained in Chapter 11).

So how do you know if you are a fast- or a slow-recovery athlete? Experience is the best indicator. How tired do you usually feel after 2 weeks of hard training? If you're still raring to go with another week of hard training, then you most likely recover quickly. If you often find yourself fatigued, and if the quality of your training drops in week 3, then you recover slowly.

Two types of athletes who typically—but not always—recover slowly are novices and athletes over the age of 50. This isn't always the case, however. I've coached over-50 and novice athletes who recovered quickly and for whom 3 weeks or so of quality training before a few days of rest and recovery worked just fine. I've also coached advanced and under-50 athletes who recovered slowly. You need to be honest with yourself in this regard. Doing very long or highly intense workouts in the third consecutive week when you are highly fatigued is counterproductive. If that frequently happens to you, I'd strongly suggest going to 3-week subperiods on your ATP. That means about 2 weeks of hard training followed by a few days of rest and recovery.

Table 9.3 shows how to do this by reducing the number of weeks in a base or build subperiod. Notice that in this table the base 3 and build 2 subperiods have been repeated so that the total training before the race isn't shortened. In using this periodization alternative while preparing

If you recover slowly, you need to schedule more frequent rest-and-recovery breaks.

TABLE 9.3 How to Adjust Base and Build Subperiods for the Slow-Recovery Athlete

PERIOD	SUBPERIOD WEEKS
Base 1	Week 1
	Week 2
	Week 4
Base 2	Week 1
	Week 2
	Week 4
Base 3	Week 1
	Week 2
	Week 4
Base 3	Week 2
	Week 3
	Week 4
Build 1	Week 1
	Week 2
	Week 4
Build 2	Week 1
	Week 2
	Week 4
Build 2	Week 2
	Week 3
	Week 4

for your first race of the season, you will train for a total of 21 weeks in the base and build periods, whereas with the standard 4-week base and build subperiods there are 20 weeks. The weekly volume shown here remains the same as was suggested in Tables 7.5 and 7.6. In other words, for each week listed below, find the weekly volume for that exact week (for example, base 1, week 4) in either Table 7.5 or Table 7.6 depending on the way you determine volume—either hours or TSS. The number of weeks in the other periods—prep, peak, and race—remain unchanged.

Another way of solving the slow-recovery conundrum is to redefine what a "week" is. So far, I've used the term to mean 7 days. The problem with that for the slow-recovery triathlete is that it spaces hard training days too closely if three such sessions are done in a week. Either there isn't adequate time to recover, or the athlete must do only two hard workouts each week in order to recover properly. Neither is a good solution. Workouts too closely spaced not only add to cumulative fatigue but also increase the risk for an injury.

An alternative is to train in 9-day "weeks." That way, there are 2 days planned for recovery after each hard training day.

Using 9-day weeks means that 6 days of hard training are included in 18 days, whereas there are a total of 5 days of hard training if a 7-day week is used with only 2 days of hard training days per week. So the 9-day week allows more quality training along with more rest and recovery. Table 9.4 provides an example of what a base or build subperiod looks like when 9-day training weeks are followed by 5 days of rest and recovery. Notice that the last 2 easy days of the second 9-day week are a part of the 5-day rest-and-recovery period.

The high and low days in Table 9.4 can be manipulated to customize training to your unique capabilities. For example, there are two high-load workouts on some days. If that load is too great on any given day, change one to moderate. The same may be done with a low workout session if you can handle a slightly greater load. Such small changes can be done on the fly if you pay close attention to how you're feeling. Such tweaking allows you to create a training week that precisely fits your needs for stress and rest. As always, if unsure, take the more conservative route. It's far better to be slightly undertrained than slightly overtrained.

TABLE 9.4 **Example of Base and Build Subperiods for the Slow-Recovery Athlete**

WEEK 1	MONDAY	TUESDAY	WEDNESDAY	THURSDAY	FRIDAY	SATURDAY	SUNDAY
Swim	High*		Low		Low		High
Bike		Low		High		Low	High
Run			Low	High		Low	
Weights	SM phase						
WEEK 2	**MONDAY**	**TUESDAY**	**WEDNESDAY**	**THURSDAY**	**FRIDAY**	**SATURDAY**	**SUNDAY**
Swim		Low		Low		High	
Bike		Low			Low	High	
Run	Low		High		Low		Low
Weights			SM phase				
WEEK 3	**MONDAY**	**TUESDAY**	**WEDNESDAY**	**THURSDAY**	**FRIDAY**	**SATURDAY**	**SUNDAY**
Swim	Low		Low				Low
Bike	Low	High				Low	
Run		High		Low			Low
Weights					SM phase		

* High and low indicate the level of duration or intensity for a swim, bike, or run workout.

These subperiods include two consecutive 9-day weeks followed by 5 days of rest and recovery.

The downside of the 9-day week is that it can be difficult for the athlete whose job demands a lot of work hours. There will be days when a high-duration workout, such as a long ride, must be done on a long workday. Consequently, the 9-day week is best for the athlete who has a very flexible lifestyle. In this regard, it's perfect for the retired athlete. (The 9-day week is fully examined in my book *Fast After 50*.)

NONLINEAR PERIODIZATION ALTERNATIVES

So far, we've examined several possible ways of altering the linear periodization plan described in Chapters 7 and 8 to better fit your training and lifestyle needs. I hope that something you've read until now closely fits your needs because linear periodization—even with the tweaks I've suggested so far—is the simplest and easiest of all the possibilities to follow. But linear periodization may not exactly suit your needs, or perhaps you're thinking about experimenting a bit to see if there's something better for your particular situation. With that in mind, let's take a look at two nonlinear planning methods. These plans manipulate workout duration and intensity, and they are the most popular of the nonlinear options used by many high-powered athletes.

We'll look first at *undulating* periodization and then at *block* periodization. Both of these approaches are considerably different from what you've read about so far. But like linear periodization, they still leave a considerable amount of wiggle room for deciding exactly what you'll do in your workouts and how you will use them to lay out a plan.

Undulating Periodization

This training method, true to its name, is based on regularly changing things around by *undulating* two of the training variables. It's not often used in endurance sports but is very popular among weight lifters. Why would you want to use this method? It could be that you have limited time to train and so you can't devote all of the time needed every week to build fitness adequately with linear periodization. It could also be that you sense the need for more variety in your training. Perhaps doing the same workouts on the same days week after week is getting a bit tiresome. Changing things around every few days may boost your enthusiasm and motivation for training. (There are also some research studies showing that undulating periodization produces greater fitness than linear periodization. But don't select it merely on that possibility; the fact is that there aren't many such studies for endurance sports. Most of the research on this topic was done with strength training used as the focal activity and may not apply to our sports.)

As mentioned, undulating periodization frequently and regularly changes things around. Those things could be our old friends duration and intensity, or even two of the three sports in a triathlon. Let's start by looking at the latter of these two options because I believe that one is the most promising alternative for most triathletes.

Sports undulation involves changing the swim, bike, or run emphasis every few days. Switching them every week is the usual way to do it. The most common method is to focus your

Sports undulation involves changing the swim, bike, or run emphasis every few days.

attention on two of the three sports and alternate the training load assigned to them while keeping the training load for the third one rather steady. There's reason to believe this works, even though no research has tested such a system. Most triathletes agree that it's very difficult to improve in three sports simultaneously. Many experienced triathletes have discovered that when they start making progress in two sports, the third one frequently takes a downturn. So how does undulating periodization solve this dilemma?

Let's look at sports undulation with an example. Let's say that cycling and running are the two sports you decide to focus on by alternating the training volume devoted to them every week. One week is mostly cycling, with a little running and a moderate amount of swimming. The next week, the emphasis on cycling and running is reversed—run more, bike less—while swimming remains the same.

This actually works out pretty well regardless of your strengths and weaknesses. Even if swimming is your greatest limiter of the three sports, focusing on the bike and run is still a good option because roughly 80 percent to 90 percent of your total race finish time is determined by these two sports. Devoting your attention to each of them every other week is likely to pay off with improved race times because you're concentrating on only two sports each week. In fact, keeping your swim training steady may also prove to be a good tactic because of the training consistency.

The plan for such an undulating system may look something like what you see in Table 9.5. This is an example of a 4-week base or build subperiod. It's merely a guide and not intended to show how *you* should train. There are many different ways to create such an undulating plan.

TABLE 9.5 First 3 Weeks of 4-Week Training Plan for Base or Build with Undulating Bike and Run

WEEK 1	MONDAY	TUESDAY	WEDNESDAY	THURSDAY	FRIDAY	SATURDAY	SUNDAY
Swim		High*		High		Low	High
Bike	Low		High	High	Low		High
Run		Low	Low			Low	
Weights	SM phase						
WEEK 2	**MONDAY**	**TUESDAY**	**WEDNESDAY**	**THURSDAY**	**FRIDAY**	**SATURDAY**	**SUNDAY**
Swim		High		High		Low	
Bike	Low		Low		Low		
Run		Low	High		High		High
Weights	SM phase						
WEEK 3	**MONDAY**	**TUESDAY**	**WEDNESDAY**	**THURSDAY**	**FRIDAY**	**SATURDAY**	**SUNDAY**
Swim		High		High		Low	
Bike	Low		High	High	Low		High
Run		Low	Low			Low	
Weights	SM phase						

* High and low indicate the duration or intensity of individual workouts.

These subperiods have an emphasis on weekly undulating bike and run training while swimming workouts remain fixed.

Notice that when 4-week subperiods are used in base and build, one of the two sports will get a greater emphasis in the initial 3 weeks. This occurs in the Table 9.5 example for biking because both the first and third weeks emphasize that sport. So this example would undoubtedly work best for the athlete who is a good runner but needs to improve his cycling. Of course, this same undulating pattern could be followed by a slow-recovery triathlete who uses a 3-week subperiod. In that case, there would be an equal emphasis on the two sports.

The other alternative for an undulating periodization system has to do with alternating intensity and duration regardless of the period—base or build. This is the most common way of using such a plan in other endurance sports when only one sport is trained. (Runners, cyclists, and swimmers have it easy, don't they?)

The most common way to alternate intensity and duration is to make one week a baselike week and the other a buildlike week—as in linear periodization. This provides a lot of variety in training that may make it more enjoyable. It also means doing both high duration and high intensity throughout most of the year. When you follow a 4-week subperiod with the last week devoted mostly to rest and recovery, there will be 2 weeks of either high volume or high intensity and only 1 week of the opposite. I'd suggest that short-course athletes do 2 weeks of high duration in the base period and 2 weeks of high intensity in build. The long-course triathlete may consider reversing that so that there are 2 weeks of high

Alternating intensity and duration provides variety that may make training more enjoyable.

TABLE 9.6 First 3 Weeks of 4-Week Training Plan for Base or Build with Weekly Undulation

WEEK 1	MONDAY	TUESDAY	WEDNESDAY	THURSDAY	FRIDAY	SATURDAY	SUNDAY
Swim		Duration*		Duration		Duration	
Bike			Duration	Duration	Duration		Duration
Run		Duration	Duration			Duration	
Weights	SM phase						
WEEK 2	**MONDAY**	**TUESDAY**	**WEDNESDAY**	**THURSDAY**	**FRIDAY**	**SATURDAY**	**SUNDAY**
Swim		Intensity		Intensity		Intensity	
Bike			Intensity	Intensity	Intensity		Intensity
Run		Intensity	Intensity			Intensity	
Weights	SM phase						
WEEK 3	**MONDAY**	**TUESDAY**	**WEDNESDAY**	**THURSDAY**	**FRIDAY**	**SATURDAY**	**SUNDAY**
Swim		Duration		Duration		Duration	
Bike			Duration	Duration	Duration		Duration
Run		Duration	Duration			Duration	
Weights	SM phase						

* Duration and intensity suggest the focus of individual workouts.

These subperiods have an emphasis on undulating duration and intensity for all three sports.

intensity in the base periods and 2 weeks of high volume in the build period. Table 9.6 illustrates a short-course plan when duration and intensity are being undulated. Simply swap these for a reverse-periodization plan.

Duration in Table 9.6 doesn't mean that all of the workouts should be equally long. Some should certainly be longer than others. Your capacity for handling high-volume training determines how long an individual workout within a sport should last and how many high-duration sessions you can do in a week. The same is true for the intensity-emphasis workouts. In this regard, such training may prove highly risky for the athlete who believes all workouts must be either very long or very intense. The rule with this method is that high-duration sessions must be low-intensity sessions, such as zones 1 and 2, while high-intensity sessions must be low-duration sessions. Trying to maintain high duration and high intensity for a given workout throughout an undulating system is likely to lead to injury, burnout, or overtraining.

> High-duration sessions must be low-intensity sessions.

Block Periodization

This is the newest periodization method. It was devised in the 1980s by Vladimir Issurin, a Russian sports scientist who created it for truly elite athletes, such as Olympians. But it has been used successfully by some who aren't quite at that level of performance.

Block periodization is designed to overcome the problem of diminishing returns in training. The closer one is to racing at an extremely high level relative to the best athletes in the world, the more difficult it becomes to make progress.

Training gains are hard to come by and can be tiny, yet they are still significant. The challenge of making even minute amounts of progress is compounded for a top triathlete on a linear periodization plan who is mixing several types of workouts into a week. There isn't a sufficiently focused stress on any single ability when one is trying to develop several at the same time.

The elite athlete is more likely to make fitness gains by focusing on only one type of workout in a subperiod, which are called *blocks* in this method. Attempting to develop more than one ability at a time dilutes the physiological effect of a hard workout. But repeatedly focusing on the same ability in a block by doing similar workouts produces positive changes quickly. For example, in one study in which block- and linear periodization methods were used, it took athletes half as many weeks to achieve the same levels of fitness when they used block periodization as when they used the linear method.

Why is this method not also best for non-elite athletes? Highly advanced athletes have a base of fitness that typically goes back many, many years. They are extremely fit relative to average athletes, even in their "off" seasons. All of their abilities are well developed. How can advanced athletes get that last 1 percent of improvement? The closer they are to their potential, the more difficult it is to make gains. That is not the case for intermediate-level athletes, and certainly not for novices. They have plenty of room to advance their fitness and performance. Highly focused training isn't necessary to make significant gains.

Were intermediate or novice athletes to focus their training on only one ability in a week for several weeks, as suggested here for highly advanced athletes, the abilities that are not being trained would fade quite badly. So this method is definitely not for those who are relatively new to serious training or who are *not* contenders in their age groups at high-level races, such as national and world championships.

Block periodization seems to work best when there is a focal-workout progression that follows a somewhat linear path. In other words, in the base period the emphasized workouts are still the basic abilities, while in the build period there is a shift toward advanced abilities.

Table 9.7 offers a suggested pattern for planning workouts throughout the season for block periodization. Here I'm using the terms *early* and *late* to describe the progression because the linear base 1, 2, and 3 and build 1 and 2 aren't readily applied in this method. The athlete progresses to the next block once the focal or "dominant" ability is determined to be well established. So the weekly durations you see in this table are rough guidelines.

Some athletes may need more or less time to achieve their objective in a given block. While the dominant ability is being developed, the secondary ability is also being maintained, which means there are fewer such workouts. What would typically be the prep, peak, race, and transition periods remain the same as described in Chapter 7.

Table 9.8 provides an example of how a week's training may be organized in the base and build weeks with block periodization. In this example, there are 18 workouts with frequent three-a-day sessions. This is obviously intended for the very high-performance athlete who is capable of managing a huge volume of training. Most advanced athletes following a block plan will do far fewer workouts in a week.

Block periodization is designed to overcome diminishing returns in training.

TABLE 9.7 **The Dominant and Maintenance Abilities**

BLOCK	WEEKS	DOMINANT ABILITY (FOCUS)	MAINTENANCE ABILITY (FOCUS)
Prep	1–4	(Preparing to train)	Muscular force
Early base	4–6	Muscular force	Speed skills
Late base	4–6	Aerobic endurance	Muscular force
Early build	4	Muscular endurance	Aerobic endurance
Late build	4	Anaerobic endurance	Muscular endurance
Peak	1–2	(Racelike workouts)	(Recovery between workouts)
Race	1	(Race-intensity sessions)	(Volume taper)
Transition	1–4	(Rest and recovery)	Aerobic endurance

Abilities to be developed and their suggested order of progression in the buildup to an A-priority race with block periodization.

TABLE 9.8 **Example of Base or Build Training Week with Block Periodization**

WEEK 1	MONDAY	TUESDAY	WEDNESDAY	THURSDAY	FRIDAY	SATURDAY	SUNDAY
Swim		Dominant*	Maintenance	Dominant	Maintenance	Dominant	Maintenance
Bike		Maintenance	Dominant	Dominant	Maintenance	Dominant	Dominant
Run		Dominant	Maintenance	Dominant		Dominant	Maintenance
Weights	SM phase						

* For a definition of dominant and maintenance abilities by period, refer to Table 9.7.

Elite athletes using block periodization are typically capable of training at a high volume—thus the high number of workouts in this example of a week.

A SIMPLE SOLUTION

Block periodization works best with a focal-workout progression that follows a linear path.

Having read this and the previous two chapters, you may well feel overwhelmed with information about periodization. There has indeed been a lot to think about for planning your season. But planning doesn't need to be as detailed and complex as these chapters make it appear. If you'd rather not wade waist-deep into all of the details of planning and sports science, but instead just want a simple way to plan, this is the section for you.

As I explained earlier, periodization can be boiled down to one simple sentence: *The closer in time you get to the race, the more like the race your workouts must become.* For the novice triathlete, this means gradually increasing the frequency of swim, bike, and run workouts in a week. For the intermediate triathlete, it means increasing the duration of the workouts to be as long as the race or slightly longer. And for the advanced triathlete, who already has the frequency and duration of training nailed down, "making the workouts more like the race" means that the intensity of key workouts becomes more racelike.

If this is all you know about periodization and you adhere to it, you'll do fine without being concerned with a complex periodization system. Because when it's all said and done, the most important question is, Are you prepared to race? If you can answer that question affirmatively—which you can if your workouts become like the race—then you will have a great performance. If you're not sure, then you haven't made your workouts enough like the race.

The simple solution for periodizing your season starts with laying out a standard week that fits your everyday schedule and then keeping it much the same as you progress through the season. That's it. Well actually, there's a bit more. Let's take a closer look.

You probably already have a standard week that nicely matches your lifestyle if you've been around the sport for some time. But let's make sure it abides by a basic principle of training that you read about in Chapter 3—reversibility. Basically, this principle says that the fitness gains you've made start to erode when you go several days without training. You start losing fitness. You can avoid this sad state of affairs by following two rules in setting up your standard training week.

The first rule is that there should be at least two workouts in each sport every week. Doing three or more is better, but only if that isn't more than you can manage. Typically, novice triathletes do two workouts per sport per week and intermediate triathletes do three. Advanced triathletes usually do three or more per sport per week. Twelve or more workouts in a week are common for a highly advanced triathlete.

The second rule is that the two or three (or more) workouts in any one of the three sports should be spread out. In other words, you shouldn't have them on back-to-back days with several days off until you do that sport again. Too many days off means that the prin-

ciple of reversibility kicks in. For example, two swim sessions in a week could be on Tuesday and Saturday, but not on Friday and Saturday. Three sessions could be on Tuesday, Thursday, and Saturday, but not on Thursday, Friday, and Saturday. The same goes for biking and running. Spread them out.

Once you have designed your standard week, all you need to do is repeat it for 2 or 3 weeks consecutively before taking several days of rest and recovery, which is discussed in Chapter 11. As the season progresses, your standard week remains largely the same. The only change the intermediate triathlete makes is to gradually and conservatively increase the durations of a few key workouts so that by race day the race duration is easy.

The planning is only slightly more complex for the advanced triathlete. At this level, begin increasing the workout durations early in the season. Make the workouts a little longer every few weeks while keeping intensity low—mostly zones 1 and 2. That's the base period. In the build period, after the basic abilities in each of the three sports are well established, increase the amount of time at a racelike intensity while decreasing workout durations. Decreasing the duration as the intensity increases keeps the workouts from being so hard that recovery is prolonged. You might do only one race-intensity workout in each sport weekly. Some advanced triathletes are capable of handling a bit more.

Note that for the advanced triathlete, increasing the intensity doesn't mean doing a "race" every week when you do these key workouts. The combination of duration and intensity is typically not as great as it will be in the race. For sprint-distance races, you can come pretty close to doing the swim, bike, or run portions at a racelike duration

The reversibility principle says that fitness gains erode in several days without training.

Lay out a standard week and keep it the same as you progress through the season.

and intensity. But this is not a realistic option as the race distance gets longer. Overtraining is a likely result.

For standard, half-Ironman, and full-Ironman training, mimic portions of the race in your workouts. For example, if preparing for a half-Ironman-distance race, you may do a bike workout that is about 60 percent to 70 percent as long in terms of time or TSS as your goal time or TSS for the race. By doing long intervals at goal race intensity for this ride, you are practicing a significant portion of the race. The same sort of thing should be done for the swim and run. Just be sure to include easy, recovery workouts between the racelike workouts every week. These will be about half as long as your longest swims, bikes, and runs and done mostly in zone 1, with some zone 2.

If you set up a standard week and follow the simple guidelines offered above based on your level of triathlon experience, all you need to do beyond that is taper your volume by reducing the durations of all workouts in the last 2 or 3 weeks before your race, as described in Chapter 7. This simplified periodization method will improve your fitness, boost your confidence, and bring you to race day ready to let it rip.

SUMMARY: PLANNING ALTERNATIVES

We have covered a lot of planning material in Part IV. By now, you should have a good idea of which periodization system best fits your individual needs. Now it's time to use that system to start planning your season. If you decide to use a linear periodization plan—the type most com-

monly used by athletes at all levels of experience—return to Chapters 7 and 8 and follow the step-by-step guidelines. Should you decide to use a modified linear plan, as described in this chapter, then make adjustments as needed along the way. It will be a little harder to work out the details for the nonlinear methods, but athletes who follow these systems are typically experienced enough to know how to plug them into a plan.

As I mentioned earlier, be aware that the plan you create initially should not be considered final. You must be flexible in your training. As you observe progress throughout the season, always keep the thought in the back of your mind that the plan may need to be adjusted. In more than 30 years of coaching, I have never had an athlete complete the season with an unaltered training plan. Something always needed adjusting. The most common reasons for change are interruptions due to illness and lifestyle conflicts, such as unexpected business trips.

Once into the plan, you may also discover that your fitness is not progressing as expected or just doesn't feel right. If so, change what you are doing to fit your needs.

The bottom line is that you must be willing to make changes. Just because your plan calls for a particular workout on a particular day doesn't mean that it *must* be done. There may be a better way. Adapt and make changes as needed. But always keep a written account in your training diary so that you have a record of what works and what doesn't when it comes time to plan the next season. A written plan for this season will prove invaluable when it comes time to design one for your next season. And it gets easier every time you do it.

You must maintain flexibility in your training.

PART V

STRESS, REST, AND RECOVERY

For all too many triathletes, training is a one-dimensional effort involving only workouts, especially hard ones. This means lots of stress, but little rest and recovery. Challenging workouts provide stress, and rest is what you do after the workouts are over. Recovery has to do with the easy workouts, the ones that also improve the advanced athlete's capacity for adapting and becoming more fit.

But high-performance training actually goes well beyond stress, rest, and recovery. Training also includes the decisions you make on a daily basis regarding seemingly insignificant things, such as when you go to bed, which foods you choose to eat or avoid, whether you take the stairs or the escalator, what books you read, which movies you watch.

The higher your goal in triathlon, the more stuff there is in your life that you must tweak to support that goal. This can include your family and friends—not that you need to find replacements, but rather that they need to be on board with your direction. High-performance training also includes your attitude about life in general. A few research studies have shown that athletes with a positive attitude tend to achieve their goals more readily than those who have negative attitudes.

You become what you do and think. For this reason, everything in your life has to do with triathlon performance. In essence, your philosophy and methodology of living determine the outcomes of your races.

I'm not going to try to change your life from the bottom up. Instead, the next two chapters will examine the balancing topics of stress, rest, and recovery in the high-performance athlete's life. These chapters will outline the totality of the concept of training. Embrace them, and you will be a better triathlete.

TRAINING STRESS

WHAT EXACTLY is training? I've used that word a lot in this book, but what is the precise definition? At its most basic level, training is the combination of stress and rest:

Training = Stress + Rest

Hard and easy. High and low. Yin and yang. Like a neutron and a proton, one without the other is unstable. Both are necessary. But simply doing some random measure of each is not enough. There must also be a balance between stress and rest. A steady diet of high-stress training without the equivalent counterbalance of rest leads only to problems, not high performance. In this chapter, we focus on the stress side of the equation. In Chapter 11, we look at rest.

So what is stress? In human biology, stress is the body's predictable reaction to an environmental stressor. This reaction can be good or bad—eustress or distress. In triathlon, the stressor is the workout, and it starts out as eustress (good stress). The product of the workout is greater fitness and greater fatigue, as explained in Chapter 3. That's healthy. But physical activity taken too far can become distress (bad stress) in the form of overtraining, which paradoxically produces *reduced fitness* along with *increased fatigue*—an unhealthy reaction. When this happens, there's definitely a problem. Distress for the overly ambitious triathlete can also result in injury, illness, and burnout. All are health-related markers of excessive stress.

How much stress you can manage without experiencing distress is determined by two factors. The one that we have little or no control over is genetics. Unfortunately, life isn't fair in this regard. Some people are blessed with genes that allow them to train at a high stress level without distress. Others aren't so well endowed, and—if it makes you feel any better—most of us are in this category.

But genetics isn't the only determiner of distress. Lifestyle factors are the other significant component—things such as experience in sports, recent levels of aerobic and muscular fitness, physical and emotional demands in your life, and of course training methodology. You do have some degree of control over these lifestyle-specific stressors. They're not always easy to change, at least not without impacting some other aspect of your life, such as relationships or finances. For example, it's doubtful that you will quit your job so that you can train more. But I can tell you with certainty that when a change in one or more of these factors results in increased stress, something must be modified to avoid calamity.

For most age-group athletes, the lifestyle aspect that is nearly always the easiest to reshape in order to avoid distress is training. If your job, family, health, finances, living conditions, or some other critical aspect of life becomes overly stressful, the stressor that you must immediately reduce is training. To continue with multiple high levels of stress is a sure way to experience disaster in both your life and your race performance.

The purpose of this chapter is to examine training stress and how you can ensure it is eustress and not distress. We will examine two related yin and yang topics—risk and reward, and overreaching and overtraining.

Reward has to do with the hoped-for benefits that result from smart training.

RISK AND REWARD

Recently, a 62-year-old athlete I was beginning to coach spent a few days with me at my home in Scottsdale, Arizona. I had him go through general physical and skill assessments, and we tested his performance in each sport. He also was assessed for potential injuries by a physical therapist and got a bike fit from a professional fitter. Along the way, we talked about my training philosophy and the direction we needed to go to achieve his very high goal of qualifying for the Ironman World Championship in Kona, Hawaii.

Tom is an analytical type who likes to dig into the details of triathlon training. One of our conversations was about the risks and rewards of workouts. Risk refers to the potential for injury, illness, burnout, and overtraining breakdowns that may occur because a workout or a closely spaced series of stressful workouts is so challenging. Reward has to do with the hoped-for benefits that result from smart training.

Tom said he had never thought of it that way before. Few athletes have, yet it is an important topic to understand in order to manage training. From having learned about Tom's recent race seasons, I was coming to the conclusion that his lack of knowledge about training balance was the root of why he had been unable to qualify for Kona in the three seasons since he had started doing Ironman-distance races. He frequently experienced physical breakdowns, mostly injuries and illnesses, which made his training inconsistent. He would no sooner start making significant gains in performance than he became injured or sick. From all of the testing I had him do, I could tell that he had great potential for long-course racing. His limiter, though, was that he was simply overly enthusiastic and aggressive when he did workouts. The stress was too great, especially the density of his training; his hard workouts were too closely spaced.

All athletes seek to improve their fitness by increasing the stress they place on their bodies.

The stress level typically varies from very low to very high. The lowest-stress sessions are short, slow, and low-effort. High-stress training is just the opposite. It always includes either very long workout durations, high intensities, high density, or a combination of these three. I gave Tom an example of this from my younger and dumber days more than 35 years ago when I would run a marathon in the morning with a friend and then come home and put in 10 more miles that afternoon. Both were slow and low-effort, but the long duration made them risky. I often paid the price for such "training" back then by dealing with extended down time due to injury and illness. That, unfortunately, is how I first came to understand the risk-reward curve.

Figure 10.1 illustrates the risk-reward curve. The difficulty of the workout increases from left to right, while the level of risk and reward increases from bottom to top. You could change the words in Figure 10.1 a bit and it would serve as a basic guide for investing in the stock market. Blue chip stocks, which have a long history of slow but consistent growth, are generally considered low-risk. While the reward of investing in these stocks increases slowly, the risk of losing your money is low. On the other hand, when a stock has a high potential for monetary reward—a young company working with new technology, for example—it also has a high degree of risk. You could become wealthy in a short period of time, or lose it all.

It's essentially the same with training: low risk equals low reward and high risk equals high reward. Just like investing in the stock market, training has the potential to go either way. The key is to find a balance. It was obvious from his pattern of breakdowns that Tom had not found the right balance.

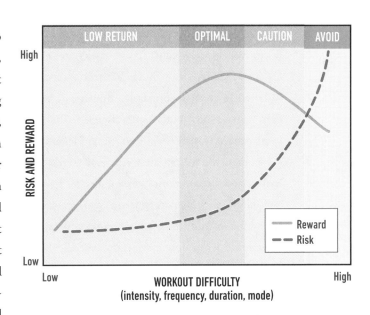

FIGURE 10.1   The risk-reward curve

Athletes who continually experience breakdowns because they "over-invest" in high-risk training are unlikely to reach their potential. They break down too often because of high-risk training. At the other end of the curve, those few triathletes who do only low-risk workouts, such as short ones at low intensity, will also never come close to their potential. Their training isn't hard enough. You have to risk something to succeed at the highest levels. However, you need to control that risk to be successful.

So what is risky training? To begin with, running is the riskiest sport in triathlon primarily because of orthopedic stress—the "pounding" of your feet on the ground. Dedicated runners without a long history of injury are rare. Soft but stable running surfaces, such as trails, grass, and dirt, reduce some of the risk of running.

Also making running risky are "eccentric" muscle contractions. In such a contraction, the muscle lengthens as you attempt to shorten it. I know this is counterintuitive, so visualize

Low risk equals low reward and high risk equals high reward.

a reverse arm curl in which you slowly lower a heavy weight. The muscle has to lengthen to allow your arm to drop, but you are also keeping the muscle short to control its movement. Your calves and quads undergo this type of contraction with every stride while running. That's why your quads are so sore after a marathon. Essentially, the muscle is being pulled apart.

On the other hand, cycling and swimming rely primarily on "concentric" contractions, meaning the muscle gets shorter as it contracts. Visualize your arm curling a heavy weight from hip-high to shoulder-high. This type of muscular contraction is very low-risk.

None of this means you shouldn't run. It just means that you must be conservative with the dose and density of run training.

For most triathletes, swimming is the lowest-risk sport. While overuse injuries certainly occur among swimmers (mostly to the shoulder), the rate of such setbacks is low compared with the rate among runners. Poor technique, paddles, and drag or resistance devices increase the risk. Once again, this does not mean you shouldn't do such training, only that you must be careful with it.

The same goes for cycling, in which the knee is the body part most commonly injured from doing too much. Risk is increased here, first and foremost, by a poor bike setup. And in probably the most common high-risk bike setups that I see, the saddle is too low and too far forward. Another risk for cyclists is high-gear pedaling, especially on a hill and in the seated position. Inadequate gearing (meaning not enough low gears) is often associated with knee soreness and loss of training time. Again, this doesn't mean you must never use high gears and low cadences when riding. There are times when this is an

Start with low-dose and low-density variations and then slowly increase the dose and density.

effective training strategy. Just be conservative with such training to manage the risk.

Plyometrics, discussed in Chapter 13, can be a risky but potentially rewarding activity. The bounding, hopping, and jumping exercises are intended to improve muscular power. The riskiest plyometrics include landing at the end of a downward jump, such as a jump over an object or off a high platform. Jumping up from the floor to land on a knee-high box, however, has a much lower risk—but also a lower reward.

In the same category of improving muscular power, heavy-load, low-repetition weight training (Chapter 13) is also risky, but again it has a high potential payoff if done correctly. Other risky activities with the potential for a nice reward include very high-speed sprints done much faster than usual, hill training of any type, and early-season racing before fitness is well established.

Note that I am *not* saying never to do high-risk, high-reward workouts. The key to being successful is to start gradually with the lower-risk (low-dose and low-density) variations and then slowly, over a significant amount of time, increase the dose and density. For example, begin your plyometrics work with upward jumping onto a platform or low-height jumping, such as rope jumping. And be patient. You must allow your body to adapt slowly and gradually. The more you try to force your body to adapt, the greater the risk for injury becomes.

Discussing risk and reward was an eye-opener for Tom. He learned an important lesson in how critical it is to err on the conservative side in order to keep risk under control while still reaping the rewards of training. He had been doing the opposite—attempting to fit in as much training as possible—and as a result his training was inconsistent.

The discussion also helped me learn more about his capacity for exercise, what had led to his frequent illnesses and injuries, and the typical early signs he experienced when the risk was too great. From this and everything else we accomplished together in those few days, we decided to follow a linear-periodization plan and use a 9-day training "week" (see Chapters 8 and 9 for details). Doing so allowed us to build fitness slowly while keeping the risk for breakdown low.

The other challenge Tom had built for himself was allowing too little time to achieve the level of fitness necessary to qualify for the World Championship. He was registered for an Iron-distance race early in the season. We had only 4 months until race day. We decided to do that race solely for the experience and in the meantime sign up for a qualifier early in the next season. That plan would allow him to train with the proper density in order to avoid breakdowns. It worked. He achieved his goal at the second race.

OVERTRAINING AND OVERREACHING

Most triathletes think of overtraining as something rather insignificant. After a few days of hard workouts, they say they are overtrained. What they mean is that they are tired. Most are a bit vague on what this condition is all about. That's all right because sports scientists are also still a bit vague about it. Overtraining is hard to define because the symptoms are a moving target—rarely the same for any two athletes.

Overtraining is actually a serious medical disorder. Very few athletes are ever overtrained, even though most believe they have been. To become overtrained, one must be extremely motivated to continue exercising while ignoring the overwhelming signs and symptoms of deteriorating health and crushing fatigue. If you are truly overtrained, merely getting out of bed in the morning is an accomplishment.

It's important to understand that fitness and health are not the same thing. It's possible to be very fit, at least relative to the general population, and yet not be healthy. In fact, the quest for fitness can easily lead to poor health. I've seen athletes become so overtrained that they have constant low-grade illnesses and yet somehow soldier on. I know of one pro triathlete whose career was cut short because he took his training to the extreme. Even after he recovered from the symptoms, which took several weeks, and raced for an additional 2 years, he was never the same. He was finally forced to retire.

Overtraining is not to be taken lightly. It's among the worst things that can happen to a serious athlete. And yet, paradoxically, in order to reach a high level of fitness, it's something you must always be flirting with. It's a risk that must be taken. The key is knowing how to reap the rewards while avoiding breakdown. Flirting with overtraining is called *overreaching*. It's the core of high-performance training. How can you overreach yet not overtrain? Let's explore the answers to that question.

Overtraining

The symptoms of overtraining are many, yet they are seldom exactly the same in overtrained athletes. That makes a precise definition difficult. Physiologically, the only symptoms that are common are poor performance and fatigue. But these can occur even when an athlete is not overtrained, which makes the condition hard to pin down.

Overtraining is a serious medical disorder.

Fatigue may be the better indicator. Every athlete experiences fatigue because physical stress is necessary to improve fitness. This process of overreaching is a necessary part of any training program. The possibility of overtraining greatly increases when an athlete ignores the fatigue of overreaching and continues to train with high stress and with inadequate rest and recovery. For young athletes, this takes several weeks of dedicated and exhaustive training. Older athletes and those who are relatively new to the sport may produce overtraining in fewer than 3 weeks.

An athlete can shed the accumulated fatigue of overreaching by resting or training very easily for a few days. After that, she can return to high-stress training. But once the overtraining syndrome has taken over the body, fatigue will not go away so easily. The athlete can become listless, grumpy, and unmotivated. These common psychological symptoms are usually best identified by a spouse and close friends. But there are other indicators that something is wrong.

Table 10.1 lists the common symptoms of overtraining. Note that not all of these will occur. In fact, an overtrained athlete may be aware of only a couple of them. Also notice that several are contradictory, such as "greater hunger than normal" and "loss of appetite." This is due to the progression of the symptoms from early to late stages. Many of the common symptoms are what might also be seen with a disease such as chronic fatigue syndrome, Lyme disease, or the early stages of infectious mononucleosis. In fact, an athlete who experiences deep and lingering fatigue along with any of the other symptoms in Table 10.1 should see a physician to be tested for these and other, similar medical conditions. The most common

way to diagnose overtraining is to eliminate possible diseases with similar symptoms.

Excessive training, which is all too common among serious triathletes, has the potential to produce overtraining. Frequent recovery for a few days is necessary to prevent it. How often and how long the recovery period should last is an individual matter that can be determined only through trial and error. We will get further into this topic in the next chapter.

Overreaching

As mentioned earlier, it's necessary to flirt with overtraining (overreach) to achieve the highest possible level of fitness. Overreaching is almost the same as overtraining. Almost. Fatigue is certainly present after a few days to a couple of weeks of serious training. And if the training continues that way long enough, you will likely become overtrained. What separate the two conditions are rest and recovery. With overreaching, backing off for a few days rejuvenates your body. If you are overtrained, though, short-term rest has no benefit. The fatigue and other symptoms continue despite easy workouts or even days off from training.

Essentially, overreaching is carefully managed overtraining. When you are training at a high workload, it's necessary to pay attention constantly to how your body and mind are responding to the stress. The single most important question to ask is, How do I feel today? If your answer is that you feel tired on consecutive days, then you need rest and recovery.

Overreaching is achieved by carefully balancing stress and rest. That is why I emphasize periodization in this book. Periodized training lays out a plan that alternates stressful days of hard

---

Every athlete experiences fatigue because physical stress is necessary to improve fitness.

Overreaching is carefully managed overtraining.

If you are overtrained, short-term rest has no benefit.

TABLE 10.1 **Common Symptoms of Overtraining by Category**

CATEGORY	COMMON SYMPTOMS
Physical	Resting heart rate higher or lower than usual Weight loss Greater hunger than normal Loss of appetite Lethargy Restless sleep, insomnia Chronic fatigue Muscle soreness Muscle and joint injury Minor cuts heal slowly Menstrual cycle dysfunction
Performance	Greatly reduced performance in hard workouts Low bike power at a given heart rate Slow swim and run pace relative to effort Inability to complete workouts Decreased muscular strength Loss of coordination Deterioration of skills
Psychological	Moody, grumpy, and emotional Apathetic Low motivation to train Poor concentration Decreased self-esteem Very high level of race anxiety Loss of competitiveness Depression
Physiological	Low level of peak lactate Low heart rate at a high power or pace High heart rate at low-to-moderate intensities High perceived exertion at a given power or pace Low heart rate variability Increased oxygen consumption during submaximal exercise Reduced maximal exercise capacity
Immunological	Increased susceptibility to colds, flu, and allergies Swollen lymph glands Bacterial infection Abnormal white blood cell differentials
Biochemical	Reduced muscle glycogen concentration Elevated serum cortisol Decreased serum ferritin Decreased bone mineral density

training with easy days of rest and recovery. Your plan completed in Part IV should include brief rest-and-recovery periods (we'll get into that topic in Chapter 11), which are usually scheduled about every 3 to 4 weeks, along with rest-and-recovery days after A-priority races and extended rest and recovery at the end of the race season. The purpose of including all of these breaks from serious training is to make sure you don't push into an overtrained state. If your training is hard enough, these breaks will come at about the right times.

Table 10.2 shows the common progression from healthy and performance-enhancing overreaching to unhealthy and performance-diminishing overtraining.

Some of the training you may do is certainly risky when it comes to overtraining. In Chapter 9, I described a training method called *crashing*. To refresh your memory, this calls for doing hard workouts daily for several days before taking a break. The reward is potentially great, but such training should be done only in a few widely separated weeks per season. While crashing builds fitness quickly, you can also end up overtrained and wreck your entire season. It's a perfect example of risk and reward at play. To avoid overtraining with such risky methods, you must learn to pay close attention to your level of fatigue and workout performance. When these exceed what experience tells you is normal, it's time to back off and rest.

INJURY AND ILLNESS

Apart from the overtraining syndrome detailed in Table 10.1, the other common training interruptions are due to injury and illness. It's usually best to stop training when you are injured or sick.

The decision comes down to severity. An injury may affect training only in one sport. In that case, you can train in the other two so long as the training doesn't aggravate the injured site. Similarly, if you have a cold that is affecting you only above the neck, such as by giving you a runny nose, and there is no fever, then low-intensity exercise may be possible. In either case, pay close attention to your condition and be prepared to cut back even more.

Knowing when to stop a hard workout is also critical to avoiding a breakdown. As a coach, when I attend an athlete's hard workout, such as intervals that push the athlete to his limits, one of my roles is to watch carefully how the athlete is coping with the stress. Besides providing encouragement and feedback, I am also there to stop the workout short of completion if I think the risk for injury or a compromised immune system is becoming too great. I can generally tell when an athlete has reached his or her limits and the risk is too high. Form begins to deteriorate. Perceived exertion becomes too great. Performance erodes. The athlete has a hard time recovering within the session. At the first sign of any of these, it's time to stop.

If you do not have a coach to do this for you, you'll need to make these decisions for yourself. Here's what I'd suggest. When in an interval session, if you feel as if you can do only one more hard effort, stop the workout and cool down. Don't do the last one. The same applies to the last few minutes of a hard steady-state workout and the last 10 percent of a very long workout. These are risky moments when you should consider stopping the session if you are in difficulty. Injury and illness may be sneaking up on you. Be especially cautious at those times when your fitness is high, as in the last few weeks before an A-priority race.

Knowing when to stop a hard workout is critical to avoiding a breakdown.

TABLE 10.2 The Progressive Stages of Overreaching and Overtraining

PROGRESSION	STAGE	COMMON SYMPTOMS
1	Moderate overreaching	High perceived fatigue Minimal change in performance Training restored by 24–36 hours of rest Performance improved following rest
2	Functional overreaching	Very high perceived fatigue Performance decline possible Several days of rest required to restore training Performance improved following rest
3	Nonfunctional overreaching	Very high perceived fatigue Performance decline apparent Several days of rest required to restore training Performance not improved after rest
4	Overtraining syndrome	Very intense perceived fatigue Performance suffering chronically More than 1 month of rest needed to shed fatigue and restore training Performance greatly diminished after recovery Competitive season over

One of the biggest challenges some athletes struggle with in stopping a workout is greed—they want all of the fitness they can get *right now*. You need patience to be a high-performance endurance athlete. It's the key to consistent training. Greedy athletes may lose more fitness than they gain over the course of a season as a result of repeated breakdowns from injuries and illness. Being patient allows your body to adapt fully and grow stronger. Regardless of how soon your race is, the body doesn't function on an artificial schedule. Fitness takes time.

Greedy training pushes your body too far beyond its current physiological limits. Its only way of stopping you is to become overtrained, sick, or injured. Those are common signs of greed and impatience.

SUMMARY: TRAINING STRESS

Balancing stress and rest in order to produce a high level of fitness is similar to growing a flower. With the right amount of nutrients in the soil and just enough water, the flower will grow and bloom. Too much of either of these otherwise good things and the plant withers and fails to achieve its potential. Using training stress to grow your fitness follows the same curve. Too much and you break down.

Getting the right amount of stress in your training depends largely on your experience. There is no one-size-fits-all formula for determining how long, frequent, or intense your workouts should be. You'll need to determine

You need patience to be a high-performance athlete.

your own formula over time. This may sound vague right now, but you will know when you've done too much in a workout or a closely spaced series of workouts. The most common symptom is that your recovery will take more than about 36 hours. You can assume your training was too hard if you are still fatigued 48 hours after a workout. In this situation, *fatigued* means you are unable to repeat the workout or another such challenging session. You've achieved stage 2— functional overreaching (Table 10.2). Of course, as your fitness increases over time, with patient training, what was once an overly hard stage 2 workout will become a moderate stage 1.

There are times when an experienced triathlete may decide to take a risk by doing a stage 2 workout or even several workouts in quick succession, as during a crash week. But the risk must be carefully calculated and fatigue closely watched. Avoiding injury, illness, and overtraining at such times still requires some degree of moderation. If you push your body just a bit too much for even a few days, your season can come crashing down. Patience is always necessary, especially with such risky training.

On the other hand, if you aren't tired after 2 or 3 weeks of training in the base or build periods, you aren't training hard enough. You've risked too little to realize a reward. As explained in Chapter 3, fitness and fatigue trend the same direction. If fatigue is never produced, then neither is fitness. You must become tired frequently if you are to become fitter. So fatigue is a good thing, not something to be totally avoided. The only issue here is how long the fatigue lasts.

Use your fatigue wisely. Don't waste it on workouts that don't fit your individual needs. The most common "wasted" workout for the serious triathlete is group bike sessions. These typically become road races similar to local criterium and circuit races that are probably familiar to you. Road racing is nothing like the bike leg of a triathlon. The outcome of a bike race is determined by frequent maximal efforts well above the anaerobic threshold. Road cyclists call these *matches*. The bike leg of a triathlon couldn't be more different. Success here demands a very steady effort at below the anaerobic threshold—not burning lots of big matches. While they may be fun, a steady diet of hard group rides with roadies greatly increases your risk for a breakdown while doing little to make you a better triathlete. Remember the most basic rule of high-performance training: The closer in time you get to a race, the more like the race your training should become.

This chapter looked at only half of what you should do in training—the stress part of the formula. Now it's time to examine the other half: rest.

REST AND RECOVERY

IN CHAPTER 10, you read about what happens when training becomes imbalanced, with too much stress and too little rest: injury, illness, and overtraining. These make up the fitness-devouring monster that frequently appears when you become obsessed with training stress. If you continually exceed what is healthy and appropriate as you prepare for your race, it's quite likely one of them will come calling. And when that happens, it will mean less fitness and a drop in performance. Nothing good comes from this. The way to keep such monstrous breakdowns at bay is with well-timed rest and recovery.

On a more positive note, rest and recovery drive fitness gains. You don't become more fit during exercise. Hard training creates only the potential for fitness. When a hard workout is followed by a few hours of rest and recovery, your body is given the opportunity to adapt to the stress and grow stronger. How many hours of recovery you'll need depends on the level of the preceding workout stress. If it was only slightly more difficult than what your body is already accustomed to, then you will probably be ready for another stressful workout in 48 hours. Workouts that are significantly harder than your current level of adaptation require a longer period of rest and recovery. But you should not do workouts like that very often. They take too much out of you and demand too much recovery time away from your training routine.

The words *rest* and *recovery* are used a lot in this book. In the context of training, what do they mean? Rest is a period of no exercise. It's downtime. A day off. There is no workout. During recovery, certain things are done to speed the body's adaptive process. This could mean a light, easy workout. As you will learn later in this chapter, light exercise actually stimulates adaptation for some athletes.

Other, similar terms you may see used are *passive* and *active recovery*. Passive recovery is another way of saying what I call rest—there is no workout. Active recovery means doing an easy session that is well below what you're capable of doing. It does not stress the body.

The best way to avoid illness, injury, and overtraining is to monitor fatigue closely, do whatever stimulates recovery after a hard training session, and rest when you need to. In this chapter, we will look at these topics more closely in order to keep your training steadily progressing toward your racing goals. Rest and recovery are just as critical as hard workouts to success in triathlon. If you are good at one but not the other, you will fall well short of your potential.

MORNING WARNINGS

How do you know when you're doing too much? In Chapter 10, I told you that in order to gain fitness, you must have enough stress in your training that you would reach overtraining if you were to continue at that rate. That's a high rate of stress, and of course you should take a break from hard workouts well before overtraining appears. But how do you know when it's time for a break? After all, other things in your life besides swimming, biking, and running can add to the stress you experience and contribute to a breakdown well before it would otherwise occur. Those other things can be related to your career, your family, your finances, or any number of other important aspects of your life. Is there any sure way of knowing that you've reached your limit and you need a break?

The short answer is no. There is nothing that tells you, with complete certainty, that you're exceeding your limits. There are only weak indicators that suggest something isn't right. I call these *morning warnings* because they are most obvious when you awaken each day. Routinely monitoring a few of these indicators every morning will provide feedback on how well you are recovering. Occasionally, you may realize that something isn't right. It isn't right because several warnings are hitting you at once. Of course, you may have one warning even when things are going well with training and you are definitely not approaching the precipice of a breakdown. It's the total weight of several warnings that tells you rest and recovery are needed.

Table 11.1 lists several common morning warnings. Select a few that you will monitor on a daily basis. Over time, you should determine which of these are your best indicators. Keep an eye on them every morning when you wake up.

Again, any one of these warnings by itself is probably not enough to warrant a rest or recovery day, unless it is extreme. But two or more warnings on awakening may be enough for you to decide to take it easy that day. Only experience will tell you which metrics are the best indicators for you and how many represent a need to decrease training. Like everything else in the realm of training, warnings of the need for rest and recovery are highly individualized.

QUICK RECOVERY

What can you do to avoid morning warnings? Rather than waiting for multiple warnings to occur and then taking a day off from training, it's better to prevent the warnings from occurring at all, or at least diminish their magnitude. In fact, for the serious triathlete, daily life is more

Two or more warnings on awakening may be enough to decide to take it easy that day.

TABLE 11.1 Common Morning Warning Indicators of Stress

INDICATORS	WARNING
Sleep	Poor quality and/or inadequate length
Overall feeling	Very fatigued, very stressed
Mood	Unusually grumpy, out of sorts
Appetite	Diminished
Motivation to train	Low
Muscles, joints	Sore
Waking pulse	High
Comparison of supine and standing heart rates	Differential increased
Heart rate variability	Low

These symptoms indicate that stress may be too high and that rest and recovery may be needed.

about recovery than stress. You may devote 2 or 3 hours daily to workouts, but the remaining hours in your day are all focused on recovery. Your training is inadequate if you aren't currently doing this. You can perform at a higher level by focusing most of your day on quickly recovering from workouts.

As you go through the nonworkout portions of your day at work, with family and friends, or whatever you may do, it's imperative that you keep recovery uppermost in your mind. This should be second nature for you. You may already be doing so. But if not, until you reach that advanced level of the serious triathlete's lifestyle, you will need to dedicate yourself to recovery consciously. By doing so, you will speed up the recovery process that allows your workouts to become even more challenging. That leads to greater fitness and, eventually, better race performance.

There's an old adage among serious athletes: Never stand if you can lean, never lean if you can sit, and never sit if you can lie down. Without even thinking about it, a serious triathlete will follow this rule throughout the day to enhance

recovery in one small way, and it's a good example of keeping recovery uppermost in your mind.

There are many ways to enhance recovery besides following such rules. As you read through the examples that follow, give serious consideration to how you can incorporate them into your daily routine.

Sleep

You already have the world's best device for recovery—your bed. Nothing is better. After all, the purpose of sleep is to rejuvenate and rebuild your muscular, skeletal, and immune systems. Sleep is your primary means of recovery from training stress.

Sleep is critical to athletic success, yet some athletes intentionally shorten their sleep time in order to fit more stuff into their daily lives. It's quite common for athletes to stay up late watching TV and then set an alarm so they will get up early the next morning in order to have time for a workout before going to work. If this describes you, you aren't getting enough sleep—or enough recovery. You can do better. Going to bed earlier

Never stand if you can lean, never lean if you can sit, and never sit if you can lie down.

and sleeping until you wake up naturally will undoubtedly improve your training and performance. That single change may improve your life in other ways, too, such as better health and a more positive attitude about life. Sleep is your most powerful recovery tool.

Sleep is so effective for recovery because it is during sleep that the body releases anabolic (tissue-building) hormones that repair damaged muscles, restore the immune system, restructure bone, heal niggling injuries, re-stock energy stores, and more. If your sleep is artificially shortened, you are potentially giving up some portion of your most important recovery method every day. And it doesn't work to try to "catch up" on sleep on the weekends. The body doesn't operate that way. It works best when you meet your restoration needs every day. Chronically shortening your natural sleep cycle is likely to have a long-term negative effect on you as a triathlete and a person.

Even if you are getting enough sleep at night, the single most important thing you can do to race faster is to get more sleep whenever possible. That's why pro triathletes frequently take naps during the day. They understand the many benefits of snoozing. You may not be able to fit in naps during the day, though; if not, your nighttime sleep becomes all the more important.

There are several things you can do to help maximize sleep time. I expect you are already familiar with the most common ones: avoiding caffeine in the late afternoon, not working out immediately before bedtime, maintaining a calm and quiet environment before going to bed, following a regular sleep schedule, and bedding down in a dark, cool room. There are others.

Some athletes take a melatonin supplement in the evening to promote drowsiness, but I don't

recommend it. When you use a supplement regularly to promote some functional change, your body typically responds by reducing or even halting its natural production of the targeted chemical. But here's an alternative solution: Studies have confirmed that drinking a glass of tart cherry juice in the evening can help. I know that sounds weird, but it seems to work. The subjects in these studies had an increase in melatonin production and improved sleep compared with those who drank a placebo.

When you eat and what your evening meal is made up of may also affect your sleep pattern. First of all, go light on alcohol in the evening because it has a rebound effect that can wake you later from an otherwise sound sleep. A late evening meal or a pre-bedtime snack may also reduce sleep quality. So you probably shouldn't eat right before going to bed. However, what you eat may matter as much as when because a study from the University of North Dakota showed that subjects who ate a high-protein meal right before bedtime had the fewest sleep interruptions. A high-carb meal produced the most restless sleep.

Indeed, food is second only to sleep when it comes to effective recovery. So let's look next at the topic of dietary protein and performance.

Food

The nutrients in food provide the building blocks your body uses for rejuvenation after hard workouts. Nearly all of this rebuilding takes place while you sleep, and the quality of what you eat is critical for recovery. The old saying that "you are what you eat" has a lot of truth to it. If you waste calories by eating low-nutrient "junk food," your body will find it difficult to repair damaged muscles, restore the immune system, restructure

Going to bed earlier and sleeping until you wake up naturally will improve your training and performance.

bone, and heal injuries. You may have gotten away with eating lots of junk food when you were a youngster, but adults experience a gradually increasing loss of health when they eat that way.

High-stress training increases the need for high-quality food. And you can't make up for a poor diet by taking vitamins and supplements, no matter how "scientific" they are purported to be. Science is still millions of years behind real food when it comes to meeting the nutritional needs of humans.

What you eat must include the macronutrients of protein, carbohydrate, and fat, and the micronutrients of vitamins, minerals, and phytochemicals. The richness of the foods you eat determines how quickly and how fully you recover from a hard workout. While junk foods may provide macronutrients, they are nearly devoid of micronutrients. That's because they are highly processed as they are manufactured, and processing food destroys its micronutrients. The closer your food is to its natural state, and the less processed it is before it hits your plate, the better it is for your health and recovery.

Relying on processed sports products in the form of powders, bars, or pills is also counterproductive to recovery. Just as with junk foods, you can get macronutrients from them, but micronutrients will be in short supply as a result of all of the manufacturing processes along the way. Even when expert nutrition scientists try to add micronutrients back into a product, it's not the way Mother Nature did it and seldom as effective. And just because a scientist was involved in its design, it doesn't mean that the thing in the wrapper is better than real food. It isn't.

The only reason to eat the powders, bars, gels, and other stuff marketed to athletes is conve-nience. For example, after a hard swim on a Saturday morning, it may be convenient to eat a sports bar on the drive home, just before you jump on the bike for a long ride. The bar will contain some macronutrients that will help you get through the second workout of the day. But even then, there are other options. A box of raisins or a piece of fruit in the car is also convenient, a lot cheaper, and denser in micronutrients. You always have options.

Nutrient density is one of the main reasons why you're better off buying your own food at the grocery store and preparing it yourself. Processed food—the powders and bars marketed to athletes—does not pack the complete nutrition per bite that you get from fresh food. Real food that is close to its original state costs much less and helps you recover more fully. Foods such as fruits, vegetables, animal products, berries, nuts, and seeds are the most powerful way you can support your training goals and general health.

Eating nutritionally dense, real food immediately following workouts is as important as it is during your regular meals, and it is probably the single thing most athletes can do to improve recovery and health. Don't waste your money on highly processed foods, even if they are marketed to athletes. Ignore the claims about how many pro triathletes are using a processed product. Those athletes are doing it for the sponsorship support, not the performance benefits.

Finding the right balance in your meals can be a challenge. Triathletes typically get plenty of carbohydrate in their diets—probably too much, especially when it comes to sugar, which is at the top of the list of ingredients in most gels, bars, and drinks. I've found that many athletes don't get enough protein and fat. Fat has been vilified in Western society since the 1970s, leading

High-stress training increases the need for high-quality food.

Nutrient density is one of the main reasons why you're better off preparing your food yourself.

many health-conscious athletes to avoid it whenever possible. But that's a mistake. Fat is necessary for health and should be included in your meals. In fact, many ultra-endurance athletes have found that a high-fat diet improves their race performances. They are less likely to "bonk" because they are burning mostly fat for fuel. Even the skinniest triathlete theoretically has enough stored fat to do a triathlon that lasts several days. And because fat-adapted athletes need less food during a race, they eliminate the likelihood of gastric distress. This is especially advantageous in races such as long-course triathlons.

But if you typically eat a high-carb diet, which is common among endurance athletes today, you need to take in some carb-rich food immediately following a high-stress workout. This could be a session that is significantly longer or more intense than your average workouts. How much carbohydrate to take in is a bit of a guessing game that depends on how hard the workout was, how big you are, when you ate your last meal and what you ate then, and what and how much you ate or drank during the workout.

Your experience plays a big role in deciding what to eat after a day's training session. Research suggests that a food with a high glycemic index, meaning that the sugar in the food is quickly released into your bloodstream, is most effective for the high-carb athlete to restore glycogen levels after a challenging session. For such an athlete, recovery food sources may include fruits (especially bananas and raisins), fruit juices, potatoes, grains, and pasta.

The research suggests that about 1 to 1.85 grams of carbohydrate per kilogram of body weight (0.016–0.03 ounces per pound) is about the right amount to take in per hour after a

hard workout. For a 120-pound athlete (about 54.4 kilograms), that works out to about 2 to 3.6 ounces (56.7–102 grams) of carbs per hour. A 150-pound triathlete (68 kilograms) may consume 2.4 to 4.5 ounces (68–127.6 grams) per hour. And a 170 pounder (77.1 kilograms) would take in 2.7 to 5.1 ounces (76.5–144.6 grams) per hour. To give you an idea of what that means in terms of food, a medium-size banana contains about an ounce of carbohydrate, or 28.3 grams. A glass of orange juice also provides about an ounce of carbs. Blend them together in a shake and you have a real-food, 2-ounce carbohydrate smoothie that costs far less than a highly processed recovery powder.

You can drink something like that starting immediately and hourly thereafter for up to 5 hours after a workout. In the real world, you don't really need to be so precise with portions, however. Exactly how much you may need and for how long is a moving target with too many variables to allow you to be so meticulous. Pay close attention to how well you recover after given workouts and what you ate as you recovered to get suggested carbohydrate recovery intakes for future similar workouts. Write it all down in your training diary to help you make good decisions in the future.

If you are an athlete who adheres to a low-carb, high-fat diet, however, post-workout food intake is not as critical for you as it is for the high-carb eater. You burn a lot of fat to fuel your workouts while sparing your supplies of glycogen, and you don't need to make a special effort to replace the fat afterward. Simply return to your normal foods to satisfy hunger, and the replenishment of fats will occur naturally.

Protein also plays a big role in your health and your recovery. There is considerable evi-

Even the skinniest triathlete has enough stored fat to do a triathlon that lasts several days.

Your experience plays a big role in deciding what to eat after a training session.

dence showing that taking in some protein following a very stressful workout, such as intervals or heavy-load weight lifting, is beneficial for rejuvenation and muscle building. Most of the research that studied the role of protein in recovery had subjects take in between 10 and 30 grams (0.35–1.05 ounces) of protein every 3 to 4 hours following a hard workout. You will get some of that protein with your meals, of course. But what about eating protein-rich foods immediately after a workout? Well, a large boiled egg contains about ¼ ounce, or 7 grams. An 8-ounce glass of milk (about 237 milliliters) also has about ¼ ounce of protein (7 grams). With 3 tablespoons of peanut butter (about 45 grams), you get about ½ ounce of protein, or 14 grams, and 3 ounces of cheddar cheese (85 grams) has about ¾ ounce of protein, or 21 grams. As with carbohydrate, how much you may need after a hard workout depends on how long and intense the session was and on your body size.

Other research has found that taking in a similar amount of protein shortly before going to bed for the night also improves the body's capability for recovery and the repair of damaged muscles following a hard training day. As we mentioned earlier, there may even be a sleep-enhancing benefit from taking in a little protein before the lights go out.

Fluids

Fluid replacement is another critical contributor to recovery after a hard workout. You are likely to come up short of a full recovery if you don't replace the water lost mostly to sweat during the session. But compared with food, this one is relatively easy. All you have to do is drink fluids steadily to satisfy your thirst throughout the post-workout hours. There is really no need to weigh yourself before and after the session and then drink that exact amount of fluids. All animals (and as *Homo sapiens* we're in that category) have a very sensitive thirst mechanism. In studies done on elite athletes who drank only to satisfy thirst over several days, they successfully replaced lost fluids and maintained body weight. You also don't need to measure and keep a record of how much you drink. All you have to do is pay attention to how you are feeling. If thirsty, drink. If not thirsty, don't drink. It's that simple. Recovery from workouts is already complex enough. There's no need to make it even more intricate.

There's one possible exception to this easy solution. It has to do with aging. There is some research showing that the thirst sensation of elderly people is decreased when compared with that of younger subjects. But none of the subjects in these studies were athletes. It may be that older athletes are more sensitive than nonathletes to changes in body fluid levels. But if you're over 60, it is probably in your best interest to pay close attention to drinking after a workout. You may need to drink just a bit beyond thirst. How much I can't say. But I can tell you that you don't want to overdo it because excessive hydration beyond thirst has not been shown to improve performance. And if you get carried away with drinking lots of fluids even when you're not thirsty, you set yourself up for far greater problems, the most common of which is hyponatremia. That's the dilution of sodium stores in the blood that leads to poor performance, collapse, and even death.

What should you drink? The best option is again simple—water. However, if you are taking in a carbohydrate-based drink, like the orange juice–

Protein after a stressful workout is beneficial for rejuvenation and muscle building.

banana smoothie suggested above, that will certainly contribute to successful rehydration.

It seems the old saw that coffee and alcoholic beverages cause dehydration is apparently not true. There is considerable research showing that both contribute positively to hydration. This doesn't mean you should necessarily use a cuppa joe or a beer to recover. I'm just setting the record straight.

Active Recovery

I mentioned earlier in this chapter that light exercise helps to speed recovery in some athletes. In the studies that have examined this method, those who experienced a speedy recovery by going easy were usually advanced athletes. Another caveat appears to be that this method works only if the athlete has a high level of fitness. What that means for you, if you are beyond 3 years of serious training in the sport, is that doing an easy workout later the same day and perhaps having another easy workout the following day works best in the base, build, and peak periods, when fitness should be high. It is likely less effective in the prep period at the start of the season or after some time away from regular training. The same would hold true if you've had time away from training because of injury or illness and lost a significant amount of fitness. If in doubt about what to do, total rest is the way to go.

Should you decide to do an easy workout, here's what to keep in mind. An active-recovery workout is one that doesn't further stress the body's systems. That means truly taking it easy. The session should be shorter than your average workout and the intensity should be zone 1 whether you use heart rate, power, pace, or per-

ceived exertion (see Chapter 4). In other words, it should be really easy. To ensure that this is the case, it's best to avoid other athletes. You're more likely to keep it easy if you are swimming, biking, or running solo.

Some types of workouts are better for active recovery than others. The best is usually swimming. An active-recovery swim is a good time to work on skills. If your legs are trashed from a hard ride or run, a pull buoy may be in order. Riding your bike on a relatively flat course or on an indoor trainer is usually the second-best option. Unless you have been running for many years and don't have a history of running-related injuries, I'd recommend avoiding active-recovery runs. For most triathletes, running is simply too orthopedically stressful for quick recovery. Even if you're one of the fortunate few who isn't prone to injury, it's still best to hold down the risk by keeping the run very short, very easy, and on a soft surface such as grass, dirt, or gravel.

Other Recovery Aids

There are several other things you can try to speed recovery. Alternating hot and cold water immersion, listening to music, elevating the legs, using a foam roller, massage, and stretching are popular recovery methods that have adherents and detractors. Research studies disagree on their effectiveness, and not all athletes respond equally well to them. And in any case, the recovery benefits, if there are any for you, are rather small when compared with those of sleep and food. But there may be something among them that you find works quite well. If so, use it whenever you have time after your most stressful workouts. Whether you have time to fit it in or not, though, remember that it is critical to pay

An active-recovery workout is one that doesn't further stress the body's systems.

attention to your nightly sleep patterns and diet. Take care of those first. Don't try to substitute one or more of these methods for the basics of good nutrition and a good night's sleep.

There are two other recovery aids involving compression that have attracted wide attention recently. Athletes strongly support them but don't entirely understand what they do or how they should be used. I've found that they do contribute to recovery when used correctly, so here's a brief overview aimed at clearing up the mystery around them.

Compression Garments

These are apparel such as stockings, calf sleeves, thigh sleeves, briefs, tights, and full-body suits worn by athletes to assist recovery. Some proponents of compression wear also say that wearing such garments, especially stockings, during exercise may even improve performance.

Compression garments have been around for a long time, used as medical devices intended to aid blood flow in people who have conditions such as varicose veins, deep-vein thrombosis, and pulmonary embolism. In the early 2000s, some triathletes began to use them during and after races to improve performance and speed recovery. By the late 2000s, they had become a common sight at races.

Do they work? Do they actually improve race times while speeding recovery afterward? While there has been a lot of research, there are no clear-cut answers. Part of the reason for this is that the studies have not focused on any single sport or activity but have instead looked at a diverse array that includes soccer, walking, weight lifting, basketball, net ball, sprinting, plyometrics, and more.

The types of compression garments studied have also varied a lot, not only in terms of the part of the body they are worn on but also in terms of how much pressure they apply to the muscles. And there are various compression ratings.

All of this has muddied the water of research considerably. Even when the sports studied were closely related to triathlon, such as cycling and running, the results ranged from positive to negative. In situations like this, when the results vary between otherwise-similar studies, it tells us that the benefits are probably quite small, if present at all. In keeping with this, my sense is that the performance benefits of compression garments during a race are minimal and perhaps nonexistent. The time it takes to put the garment on in the transition area is probably greater than the amount of time gained by wearing it, if there is any time gain at all.

When it comes to recovery, however, I believe there may be some benefit. Most of the research suggests this also. I've talked with many athletes who have used different types of compression garments both during workouts and in recovery. Their opinions are divided when it comes to performance, but most sense that they help to hasten recovery. Could this be a placebo effect? Possibly. And that may well be all right. It all comes down to what works for you.

So there may be something beneficial in using compression garments in the hours immediately following a workout to assist recovery. This recovery aid is worth a try.

Pneumatic Compression Devices

Pneumatic compression devices are basically more powerful versions of compression garments and are meant to be used after a stressful workout

It is critical to pay attention to your nightly sleep patterns and diet.

There may be a benefit to using compression garments immediately following a workout to assist recovery.

to speed recovery. Commonly used compression devices as of this writing are NormaTec, Recovery Boots, and RevitaPump. They usually fit over the legs from toes to hip. These devices provide both compression and a small degree of something similar to massage. They are made up of chambers that are sequentially inflated by a pump from toe to hip and then deflated to (theoretically) help the body's circulatory system remove metabolic waste from the muscles.

They are rather pricey, so most are commonly used at "recovery stations" in health clubs or in bike, running, and triathlon shops, where customers pay a fee to use them.

Do they work? The consensus seems to be that they do. Then again, like other recovery products, they may simply be a placebo. The research on their effectiveness is generally positive. My impression from having used one of these brands considerably is that they are beneficial. Not everyone agrees.

PLANNED RECOVERY

Let's refresh. The most important lesson of this chapter is that your body adapts to hard workouts through rest and recovery. I can't emphasize this enough. It's the major take-home message and one that you *must take to heart*.

The adaptive benefits of rest and recovery are many. Muscle strength and endurance improve. The heart's stroke volume (the amount of blood pumped per beat) increases. The tiny blood-delivering capillary beds in muscles grow to allow your heart to deliver more oxygen and fuel. Blood volume increases, which also enhances oxygen delivery. Aerobic enzymes increase to contribute to your endurance. Glycogen stores

Your body adapts to hard workouts through rest and recovery.

are re-stocked, allowing harder workouts in the following days. These are only some of the physical changes that result from recovery, and with frequent and regular rest and recovery the physiological gains are enormous.

Consequently, the biggest mistake you can make is to continue to train through what was planned to be a rest-and-recovery week. Athletes often do this because they feel a need to gain more fitness in the last few weeks before an important race. This is a huge mistake. Even if you manage to avoid a breakdown, the quality of training will decline as fatigue continues to accumulate, and the result will be an even worse race performance.

Another common mistake is to make the workouts too hard on what were supposed to easy days. Instead of doing them in zone 1, as called for in the training plan, they become zone 3. Or what was supposed to be a short active-recovery session becomes a long one. Making such adjustments seems like a good thing because raising the average workload improves fitness. And that general concept is true, but the workout should not be made slightly harder on a recovery day. These days *must be easy*.

Keeping easy workouts truly easy is especially necessary during periodic rest-and-recovery weeks. In Chapter 7, I walked you step by step through the process of building an annual training plan. One of the steps involved was to include breaks from training every third or fourth week. This is evident in Tables 7.5 and 7.6, where in every period's week 4 the hourly volume or training stress score is decreased considerably compared with that of previous weeks in the same period. These are the planned rest-and-recovery weeks.

Rest-and-Recovery Weeks

Rest-and-recovery "weeks" are seldom 7 days long. Most advanced triathletes can recover and be ready to go again in fewer than 7 days. Reducing the training load for 3 to 5 days is usually enough. It's during these periodic breaks from hard training that you shed accumulated fatigue so that the next period starts at a high level of readiness.

What should a rest-and-recovery week look like? As you can imagine, this is determined by factors that include your level of experience, current fitness, and how hard the preceding weeks of training were. You may, for example, decide to make it only 3 days long because the preceding 2 or 3 weeks of training weren't all that hard. Or you may be really fatigued and decide on a 5-day break. You can decide for yourself during the rest-and-recovery week as you gauge how your body is responding.

Regardless of how long the break is, planning the week generally follows a pattern. Table 11.2 illustrates what a 5-day rest-and-recovery week may look like. This could easily be made into a 3- or 4-day break from serious training.

Note that an "optional second workout" is listed for most days. If you frequently do three workouts a day in a "normal" training week, do no more than two a day in a rest-and-recovery week. If two-a-day sessions are your common way of training, then do only one workout per day in a rest-and-recovery break. If one session per day is what you usually do, then do that in a rest-and-recovery week, but also be sure to take at least 1 day off from training altogether. I recommend some single-workout days regardless of your usual schedule. Those who usually work out more than 14 times in a week may opt to do a very light workout on Monday. But if in doubt, leave it out. You'll likely recover faster this week if one of the days is a day with no exercise.

In Chapter 9, I mentioned that the 2 or 3 weeks building up to a rest-and-recovery break may last 17 to 25 days. That's because the rest-and-recovery week seldom lasts a full 7 days. If you train in 3-week periods, meaning about 2 weeks of focused hard training followed by rest and recovery, and your training break lasts 4 days, then the next period of serious training will last 17 days (21 minus 4). If you take a 5-day break, the focused training lasts 16 days. If you typically train in 4-week periods and your rest-and-recovery break lasts 3 days, your total time for serious training is 25 days (28 minus 3). What all of this means is that the number of days devoted to quality training may vary from period to period depending on how long you decide to make your rest-and-recovery breaks. You can make that decision during the break as you gauge how well you are recovering.

Rest and Test

Notice in Table 11.2 (page 184) that the last 2 days of the week are dedicated to testing. This is the perfect time to measure your progress, because you are rested and ready to go. The number and type of tests you do are entirely up to you. You could, for example, decide to test all three sports. That's what is assumed in Table 11.2. Or you could decide to test only one or two sports. There may even be times when you decide not to test at all and get right back into serious training. As for which ability to test within a given sport, see the test protocols in Appendixes B, C, and D.

Most advanced triathletes can recover and be ready to go again in fewer than 7 days.

TABLE 11.2 **A Typical 5-Day Rest-and-Recovery Week**

	MONDAY	TUESDAY	WEDNESDAY	THURSDAY	FRIDAY	SATURDAY	SUNDAY
Purpose	Rest/recovery	Recovery	Recovery	Recovery	Recovery	Test	Test
Workout	Day off	Swim	Bike	Run	Swim	Run test	Bike test
Optional second workout	Strength	Run	Swim	Bike	Bike	Swim test	(None)

Recovery on Demand

Making rest-and-recovery periods part of an overall training plan works best for most athletes, but breaks don't always have to be planned in advance. Athletes who have been around the sport for many years and are good at sensing when they need a break from serious training can take a break based strictly on their experience. This is called *recovery on demand.* When the morning warnings indicate you've reached your limit, you simply assume that you need a break. This can happen at any time and is not based on a planned schedule.

Heeding these warnings accurately is a skill most of us don't have because it involves paying very close attention to how all of the body's systems are responding to training. Most of us are far too goal-focused and linear to decide suddenly that it's time to rest and recover. Without days set aside in advance for regular breaks from training, we're more likely to press ahead regardless of how tired we may be and end up sick, injured, or overtrained.

Recovery on demand is the ultimate method for managing recovery. It works best for coached athletes, when athlete and coach have daily, face-to-face contact. An experienced coach can tell when an athlete needs a break merely by seeing and talking with her or him. Most self-coached athletes, however, are emotionally attached to their goal to the point of disregarding their physical condition and are not good at stepping back to take in the big picture. So if you are not good at this and don't have close contact with a coach, it's best that you pre-plan your rest-and-recovery weeks.

RACE-WEEK REST AND RECOVERY

It seems that athletes sometimes train much harder than is necessary and rest less than they should, even right before A-priority races. Take Emil Zatopek, for example. This Czech distance runner of the 1940s and 1950s is considered one of the greatest runners of all time. He was relentless when it came to training intensity. He did not believe in running slowly. In fact, he is often credited with being among the first endurance athletes to train with highly intense intervals. This approach helped propel him to 18 world records and five Olympic medals. In the 1952 Helsinki Olympics, he won the 5,000- and 10,000-meter races and broke the Olympic records at both distances. Then he decided at the last minute to run the marathon, which he had never done before. He won it, too, again breaking the Olympic record.

Recovery on demand is the ultimate method for managing recovery.

Zatopek is often referred to as the hardest-training runner of all time. Like most athletes of his era, he didn't believe in resting before racing. But Zatopek is also a good example of how rest at the right time can elevate an athlete's race readiness—what we called form in Chapter 3. As Zatopek discovered at his career breakthrough event, sometimes a forced rest is exactly what is needed.

In 1950, Zatopek was training for the European Games when he became sick 2 weeks before the competition. Food poisoning was diagnosed and he was hospitalized, spending several days in bed. Just 2 days before the Games, which at that time were considered second only to the Olympics in terms of sports prestige, he was released from the hospital. Against the advice of his doctors, he raced both the 10,000 and the 5,000 meters. Despite having not trained for several days, he won both races, lapping the field in the 10,000 and winning by 23 seconds in the 5,000. In each race he ran the second-fastest time ever recorded for the distance. This was 2 years before his career peak at the Helsinki Olympics. Could the forced rest have had something to do with his success that week? Given his propensity for hard training right up to race day, I suspect so. He learned a valuable lesson and rested before all later races, including the 1952 Olympic Games.

In a similar manner, I've known of athletes in a variety of sports who were slightly injured or became sick a few days or weeks before a competition and then turned in a personal-best performance. They were forced to rest. I call this the Zatopek effect. Sometimes the body must say "enough" in order to come into form.

Rest is a miraculous cure for too much training. Left to their own devices, athletes will almost always opt to put in more volume, go faster, and train longer right up to the last few days before an important race. Most are ultimate examples of the Puritan work ethic. More is always better. Seldom do they consider the need to allow the body to "catch up" with all of the accumulated fatigue of training.

If you're a self-coached, advanced-level athlete, chances are you don't allow enough rest and recovery before A races. I see this all too often. But this is when you must rest and recover. How much of a taper do you need? A taper typically lasts 1 to 3 weeks, depending on many variables. The more important the race, the more likely your taper period should be long. The more fit you are, the longer the taper may be. The longer the race, the longer the taper. Races late in the season may benefit more from a longer taper than those earlier in the year. Taper length also varies by sport. Running, for example, demands a longer taper than cycling because the body is subjected to more orthopedic stress during running. Cycling generally requires more tapering than swimming. All of this is explained in detail in Chapters 7 and 8.

A bare-bones, minimum taper is about 2 to 3 days of greatly decreased activity. That's the sort of thing you do right before a B-priority race. It's just enough to shed a bit of the fatigue. But for an A-priority race, you need a longer taper. It might consist of 2 to 3 weeks of stair-stepped training reduction—especially a reduction of workout duration and therefore training volume. Table 8.2 provides guidance on how to organize a taper during the peak period that ends about a week before a race. Table 8.3 suggests how you may train in this last week leading up to the race. The example in Table 8.3 represents a greatly reduced

Sometimes the body must say "enough" in order to come into form.

A bare-bones, minimum taper is about 2 to 3 days of greatly decreased activity.

training volume from what you had probably been doing for training back in the base and build periods because this is your final opportunity to shed performance-detracting fatigue. Take full advantage of it to get rested up.

The night before the race, go to bed at a time similar to when you normally bed down. You may have trouble falling asleep. That's not unusual for athletes of all abilities, but somewhat more common for those who are less experienced with racing. You need not be concerned if you have a sleepless night. One research study conducted at the University of Texas showed that 25 to 30 hours of sleep deprivation did not cause a loss of aerobic performance in male and female cyclists. It's likely the same for swimming and running.

TRANSITION-PERIOD REST AND RECOVERY

After a race, you also need a break from highly focused, physically and mentally demanding workouts before you ramp up the training for your next race. This is the transition period—a time of greatly reduced physical activity. How long it lasts depends on when it is in the season and when your next race is scheduled. After an early or midseason A-priority race, this brief break from training usually lasts 3 to 7 days, depending on how much the race and your race prep took out of you. After the last race of the season, you should take 2 to 6 weeks for a transitional break.

The transition period isn't a time to become a couch potato. Much like the rest-and-recovery breaks you took every third or fourth week throughout the season, this is a stretch of greatly reduced intensity and volume. The purpose is to rest your body and refresh your mind.

It is a great time to spend with your family or do things you enjoy but can't fit into your busy days when training hard.

Some low-key workouts during this period, along with occasional days off, are good for maintaining a bit of aerobic fitness while satisfying your need to be active. This is the time of the year when it's best not to have a plan. Decide each day what you will do for exercise, if anything at all. You could go for an easy ride with a buddy. But exercise now doesn't have to be swimming, biking, and running. You might hike in the hills with your family. Perhaps you play a pick-up basketball game with friends. Or maybe you decide to try your hand at tennis. Don't become totally inactive. Do something on most days, but don't make it more of the same focused training that you've done throughout most of the preceding season.

How long should your season-ending transition period last? You will know it's time to get back to training when there are no more aches or pains, when you're so well rested you are perhaps starting to gain weight, and when you start craving focused training again. This is when it's time to begin a new season.

SUMMARY: REST AND RECOVERY

The key message of this chapter is that you need periodic rest-and-recovery breaks in order to train for high-performance racing. Without these breaks, you are likely to experience a breakdown that derails your season. There are several times throughout the year when it's critical to cut back on training and even take complete days off from any exercise at all. The most frequent of these,

You need not be concerned if you have a sleepless night.

and perhaps the most critical, are the rest-and-recovery weeks that come after 2 or 3 weeks of hard training.

Recall that a rest-and-recovery "week" should not literally be taken to mean 7 days. Some athletes recover very quickly and may find that they are ready to go again in 3 days. Others need 5 days or more. Older athletes are more likely than younger athletes to need longer recovery breaks. Less fit athletes also need more time than those who are highly fit. Experience is the only way to know what works best for you. But also realize that recovery is a moving target, and fatigue won't always require the same number of days to shed. Although 3 days may work after one training period, the next time you may find you are still tired after 3 days and so need more.

When your training is laser-focused, as in the base and build periods, fatigue is slowly but surely building. After an easy training day, which may occur several times in a week, some of this short-term fatigue is shed, but not all of it. What happens over one of these training periods is that fatigue slowly ratchets upward. It accumulates so slowly that you may not even be aware of it. This is especially true if you are concentrating on an important race and feel the need to fit in a few more workouts. At such times, you may decide to delay or even skip a planned rest-and-recovery period. That can easily prove to be the mistake that wrecks your season. Don't skip these breaks from training in order to do more hard training. It will likely come back to haunt you.

You must consider how many daily workouts to do in these extended rest-and-recovery breaks. The starting point is to do one less workout than you normally do in a day. So if you normally do a daily session in each sport—three-a-days—leave one out on each recovery day and vary which two you do each day. If you usually do two sessions a day, do only one. If you typically do only one, take a couple of days off completely. If you are not recovering quickly during these days, then do even less. The purpose is recovery from fatigue—not more fitness. Less is better now.

Second in importance are the easy days that are included every week throughout the season. These can be planned, as when a hard training day is routinely followed by an easy one or even a day off. Or, for the experienced and highly self-aware athlete, easy days may be included based on demand. In other words, when sensing that recovery is needed, the perceptive triathlete decides to have an easy day regardless of what is called for in the plan. The suggested morning warnings listed in Table 11.1 may prove helpful in making a decision.

What exactly an "easy" day of training consists of depends on the athlete. Recall from Chapter 3 that the only two training variables you can manipulate to make a workout easy or hard are duration and intensity. When it comes to intensity, defining an easy day is simple. It's a zone 1 workout. Duration is a bit harder to be so precise about. If you're an elite athlete who trains upward of 30 hours per week, a workout with an easy duration may be a 2-hour ride. But if you train 6 hours in a week, then an easy duration may be something more like 20 minutes.

Two other times in the season when rest and recovery are critical are in the week immediately preceding an A-priority race and the week after. If you don't cast off a significant amount of fatigue before an important race, you are likely to have a poor performance. Table 8.3 suggests one way of doing this while maintaining a high level

What exactly an "easy" day of training consists of depends on the athlete.

of fitness. You need to find a race-week pattern that works for you and then use it every time.

Taking a rest-and-recovery break the week after a hard A-priority race, especially one that came at the end of several weeks of highly focused training, will allow you to rejuvenate, both physically and mentally, before starting the buildup to your next race. A post-race break typically lasts 3 to 7 days during the season. After the last race of the season, this break can be as long as 6 weeks. But even that may not be long enough. I once coached an athlete who trained with great focus for her first Ironman, broke the course record for her age group, and then needed 6 months off from serious training. She was fried.

Adequate rest and recovery, regardless of when in the season you do it, is largely the result of trial and error. The key to getting it right is to be conservative. It's more beneficial to do too little training than too much. You're much better off being slightly undertrained but enthusiastic than to be constantly tired and apathetic.

THE COMPETITIVE EDGE

In Part VI, we consider three areas of training that triathletes often neglect—speed skills, muscular force, and the training diary. I suspect the reason why they are overlooked usually has to do with time constraints. Most triathletes are busy people who try to fit in two daily workouts around family, career, and other obligations. They feel as though something has to give, but my goal here is to show you how you can fit all three of these training tools into your busy life.

There's no doubt that refining your swim, bike, and run skills will result in faster racing, and you don't need to add more workouts to your training week to accomplish this. In Chapter 12, I'll teach you how to periodize your training early in the season to become more skilled, then show you how to maintain those skills as the season progresses. You'll be glad to know that it doesn't take nearly as much workout time to maintain a skill as it does to develop it in the first place. For maintenance, warm-ups at the start of a workout are a perfect time to enhance your skills. If you follow the skills development guidelines here and create a training plan as suggested in Chapters 7, 8, and 9, you will not place any greater demands on your sparse time available for training.

In much the same way, I'll teach you in Chapter 13 how to build strength by following your periodization plan from Part IV. Muscular force workouts in the gym are generally the most time-consuming sessions aside from swimming, biking, and running. But it doesn't have to be that way. Although it's beneficial for performance for you to improve strength by lifting weights, there are sport-specific alternatives that don't require you go to a gym. As you'll see, you can do slightly altered swim, bike, and run workouts to accomplish much the same outcome.

In Chapter 14, you'll see why a training diary is your most valuable tool as a serious triathlete. I'll show you how to use it to plan your season. To limit the time spent poring over training numbers, you'll also learn what to record in terms of critical workout and race information. Your diary will prove valuable in keeping you on track for your season's goals.

Part VI is all about gaining a competitive edge by learning how to do those seemingly small things that are so critical to high performance.

SPEED SKILLS

CHAPTER 6 introduced the concept of six physical abilities that you need to train for high-performance racing. The three basic abilities are aerobic endurance, muscular force, and speed skills. The three advanced abilities are muscular endurance, anaerobic endurance, and sprint power. The workouts you see described in Appendixes B, C, D, and E are based on these abilities. Given the nature of nondrafting triathlon, which is the primary focus of this book, sprint power is not included in the workouts because it's rare that a race comes down to a sprint at the finish line.

Of the five other abilities, triathletes most typically shortchange speed skills. And yet that's the ability you most likely need to improve. I generally see triathletes working on their speed skills only when they are in the pool doing drills. But even then, many don't understand what the drills are intended to accomplish. And they commonly use poor technique when doing them. You must perform a swim drill precisely, or it's a waste of time.

Beyond swim drills, I seldom see triathletes working on skills that will improve their biking and running. Most seem to believe that these sports are devoid of skill. But if you look around at the athletes during your next group ride or run, it'll be apparent that some have good skills while others waste a lot of energy because their skills are so poor. The movements of skilled cyclists and runners are smooth and effortless. It's apparent that they are not wasting energy. Those with poor skills look sloppy and appear to be working very hard. It's apparent they are wasting a lot of energy.

Fast athletes typically have good skills that conserve energy during movement. They're efficient. Slow athletes are slow, in part, because their skills are poor. They waste energy and are inefficient. Improving speed skills, and therefore efficiency, presents a great opportunity for performance enhancement for most athletes.

EFFICIENT MOVEMENT

You may recall from Chapter 6 that there are three physiological determiners of fitness: aerobic capacity (VO_2max), anaerobic threshold, and economy. One of your most important training goals is to build a high aerobic capacity so that you are capable of using a lot of oxygen to produce the energy needed for movement. You want your anaerobic threshold at a high percentage of VO_2max. And you need to be economical so that you waste no energy while swimming, biking, and running. (We're discussing skills in this chapter, but we're really focusing on economy.)

Chapter 6 described economy in some detail. Some of its determiners are completely outside your control, such as the size of your torso, the length of your arms and legs, and the size of your hands and feet. Triathlon is particularly demanding because your body can be nearly perfectly proportioned for one of the three sports yet poorly sized for the others. For swimming, you'd like to have a long torso and long arms to make you economical in the pool. But for the run, a short torso and long legs (especially long shin bones) are preferable. The long arms that serve so well in swimming are a disadvantage in running. And of course the bike has a completely different set of physical preferences, one of them being long thigh bones to improve pedaling performance. Obviously, there is no perfect body for triathlon, and you're likely to be more economical in one sport than in the other two. It's the same for all triathletes.

You're likely to be more economical in one sport than in the other two.

You do have some control over these physical determiners of economy, however, and the most adaptable one is movement skill. An athlete who wastes energy because of poor movement skills lacks efficiency. Regardless of how well your body may be designed for swimming, biking, or running, if your movement skills are poor, you will waste oxygen and fuel. You'll be inefficient. That means eating more food during races to meet the body's demand for energy, especially during a long-course race in which refueling is critical to performance. As food intake increases during the race, the risk for a digestive system failure marked by bloating and nausea increases. The longer the race, the more important movement efficiency becomes. You can waste a lot of energy in a sprint-distance race and get away with it—but not in an Ironman.

What I want to teach you in this chapter is how to improve your movement efficiency in each of the three sports by improving your speed skills. We'll start with the swim because it is the sport in which movement skill is most critical. But before getting into that, I want to show you a process for improving a skill that you can follow to make sure it is properly developed.

SKILL DEVELOPMENT

In this chapter, I will introduce several new swim, bike, and run skills. Some of these may be counter to what you've been taught before and may present completely new movement patterns for you. Some are likely to challenge you not only physically but also mentally. Over many years, I've come to understand that they are both effective and efficient. Once mastered, they have the potential to make you not only faster but also more efficient.

Mastering these skills is mentally challenging because you may have to give up old ideas of what you've been taught for many years. If you are already fast and efficient at each of the sports, there is no reason to change. But if your race performances are well below what you think you're capable of, then I highly recommend that you consider a change in your sport techniques. It will take several weeks to accomplish this.

The best time to make changes is at the beginning of a new season, during the prep period. Learning new skills may well spill over into the early base periods. As you make skill changes in a sport, you are likely to slow down and even become less efficient for a while. That's common. When changing old, well-ingrained movement patterns, your body will at first resist. It will feel strange, and your heart rate is likely to be higher than normal. Stay with it. Eventually, things will turn around and you'll become faster and waste less energy.

When you develop a new skill, there is a procedure you should follow that will help you hone the skill. You need to master each step in this procedure before going on to the next one. Some of these steps will come to you very quickly in a single practice session, while others will take several sessions. Start each session of skill development by repeating the previous session to remind your muscles and nervous system of what you're trying to do.

Step 1: Observe. The first step in learning a new skill is watching other athletes who have already mastered it. Watch good swimmers, cyclists, and runners. Notice how they move. Pay special attention to their movement during the particular skill you're trying to develop. A great time to do this is immediately before you work on that skill. For example, before you get into the pool, stand on the deck watching a good *open-water* swimmer for a few minutes (I'll explain the emphasis on open water shortly). Notice the joint angles, and pay attention to the rhythm. Keep this image in your mind as you get in the water and start work on developing your skill. Another way to do this is to make short videos of athletes performing the skills as you want to do them. Watch the appropriate video right before you start your workout. Keep that image in your mind as you practice.

Step 2: Move slowly. The second step is to make the movement slowly while watching yourself move. Isolate the movement and do it outside the context of the entire body's movement. You're moving only one body part while the rest of your body remains stationary. If it's the arm or leg, alternate sides. If you're working on a swimming skill, do this on the deck, not in the water. For running skills, you may need to hold onto something for balance while watching your foot and leg slowly go through the running motion described later on. This stage in the learning process may take only a single session to master, but for several weeks it should be a part of the warm-up for that particular sport each time you do a workout.

Step 3: Assimilate. Once you've honed the skill by isolating and slowly doing it over and over while watching, it's time to do it in the context of the sport. Now you swim, bike, or run while staying focused only on making the critical movement of the single body part. For example, pay close attention to only one arm and hand or one

As you make skill changes in a sport, you are likely to slow down and even become less efficient for a while.

The first step in learning a new skill is watching other athletes who have already mastered it.

leg and foot. Disregard anything else your body may be doing at this stage. Get that one body part moving correctly before you work on anything else. In the pool, when you work on the arms, use a pull buoy so you can focus your attention. Make the movements slowly in this step. Watch the body part while moving if you can. Eventually, you must learn to sense what the focal body part is doing without watching. This stage in skill development can last for a few days. Once you have mastered it, you will still do this slow-motion movement with a single arm or leg focus during warm-ups.

Step 4: Speed up. After you've mastered the movement in slow motion, which may take a few sessions, you can slowly add speed. Now you need to divide the workout into short segments lasting only a few seconds at first, building eventually to a few minutes. After each of these brief repetitions, you must rest (stand at the pool wall, coast on the bike, or walk in the run) in order to prevent fatigue from setting in. Fatigue is the enemy of skill development. If you do long, continuous swim, ride, or run sessions at this stage, the skill will fall apart. You'll revert to your old movement patterns. Brief repetitions while staying focused on the skill with long recoveries after each repetition are essential. It may take several weeks at this stage of skill development to become accomplished.

Step 5: Go long. Now that you've spent several weeks mastering the movement with brief repetitions and long recoveries in between, you begin to add endurance and therefore fatigue. Now you do long swim, bike, and run workouts. At this stage, you must stay focused on proper move-

> Fatigue is the enemy of skill development.

ment when you become tired. At the first sign of the new movement pattern breaking down, take a recovery break to shed some fatigue. Then return to the endurance workout while again staying focused on the skill. This stage may also last several weeks.

Step 6: Add pressure. This is the ultimate gauge of skill development. Can you make the desired movement patterns in a race? To test yourself, do a C-priority race with the goal of maintaining your newly developed skill during a high-effort performance. Pay close attention to your new skill throughout that portion of the race. After finishing, evaluate how you did. Were you able to maintain the new skill throughout the race? If so, you have completely mastered it. If you broke down and reverted to your old patterns, you need to take a step back and continue working on it.

SWIM SKILLS

I've been arranging weeklong camps for triathletes for several years. What's been apparent at these camps is how poor nearly all triathletes' swim skills are. In swimming, skill is more important than "fitness." If your skills are mediocre, you can spend hours in the pool doing interval sets and long-tempo swims and never get much faster. For most triathletes, the key to swimming faster is economy and, more specifically, their skills.

In my camps, we spend the entire week working only on swim skills. The week starts with a 500-meter time trial to establish a baseline. On the last day, after several sessions focused on skills, we repeat the time trial. About 90 percent of the campers swim faster on the last day without ever having worked on their aerobic capacities or anaerobic thresholds. And that's at the end of what typically is about a 25-hour training week, so the level of fatigue is high. I suspect that the 10 percent who don't swim the time trial faster are simply pooped. They sometimes tell me later that after they returned home and rested, their swimming had indeed improved. So I know what I'm about to teach you works.

Now is when the mental challenge I mentioned to you earlier becomes an issue. I'm going to teach you skills that are likely contrary to what you've been taught. You're going to have to make a decision: Do I keep on doing what I've been doing, or do I make a drastic change in my swim technique? If you've made good progress with your old method—if you are already fast and efficient—then there's no need for change. But if you've been training in the pool for years without becoming appreciably faster, then it's time to reconsider your skills.

What I will teach you in this section is how to become a good *open-water* swimmer—not a pool swimmer. There's a difference between the two that we will delve into shortly.

Your purpose here is to swim faster in a race. Will you suddenly become the fastest swimmer in your masters group? Probably not. Will you break age-group records in the pool? Not likely. What you will do, however, is swim faster in a triathlon without training any harder. Swimming faster depends much more on your technique than on how fit you are. You may not be first out of the water in a race, but you'll have a faster split. I've seen it happen with many triathletes.

You may feel conspicuous, and you may even be told that what I'll soon describe to you is wrong. If you can't get past this mental chal-lenge or if you're satisfied with your swimming as it is now, then skip this section and go straight to the bike skills section. But if you want to swim faster in triathlons without training harder, then read on.

PDLC

Coaches often get bogged down in the details of training, especially skill development. We know a lot of stuff and want to impart this knowledge to our athletes. I've certainly been guilty of that. When it comes to swimming, we try to point out every stroke flaw an athlete may have and try to correct it—no matter how small and insignificant the change may be. For example, should your fingers be open or closed during a stroke? I've heard coaches emphasize this in a session—one way or the other—and then spend an entire workout on it. Yet this is at best a 2 percent change. It's not worth the time spent trying to "correct" it. You need to devote your valuable training time to making changes that will make you much faster—20 percenters.

How about the kick? How many hours do you spend on a kickboard in a season? The only time a powerful kick matters is when you are accelerating. In a pool, that happens every time you come off the wall. But in an open-water swim, the only times the kick matters are at the start and when you go around a buoy. That amounts to seconds, even in an Ironman. In open-water swimming, the kick is done primarily to balance the body, much as the arms are used in running. Kicking in a triathlon is not for steady-state pro-pulsion. The time spent on a kickboard could be better spent working on what will help you shave several minutes off your race times. That's what I will teach you next.

Swimming faster depends more on your technique than on how fit you are.

In open-water swimming, the kick is primarily to balance the body, much as the arms are used in running.

There are only four skills you need to master to become a faster and more efficient open-water swimmer. I call them collectively *PDLC*:

- Posture
- Direction
- Length
- Catch

If you master these four skills and don't concern yourself with *any* of the other stuff that you could possibly devote valuable training time to, you will become a faster open-water swimmer. More than likely, you are already doing at least one or two of these four correctly, which means you will probably have only two or three to skills to master to become a better swimmer.

In what follows, I'll take you through the four basic open-water skills. As you read about each, consider whether it is a skill that you have already mastered. If you're unsure, have someone shoot a video of you swimming, both from the front and from the side, so that you can better judge your mastery of the skill. Underwater filming is best, but have the filming done above water if that's your only option. Shooting a video is quite beneficial and should be done frequently. In my camps, we do it in every swim session for every athlete.

You need to master the four PDLC skills in the order I present them here because each builds on the previous one. They also become slightly more difficult to master as you progress through the list.

Posture

In the pool, most triathletes swim with their head up and eyes focused on the approaching wall. As they do this, the hips are lowered in the water because the spine is extended. Drag increases as the hips get lower. The water drag is like the air drag you experience when you sit up on your bike. It will slow you down considerably. But just as you go faster when you get into your aero bars on the bike, so will you immediately swim faster once you master proper swim posture.

The head-up posture not only increases drag, it also restricts air intake, makes it more difficult to take a breath when you are swimming freestyle, and increases the stress on your neck and shoulder muscles. To see what I mean, stand up now and look at the ceiling for a few seconds. The higher up you look, the more you will feel forward movement of your pelvis along with restricted air intake and muscular tension. All of this will make you a slower swimmer. It's a big deal.

To improve your posture, point your nose toward the bottom of the pool. Figure 12.1 shows you how to do this. The lane line will keep you swimming straight. At first, you will be very uncomfortable looking down because we like to see what's ahead of us. To see where you're going, roll your eyes up with your nose still pointing down as if you are trying to look over a pair of glasses. In open water, of course, you will take quick and frequent looks at landmarks with your eyes above the surface of the water. You would do that regardless of your head position. So there's nothing to be gained and a lot to be lost by looking forward. Keep your nose pointed down. It will probably take only one swim session to get the hang of proper swim posture. Start working on it before you get into the pool by standing on the deck, bent over at the waist, with your nose pointed down while you reach out to take a stroke through the air. You will need to repeat this on-deck drill before each swim practice to

You will immediately swim faster once you master proper swim posture.

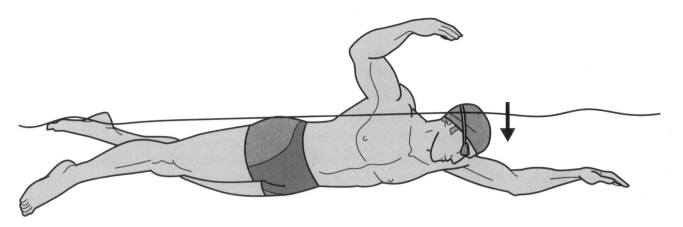

FIGURE 12.1   The nose-down head posture in swimming

ingrain it. More than likely, by your next swim session, you'll be able to advance to the next PDLC skill—direction.

Direction

Don't start working on this skill until you have mastered posture. For most triathletes, direction is a bit more difficult than posture to master. It has to do with the angle at which your hands and arms enter the water relative to the intended swim direction. On entry, they should be aimed in the direction you are swimming. Many triathletes cross over— that is, their arms cross the line of their intended swim direction. This is much like running with one foot and leg crossing over in front of the other foot and leg just before footstrike. That would be ridiculously inefficient, yet many triathletes do something very similar when swimming. This is another big deal—a 20 percenter.

You won't come close to your potential for fast swimming until your hand and arm point in the right direction on entering the water. For this to be done, the hand should enter in front of the shoulder, not the head. Most triathletes who make this mistake don't know they are crossing over. To them, it feels as if the hand is in the right place simply because they've done it that way thousands of times. To find out if you are crossing over, have someone record a video of you swimming from a head-on position. Notice where your hands are entering the water. You may be crossing over with both arms, or only one arm. If just one, note which arm it is. If you're not crossing over at all, then go on to the next skill—length.

The on-deck drill for learning the direction skill is simple. Stand bent over at the waist with a proper head posture and slowly reach out with one arm in front of your shoulder as if taking a stroke. Peek up to see where your hand is. It should be in front of your shoulder and not crossing over. Do this individually with each arm. A variation on this deck drill starts the same way while you are bent over at the waist. Take a stroke through the air. But now, without looking up, have a training partner correct your hand and arm position. Get the feel of where the correct position is. Once corrected, try it again slowly to see if you can put it back in the same *corrected* position. Do this on both sides. Repeat several times while being monitored by your training partner. Once you've mastered the deck drill, it's time to take this skill to the water.

A simple in-water exercise for learning good direction is the "penguin" drill. Swim one length

Your hand and arm must point in the right direction on entering the water.

of the pool while trying to put your hands and arms into the water much more widely apart than your shoulders. Have someone shoot a head-on video again while you swim like a penguin. Watch the video to see where your hands now enter the water. Most athletes with poor direction skills will find that their hands are now exactly where they are supposed to be on entry—in front of their shoulders. If this is what you find, the fix is easy—swim the penguin drill all of the time. It will feel weird for a few workouts, but you will soon adapt. You'll swim faster as a result.

Length

Once your posture and direction skills are well established, it's time to go to work on stroke length. This is a bit harder to master than posture and direction, but it's a necessary skill for swimming faster. Few triathletes have good length when they swim. It's a common efficiency flaw.

As the name implies, this skill has to do with how long your body is in the water from fingertips to toes. Fast swimmers are very long and narrow on each stroke, much the way a speedboat is long and narrow. Many triathletes, unfortunately, swim like tugboats—which are short and wide. They have an insufficient hand and arm reach and therefore experience a lot of water resistance. That's a double whammy. The resistance is a result of never being streamlined; instead, the shoulders are held in a square position or parallel to the pool wall toward which you are swimming. Because the shoulders stay in this square position, the hips do too. The body is thus short and wide like a tugboat.

To swim more like a speedboat, you need to become long and narrow in the water. Let's once again start on dry land to learn what this means. Stand on the deck facing a wall that is just a few inches away from you. With one arm at your side, reach up over your head with the other arm as if taking a stroke and place your hand on the wall. Try this individually with each arm. If you're like most triathletes, when you reach up with one arm you automatically go into the tugboat position with the hips and shoulders still square to the wall.

Now let's adopt the speedboat position by reaching even higher with one hand and getting as long and narrow as possible. To do this, get up on your toes and reach as high as possible with your hand. This will cause your shoulders to tilt and your hips to rotate. (Don't look up. Remember your posture.) You are now a speedboat. Notice that your hips rotate without your even thinking about it. There is no conscious rotation of the hips; instead, they rotate because you are reaching high with your hand and arm. It's like a baseball pitcher whose hips rotate while he is throwing a fastball. The pitcher doesn't think about his hips in order to throw the ball. He is focused on extending his arm. The hips follow the arm movement. It's the same for swimming. Your hips will rotate properly and your shoulders will tilt if you get your arm fully extended. That will produce the speedboat length we are aiming for in the water.

Now take this skill to the water by doing two length-focused drills while swimming. I'd recommend using a pull buoy so you can keep your attention focused on your upper body.

The first one is the "slap" drill. You're going to simulate a baseball pitcher's arm and hand motion. Swim one length of the pool by reaching out *over the water* and slap the water with your

Fast swimmers are like speedboats: very long and narrow on each stroke.

Your hips will rotate properly and your shoulders will tilt if you get your arm fully extended.

hand as if throwing a ball. When your hand slaps the water, your arm should be fully extended, as a pitcher's arm is. You're not trying to swim prettily. This is not synchronized swimming. Be aggressive with the throw and slap. If you get the slap out far enough beyond your shoulder—if you are truly long—your shoulders will tilt and your hips will rotate. Head-on and side-view videos should tell you. If they don't, we need to go on to the next drill.

This one is the "belly-to-the-wall" drill. Again, swim a length of the pool trying to get a long reach with each stroke. To become more aware of what your shoulders and hips are doing, concentrate on pointing your belly button toward the pool's sidewall on each stroke. You'll alternate pointing your belly button toward the right wall and then the left wall, back and forth, all the way to the other end of the pool. Keep your breathing pattern as it usually is. You should now be rolling from side to side with your hand way out in front with each stroke.

Once you have mastered the long stroke, you won't be slapping the water or pointing your belly button at the sidewalls. These are merely exaggerated movements to help you learn what is for most a fairly difficult skill to master.

Again, have a training partner record a side-view video of you swimming to see if you are truly reaching and rolling with each stroke. The more frequently you shoot and analyze videos, the sooner you will master the skill.

Catch

You've probably been told many times by masters coaches to work on your catch. A poor catch is a common flaw of triathletes. Unfortunately, when it comes time to develop an athlete's swim skills, many coaches teach a technique that makes it very difficult to get a catch. I used to be guilty of this, too. It was, and continues to be, "group think": If others are doing it, it must be OK.

With the traditional pool-swim technique, what makes the catch so hard to do is the place where your hand enters the water—near your head. The next thing you're typically told to do with this technique is to extend your arm in the water as if putting it into a sleeve or reaching into a mailbox. You've undoubtedly been taught that the way to get to that entry position by having a high, bent elbow. I used to have triathletes do a "fingertip-drag" drill to get the elbow high, or to act as if they were pulling up a zipper along the side of the body. All of this teaches a poor technique for open-water swimming.

So what's wrong with doing all of this? Had you started learning this movement when you were 7 years old and on a competitive swim team, you probably would have figured out a way to produce a catch with it. But because you probably started swimming later in life, the whole business of a catch remains a great mystery that somehow you're unable to figure out.

So what is a catch? It's simple. When you are swimming in a pool, a catch occurs when the palm of your hand is pointing at the wall you're swimming away from. Trying to pull that off when your hand enters the water close to your head and your arm extends with your fingers pointing at the wall you're swimming toward is a challenge. A lot of fairly complex movements have to happen throughout this maneuver in order for you to catch the water.

The biggest problem with the traditional hand entry and reach maneuver is that once the arm is

In a pool, a catch occurs when the palm of your hand is pointing at the wall you're swimming away from.

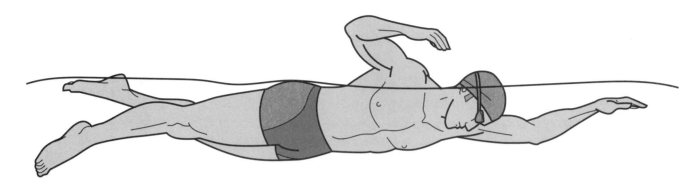

FIGURE 12.2 The "death move." Note the left elbow is below the wrist and the left fingers are pointed at the forward wall.

extended with the fingers pointing at the forward wall, the elbow is lower than the wrist. I think of this as the "death move" because once you get into this position—elbow below wrist—you're dead in the water. Figure 12.2 illustrates the death move. The only way to propel yourself while in this position is with a kick. That's a huge energy waster. And if you work on trying to increase your length per stroke, as you've probably also been taught to do, it only complicates the attempt to learn the catch by magnifying the death move.

Learning the catch is not difficult. The challenging part is overcoming the ingrained movement pattern that results in the death move. Begin by forgetting about high elbows and hand entry close to the head. That's how the death move starts. Very few good open-water swimmers do this. Most use a stroke that has a high hand, not a high elbow, during the above-water recovery phase. The next time you go to a triathlon as a spectator, watch how the pros swim. You'll see lots of high hands with extended elbows above the water.

Why have your hand high? Because when you combine that with a long reach over the water (not *through* the water; remember the *L* in PDLC) and the fingertips entering first, you eliminate the death move and *immediately* get a catch. When you do this, a strong kick is not necessary for propulsion as it is with the death move. Forward movement comes from the catch, as it should.

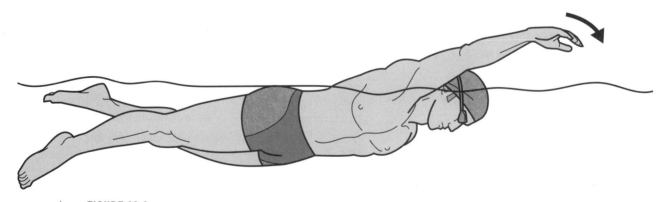

FIGURE 12.3 The catch starts before the hand enters the water. Notice the fingers are already starting to point down. Once your fingers enter the water, pull down and back with your fingers pointed at the bottom of the pool.

Figure 12.3 shows how combining length with a fingertip entry produces a catch. As soon as the hand enters the water, the palm is facing the wall behind you, not the bottom of the pool. As you pull the hand and arm down and back, you have an effective stroke that is as long as your entire arm. Triathletes with a death move typically have a stroke that is only a few inches long because they don't get the palm to face backward until it's under the chest.

Highly experienced and advanced pool swimmers learned to overcome their death move as youngsters. So can you once you learn how to do it, but it's a much more advanced skill than simply reaching over the water, not through it, and having the fingers enter first.

So how do you develop this skill of reach over the water and then catch? Let's start on deck again. Stand bent over at the waist with both arms at your sides. Take a stroke with one arm while keeping the elbow straight. Reach. The shoulders should tilt during the stroke to maximize length. As the arm is reaching its full extension, point the fingers down at the deck. You now have a catch. Pull the arm down and back. Look up to see where the hand and arm are to confirm your catch. Try this with the other arm. Then keep your good posture position and have a training partner assist to ensure that you have the fingers pointing down at extension. Slowly repeat this several times on the deck with each arm so that you start to ingrain the skill. Now get into the water.

Here's a quick position reinforcement you can do as soon as you are back in the pool. If your pool has starting platforms for racing, reach up with both hands and place your palms on the platform. That's the catch position, and you can use it to lift your body up a bit out of the water as though you were going to get out of the pool. Feel the power you can generate from this position. Now point your fingers toward the ceiling instead of putting them on the platform. That's the death move position. It's obvious there's no way you can lift yourself out of the water without putting your hands on the platform. It's the same when you swim. There's no way you can propel yourself forward in the water with your fingers pointing straight ahead at the next wall. You must catch the water to go forward.

Now it's time to develop the drill while swimming. By this time, you should have mastered posture, direction, and length. Sometimes at this stage in swim skills development, I find that athletes begin to revert back to their old habits, especially when it comes to length. A short stroke makes a more feeble catch. So we're going to start with a drill that combines length and catch—the "windmill" drill.

Use a pull buoy at first as you learn this drill. Your goal is to swim like a windmill. In other words, your arms will be straight with the elbows *never* bending, whether above the water or in it. As your hand and arm are swinging high over the water, reach out, much as you did with the slap drill. Only instead of slapping the water, point your fingers down as shown in Figure 12.3 in order to create a catch. You should have good posture, be reaching in the direction of the forward wall, and have tilted shoulders with a slight hip roll as you catch the water.

Once you have mastered the windmill drill, along with posture, direction, and length, you will be swimming faster than when you used the all-too-common death move. I've found some triathletes swim so much better doing the wind-

You must catch the water to go forward.

The key to speed is to commit fully to improving PDLC.

mill drill that I tell them to just swim that way all of the time.

Swim-Skills Training

You now know how I teach triathletes at my camps to improve their swim times by working only on skills. Most do improve. The key is to commit fully to improving PDLC. The starting point for this is knowing which of these four skills you already do well and concentrating on the remaining ones by working your way through them—from *P* to *D* to *L* and finally to *C*. For example, if you already swim with good posture, you should focus your attention on getting the direction skill mastered before moving on to length and finally catch. Don't progress to the next skill until you've mastered the previous one.

This will take some time, perhaps a month. If I were your coach, I'd have you devote 4 weeks—about 12 to 16 swim sessions—just to mastering PDLC by doing the drills described above.

You want to do each of these sessions the same way. Before getting in the pool, work on the session's focal PDLC skill for that day on deck. Once you have the feel for it, get into the water. What you will do now is swim one length of the pool at a slow pace. Over the duration of the session, swim each length more briskly, but not all out. While swimming a length, focus your attention only on the one skill you are trying to improve. Think of nothing else. Don't concern yourself with how fast you are swimming. There's no need to time it. Let that wait until you've mastered PDLC by the end of the month.

When you finish a length, stop and rest at the wall. Take as long as you want. Don't make the rest stops brief in order to improve your endur-

ance. That will only inhibit your development of the new skill. Resting at the wall is the time to let your mind wander. Look around at what's going on with other swimmers. Think about anything except your swim performance. Your thoughts can be on what you'll have for supper tonight, a project you are working on, or how your bike ride went yesterday. Rest and relax. Your breathing should become calm. When you're ready to swim the next length, bring your mental focus back to the PDLC skill you are working on. Nothing else. Again, swim another length while focusing only on making this movement correctly. Then stop again and fully rest. Think about anything but swimming. Repeat this over and over for the entire session. This workout is called *fast-form 25s* and is described in Appendix B in workout SS1.

When doing a PDLC swim session, don't concern yourself with whether your fingers are open or closed, kicking, "finishing" your stroke, putting your arm in a sleeve, or anything else you've been told is "important." Once you've fully mastered PDLC, you can return to any of these 2 percent skills to achieve the small gains they'll give you. For now, though, work only on the 20 percent skills: posture, direction, length, and catch.

The perfect time to do this PDLC workout is the base 1 period at the start of your season. That's usually in the winter months. But regardless of where you are in your season, developing better swim skills will pay off with faster times. By swimming only brisk single lengths of the pool for 12 to 16 consecutive sessions, you'll be able to focus completely on the skill you are trying to develop. As soon as you master the PDLC skill you are developing, go on to the next one.

Resting at the wall is the time to let your mind wander.

Greatest gains come from the skills of posture, direction, length, and catch.

You may double back from time to time just to make sure you aren't reverting to old habits.

Frequent videos will tell you how you're progressing. After 4 weeks of PDLC-focused sessions, you will be swimming faster without ever having done anything longer than a single length and without having done any strenuous intervals. You will have also learned a valuable lesson: When it comes to swimming, skill mastery is more important than what we typically call *fitness*.

BIKE SKILLS

While swimming is highly skill-based, cycling is the least skill-oriented of the three sports. This doesn't mean that skill in riding a bike is unimportant. It's just less critical to performance than in swimming. On the bike, there are four primary skills to master—pedaling, cornering, climbing, and descending. The good news is that this is going to be easy. There are two things you can do that will help with all four skills.

Bike Fit

The starting place for developing these skills isn't drills, it's getting a bike fit. This is the PDLC of cycling. Just as with swimming, the time to do this is early in the season; the base 1 period is the perfect time. There's nothing more important for your riding for the remainder of the season. A proper bike fit will greatly improve not only your skills but also your hard workouts so that you reap greater fitness benefits.

The bike fit is so important that you should get one every year even if you are riding the same bike from last year on which you already had a fit. Things change. You may become less flexible as you age, and also as your muscles develop from strength training. Or you may be more flexible because you spent a lot of time working on range of motion or taking yoga classes. Perhaps you recall from last season that your back got tight when you were doing long-course races and you had to sit up frequently. You may have developed a niggling injury or gotten rid of one. Perhaps the distance you are racing this year for your A-priority races is different from last year's. Your butt may be getting sore on long rides. You may have purchased a new saddle or stem last year. Lots of stuff can have changed. Even if you can't come up with a good reason to do so, get a bike fit anyway. A good bike fit will save you more time in a race than all of the expensive bike equipment you could possibly buy. It's well worth the time and cost.

You may unfortunately learn from the fitter that the bike you are riding simply doesn't fit you. The frame is too big or too small. I hope that isn't the case because new frames are expensive. I see riders in this sad situation in almost every race I go to. If you do get a new bike, ask your fitter to take a look at the ones you are considering, just as you might have your auto mechanic look at a car you are thinking of buying. Getting a good deal on a new bike isn't a good deal if the bike doesn't fit you properly.

The fit should be done by a professional. Don't ask your spouse or training partner to do it for you (unless he or she is a professional bike fitter). Also, search for someone who knows about fitting triathletes, which is different from fitting road racers on time-trial bikes. Roadies don't have to dismount and run. Most shops that specialize in triathlon either will have someone on staff who does fits or can refer you to someone who does.

Bike fitting used to be primarily an art; now it is mostly a science. A good fitter will put you in

A proper bike fit will greatly improve your skills and hard workouts.

a position that optimizes your physique, physiology, and race purpose. He or she will consider your unique balance for safety, comfort, power, and aerodynamics. You'll learn how to sit on a saddle (many do it incorrectly); what your head, spine, and hip posture should be; and how simply to ride faster. It's money well spent.

The bottom line is that all of your bike-handling skills will improve after a good fit, even before you have worked on them. You'll waste less energy when riding and be more powerful. And your risk for a bike-related injury in the coming season will be greatly decreased. If you are truly serious about improving your performance on the bike, money spent on a bike fit is some of the best money you'll spend. You'll come away after an hour or two as a much better cyclist.

Off-Road Riding

When it comes to pedaling and the bike-handling skills of cornering, climbing, and descending, one of the best ways to refine those skills is by riding off road on a mountain bike or cyclocross bike. The best times to do this are in the prep and base 1 periods at the very start of your training year. For most triathletes, that's also during the late fall and early winter months, when the days are short and the weather more unforgiving. That's a good time to stay off the roads. And even though you go more slowly when riding off road, you can accomplish a whole lot more in less time, especially when it comes to skills.

Why is riding off road so good for bike skills? It's because all of your movements are exaggerated and done at a slow speed. Let's look at pedaling skills during hill climbing as an example of this. On a triathlon bike, you can be pretty sloppy when pedaling uphill. You'll still get to the top just

fine. But off road, especially when you are riding on a loose surface material such as gravel or sand, your pedaling must be precise. If you only push down hard on the pedals, the rear wheel will slip on loose terrain. You're likely to have a slow-motion fall as a result. So you have to learn to keep fairly even pressure on the pedals through the entire pedal stroke. That's a skill that will pay off when you get back to the roads in base 2.

The same sorts of benefits are reaped for the other skills, such as cornering and descending. By working over loose terrain and around obstacles at a slow speed, you'll become more skilled at handling a bike. Without doing even a single drill, your skills will tremendously increase from riding off road. You'll also have fun and will enjoy a nice break from your normal cycling routine.

RUN SKILLS

Running is in the middle when it comes to the importance of movement skills in the three sports. Skill isn't as critical here as it is in swimming, but it's more important than what's required for cycling. Like developing swimming skills, developing run skills can be narrowly focused. There are lots of skills we could talk about here, but most would produce at best 2 percent improvements in performance. The 2 percenters include how much bend you have in your elbow while running, how your arms swing relative to the center line of your body, how straight or curved your spine is, how far ahead your eyes are focused, and many more that we coaches often get bogged down in when we teach running technique.

Only one skill when mastered can produce a significant improvement in performance. That skill is how you place your foot on the ground.

A mountain or cyclocross bike will refine your cornering, climbing, and descending skills.

Developing run skills can be narrowly focused.

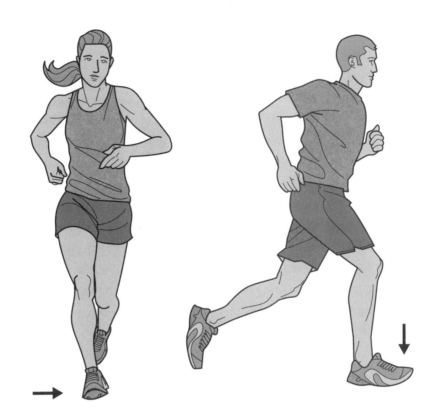

FIGURE 12.4 (left)
Head-on view of good foot placement

FIGURE 12.5 (right)
Side view of good foot placement

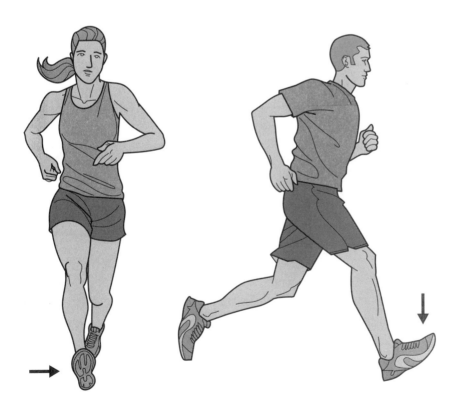

FIGURE 12.6 (left)
Head-on view of poor foot placement

FIGURE 12.7 (right)
Side view of poor foot placement

There are lots of opinions on how to do that—and even on how critical it is for run performance. But just as we see most good open-water swimmers use a PDLC stroke, most good triathletes place their feet on the ground in a similar way when running. Let's see how they do it.

Figures 12.4 and 12.5 illustrate from two angles good foot placement during running—head on and from the side. Notice that the lead foot in both figures is just about to make contact with the ground. The feet in both instances are also nearly parallel to the surface. These two have nearly perfect foot placement. Yours doesn't have to be so close to perfect. The heel can strike the ground first so long as the ball of the foot makes contact at almost the same time. In other words, a rear-foot strike is fine as long as the forefoot is perhaps an inch (2 cm) or less above the surface at heel strike.

Figures 12.6 and 12.7 show how some triathletes run—with a pronounced heel strike and the forefoot considerably above the ground. The time differences in forefoot contact in the four examples are only in milliseconds, but those milliseconds are important when it comes to running efficiency. When the foot makes contact with the ground in a nearly flat position, potential energy is stored in the calf muscle, much as it is when a rubber band is stretched. From the flat foot position, this energy is quickly released, helping you run somewhat more efficiently than if your forefoot strikes the ground somewhat later. The exaggerated heel strike, with the foot angled so that the toes are pointing at the sky, as in Figure 12.7, stores no potential energy because the calf muscle isn't quickly stretched. In this case, the foot performs more like a rocking chair, preventing the calf muscle from acting like a rubber band.

You can get a sense of what this feels like by doing a simple drill. Stand with a good running posture—your knees slightly flexed and your weight toward the balls of your feet. Now bounce up and down, getting just a couple of inches off the ground and landing with a flat footstrike. Notice how effortless this is. Now do the same bouncing drill, only this time put your weight back on your heels. The difference is remarkable. It takes considerably more effort when you land on your heels than when you land on flat feet. Most of the difference you experience in this simple drill has to do with stored energy being released (flat footstrike) or lost (heel strike).

What I've noticed in more than 30 years of coaching triathletes is that footstrike is improving. In the early days, most of them had a pronounced heel strike. Now, most run with a relatively flat foot placement. But that doesn't necessarily mean *you* have a good footstrike. To find out, have someone shoot a video of you both running toward the camera and in side view. Head on, you should see very little of the bottom of the shoe of the lead foot (Figures 12.4 and 12.6). In the side view, the lead foot should be nearly parallel immediately before footstrike, not with an exaggerated heel strike (Figures 12.5 and 12.7).

Foot-Drop Drill

If your videos show you have an excellent foot position, your running efficiency is probably quite good. But if you do see poor foot placement, you need to do something to correct it. As with swimming, we start with "on-deck" drills and gradually progress to faster, racelike movement.

The first drill is simple. Stand facing a wall and about 20 inches (50 cm) away from it. Put

The heel can strike the ground first so long as the ball of the foot makes contact at almost the same time.

To improve foot placement, start with on-deck drills and progress to racelike movement.

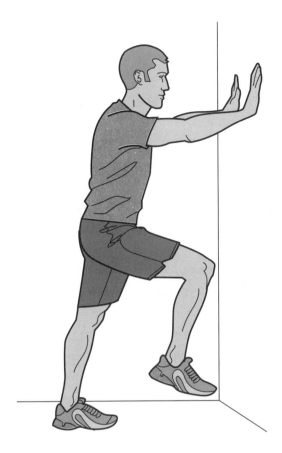

FIGURE 12.8 The foot-drop drill

your hands on the wall so that you are slightly leaning onto it. Now lift your right foot off the floor as if taking a running stride and let it drop back to the floor (Figure 12.8). The right foot should drop straight down and land *in front of* the left foot—not beside it. Repeat this several times with both feet. Closely observe what your feet and knees do. Notice that the wall doesn't allow you to reach out with the right foot, which would set you up for an exaggerated heel strike. When the foot is lifted off the floor, the knee bends considerably, with the raised foot hanging directly below the knee—not in front of it. Those are the foot and leg positions you see illustrated in Figures 12.4 and 12.5. Reaching with the foot is what sets you up for an exaggerated heel strike, as is quite obvious in Figure 12.7.

Strides Drill

Once you've mastered the foot-drop drill, you should progress to a "strides" drill, which is very similar to doing single lengths of the pool in swimming. This drill is best done on a soft surface, such as grass. A park or football field where you can run in a straight line for about 120 yards (130 m) is about right. Terrain that is slightly downhill is perfect. Start the drill by running the length of the field at a comfortable, warm-up speed. Pay close attention to your lead foot and knee. The foot should be rising and falling below the lifted knee just as with the foot-drop drill. Concentrate on nothing else but this. Turn around and walk back to the starting point. Yes, walk! Do *not* run. This is a long recovery, just as you did in the pool.

Once back to the start point, turn around and run another length. Do four to eight such strides in a session. Each should be slightly faster than the previous one, so start slowly. Stay focused on your foot position—below the knee and flat as when leaning on the wall. Have someone shoot a video of you doing this drill from the side. Analyze it to see if you have a nearly flat foot placement. You should not be reaching with your feet. The video is critical feedback for making progress, so have one made frequently.

In an advanced version of strides, you run as described above, only now you count your steps for one leg only. For example, count every time your right foot strikes the ground. Use your watch to time each stride and count steps at the same time. Run for 20 seconds on your same grassy surface while counting. The goal is to count 30 steps in 20 seconds. That's a cadence of 90 revolutions per minute (RPM). Continue to focus on a flat foot landing when doing this timed drill.

The strides drill is similar to doing single lengths of the pool in swimming.

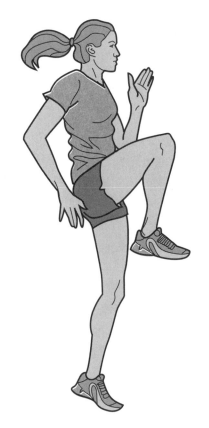

FIGURE 12.9 The skipping drill

Skipping Drill

Now let's add another drill to be combined with the strides drill—the "skipping" drill. Chances are you did this a lot as a kid. Every kid skips because it's fun. It came naturally when you were young, but it's probably been a while since you last skipped, so it may take some time to get the movement pattern back again. This drill is worth the time investment. Skipping teaches you how to keep your feet in the flat position and under your knees without looking, which athletes tend to do when running strides. That's all right at first, but eventually it needs to be avoided. Figure 12.9 shows how to skip. This is essentially a hop on one foot with the other foot elevated. Alternate legs so that you do a single hop on one leg

and then a hop on the other. Do about 20 seconds of skipping after each stride before you begin to walk back to the strides starting point.

Advanced Strides Drill

After a few timed strides plus skipping sessions, you will be ready for an advanced running drill to build power. Just as before, run a length of your grass course and time the run as described above. As you turn around to head back to the strides starting point, start skipping. Only now, let's modify the skipping. There are two advanced variations of this drill you can do. On one of your 20-second skipping drills, try to get as much height as you can with each skip for the entire 20 seconds. The other variation is to get as much length as you can with each skip. These are a form of plyometrics, which we'll describe in much greater detail in Chapter 13. For now, the bottom line is that plyometrics build running power.

The final stage of the skipping drill progression is to do the workout barefoot. This will strengthen your feet and lower legs to help you run faster, and it will also reduce the likelihood of a running-related injury. Be aware, however, that this highly advanced running drill can also *cause* injury. We're back to the risk and reward of training, discussed in Chapter 10. Approach barefoot running with caution. The first concern is about stepping on something sharp. Closely inspect the strides run course to make certain there is nothing that can injure your feet while you are running barefoot. Also check for dog droppings. And don't run barefoot if you have a cut on your foot, no matter how small.

This last iteration of the strides drill should not be attempted until you have done several such workouts with shoes on. The last few such sessions before you do them barefoot should be done in minimal running shoes, such as racing flats or even water walkers. The idea is to strengthen your feet gradually rather than try to make them stronger right away and end up injured. Patience! When starting to use minimalist shoes and when doing the first barefoot sessions, start with a low number of sets. If you've been doing eight of them with your regular running shoes, do only four the first time you use lightweight shoes. Build back up to eight with them before going barefoot. Then do only four stride-skip plyometrics sets when starting the barefoot drills.

SUMMARY: SPEED SKILLS

All triathletes can stand to improve their speed skills, no matter how advanced they may be. In the late 1990s and early 2000s, I coached Ryan Bolton, a pro who was one of the fastest runners in the sport at the time. In addition to his swim and bike skills work, I had him do strides drills every week. You can always get faster, but as long as your skills are lacking, your odds of improving through hard training sessions are greatly reduced.

Good speed skills start with the most basic movements of the sport. This is especially true for swimming. Devoting your valuable pool time to working on tiny improvements is all right if you are a national- or world-class swimmer. If not, you need to master the basic skills of open-water swimming before you move on to the most advanced skills. The basic skills are posture, direction, length, and catch—PDLC, as you learned to call them in this chapter. Once you have mastered these, you can then advance

to the minute changes that may take you to the highest level in swimming. Until then, focus only on mastering PDLC. The best time to do this is in the base 1 period at the start of your season. However, it's never too late to start.

As the least "skill-centric" of the three sports, cycling is relatively easy to master. The starting point is to have a bike fit done by a professional who works with triathletes. Do this before starting each new season even if you are using the same bike as in the previous season and even if you were fitted to it then. Things change. The athletes I coach get a bike fit every season. Base 1 is a great time to do this. And ride off road as much as you can in the prep and base 1 periods to refine your pedaling and bike-handling skills. Besides being an effective way to improve skills, it is also lots of fun and a nice break from road riding at exactly the right time in the year.

The most basic speed skill in running is foot placement. Fast runners all make foot contact with the ground in much the same way. Their feet either strike flat on the ground or with a very slight heel-first landing (some land on the forefoot, but I wouldn't recommend that unless you've been running that way for many years). None of them run with the toes of their lead foot pointing at the sky because that foot is well in front of the knee. If you run with such an exaggerated heel strike, then you must correct this before you'll be able to advance as a runner. Hard training sessions are of little value if you make ground contact with your foot forward of your knee. That's a braking motion, and it will cause you to run more slowly and use more energy than is really needed. As with the swim and bike skills, the optimal time to work on running skills is the base 1 period. As with the other sports, though, refining your

All triathletes, no matter how advanced, can improve their speed.

running skills can and should be done no matter where you are in the race season right now.

Once you master these swim, bike, and run speed skills, you're not done. Skills have a way of eroding over time. You're likely to shift back to your old habits gradually without even being aware of the change. Skills work should continue as a part of every week and every workout year-round. Skill refinement never ends. Continuing to work on refining them will add greater benefit to your other hard training sessions. In training, never allow your form to break down while you are trying to go faster. Technique is critical to performance.

MUSCULAR FORCE

TRAINING IS NOT ONLY for your heart and lungs. It's ultimately muscle that makes you fast. Your training should first and foremost be about muscle, not only when you've got the pedal to the metal but also when you're doing an easy, aerobic effort. Research consistently shows that when muscular force is improved, speed increases at the anaerobic threshold. That's one of the three markers of fitness described in Chapter 6. The other two, you may recall, are aerobic capacity and economy.

Economy also improves with greater muscular force. In the last chapter, you read about how improving speed skills makes you more efficient by reducing the energy cost of swimming, biking, and running. Skill is one of those things over which you have some control when training to be more economical. Another one of those controllable elements is muscle power.

In this chapter, we'll study some other methods for improving speed and economy—plyometrics and strength training. I've used these training methods with many triathletes over the years and seen consistent improvements in fitness and performance. Training with both of these benefits your neuromuscular system in ways that traditional endurance training can't do.

NEUROMUSCULAR TRAINING

Your neuromuscular system is made up of nerves and muscles. It functions much like a computer. Muscles—the hard drive—get the work done, but they do only what the nerves—the software—tell them to do. It takes both for either the computer or your body to work properly. The brain sends signals to the muscles through the nerves and you move in a certain way. The more often a few select nerves stimulate certain muscles, the better you get at a given movement. It's much like a walking path through a vacant corner lot that gets worn over time. At first, you can walk any direction you want through the lot. But the best possible path will eventually be established if a lot of people take the short cut through it frequently. The more times it's used, the better the path becomes. That's basically what I was telling you to do in the last chapter when I described doing single-length intervals in the pool while focused only on PDLC with long recoveries after each lap. You were building nerve pathways to fire certain muscles at the right times and in the right ways. Repetition increases your skill for a particular movement.

The same thing happens with muscle power, which involves how many muscle fibers are being stimulated at the same time. The more times you use certain nerves to cause the muscles to contract powerfully, the faster and more economical you become. The path becomes very wide and well worn. Poorly trained athletes can activate only a small portion of their available muscles, and those fibers are weak. The path is narrow and not well worn. This makes them slow. They lack the muscular power that comes with being able to call on many strong muscle fibers to contract in the proper sequence at just the right times.

Sports scientists used to believe that only muscle size determined a person's strength. Strength training then was built around producing big muscles. But since the 1980s, strength training research has shown that the nervous system plays a major role in how powerful an athlete is. While you can still expect large muscles to be strong, size is not the only determiner of power. Strength training, when done correctly from an endur-

ance athlete's perspective, also improves power by teaching the nervous system to work effectively.

Furthermore, the coordination and timing of the innervation (nerve stimulation) of the various muscles involved in a specific skill, such as pedaling a bicycle, have to do with how well trained the nervous system is. To improve the power produced for the skill requires doing strength- and power-building exercises that closely mimic the sport-specific movement you want to improve.

There is perhaps even more happening in the nerves that determines how well you do in a triathlon and that can be improved by weight lifting. The neuromuscular system can become tired during extended endurance. I'm sure you are well aware of this. We typically blame such fatigue on tired muscles. They resist innervation. But it is just as likely to be the nerves—or even the brain—that is becoming fatigued. You're simply more aware of fatigue happening in the muscles. Sports science is still trying to figure out exactly what fatigue is. Something we do know is that a muscle with strong endurance is capable of resisting whatever the cause of fatigue may be.

What I want to show you in this chapter is how to use two training tools to strengthen your neuromuscular system and ultimately make you more powerful and capable of going fast for a long time. These tools are plyometric training and strength training. They have the potential to produce great performance rewards. Recall, however, from Chapter 10 that when there is a great reward from something done in training, there is most assuredly a great risk associated with it. That is certainly true of plyometric exercises and weight lifting. While they have the potential to improve your performance, you can very easily be injured when doing either one. The most com-

Repetition increases your skill for a particular movement.

The nervous system plays a major role in athletic power.

mon cause of such breakdowns is impatience—the athlete rushes into these types of workouts and does too much. Workout dose (how hard) and density (how frequently) are too often accelerated beyond what is safe, resulting in an injured knee, back, foot, or some other body part that is vulnerable. You must be cautious and conservative when doing either of these types of training.

Although the training is risky, you will likely avoid injury if you follow the plyometric- and strength training guidelines in this chapter. But you need to be aware of what you are experiencing when doing them regardless of what I suggest. At the first sign that the physical stress and strain in one of these workouts are too great, you need to stop and evaluate what you are experiencing. Signs of stress and strain usually mean that you are getting ahead of your body's ability to adapt. You're doing too much too soon. It takes several weeks to realize the gains from doing these workouts. Rest, then start back at a lower level of effort and allow your body to adapt slowly.

MUSCLE

There are several muscle types throughout your body. At the most basic level, these are divided into fast-twitch and slow-twitch muscle fiber types. The slow-twitch fibers are your endurance muscles. They aren't very powerful, but they can contract over and over before fatiguing. Fast-twitch muscles are just the opposite. They contract very powerfully but fatigue quickly. Every triathlete has a unique mix of these two general muscle types. Some of us have lots of fast-twitch fibers and therefore are quite powerful, but typically with poor endurance. Others have more slow-twitch fibers and so can keep going a long

time. We have different blends of muscle types throughout the body.

Your blend of muscle types was determined at conception by your parents. But you can change them slightly. By doing a lot of long, moderate-intensity workouts, an athlete with mostly fast-twitch fibers can cause some of them to take on the endurance characteristics of slow-twitch fibers. The opposite is also possible. With strength and power training, some of the fibers will take on more of the power traits of fast-twitch fibers.

What all of this means is that you need to decide what is best for your triathlon performance when it comes to strength training. I've coached a few triathletes who came to the sport from a bodybuilding or power-lifting background for which they were well suited physically. They certainly did not need to develop their strength further by lifting weights. What they needed was more endurance training. Most of the triathletes I've coached over more than 30 years, however, benefitted considerably from improving their strength and power.

Into which category do you fall? Are you a natural-born power athlete with big muscles and a propensity for adding bulk easily when following a strength building program? If so, then high-load strength training is not for you if you want to improve your triathlon performance. If you decide to lift weights, which isn't necessary in this case, use only light loads with many repetitions. If, on the other hand, you are an "ectomorph" with a thin body structure and relatively small muscles, strength training is likely something that will make you faster.

Speaking in very general terms, the triathletes who will commonly benefit the most

You must be cautious and conservative when starting your weight lifting and plyometric programs.

from strength training, besides ectomorphs, are women and those over the age of 50. But don't assume that this is true in your case just because you fall into one of these categories. I've worked with many athletes who were not easily placed in a category. If you're unsure, all you can do is to try strength training and see what happens. You may be pleasantly surprised that you become faster and more powerful, or you may discover that lifting weights builds too much bulk.

Now let's get started studying the details of plyometric and strength training and how you can use them to improve performance.

PLYOMETRIC TRAINING

Plyometric training consists of explosive bounding and jumping drills. It was briefly introduced in Chapter 12 when I told you about the strides workout. Perhaps the perfect workout for improving your running efficiency, plyometric training combines fast running with a focus on form on a fairly soft surface, such as grass, and bounding drills between the fast-form runs. While there is some research showing that plyometric training improves cycling, it's most effective in improving running power and speed. It trains the neuromuscular system to make quick and powerful contractions. This benefits your running by making you faster.

Looking at running from a strictly biomechanical perspective, there are three things you can do to run faster. One is to increase your stride length. Another is to quicken your cadence. The third is to reduce your ground contact time. This last one has to do with how long the foot remains in contact with the ground after the initial footstrike. We're talking milliseconds here, but fast

runners stay on the ground for a much shorter time than slow runners. In fact, each of these three contributors to fast running is individually quite small, but taken together over a long run, they can amount to several minutes.

You could devote a great deal of your valuable running time simply to doing plyometric drills, but that isn't necessary. Because the changes you're making to the neuromuscular system are tiny and it will take several weeks before you see noticeable improvements in stride length, cadence, and ground contact time, I'd recommend taking a long-term approach. Trying to force your body to adapt quickly is a sure way to end up injured. Doing strides with plyometrics two or three times each week along with about eight strides in a session (each stride takes about 20 seconds), especially in the early base period when you're working on running efficiency, will keep the risk low and allow a thorough adaptation. After 6 to 8 weeks of such training, you can go into a maintenance mode with one or two such sessions per week for the remainder of your preparation for the next A-priority race.

The combination of strides and plyometrics can be a workout on its own when preceded by a long warm-up and followed by a long cooldown, or you can use it as part of the warm-up for another run workout. Such training should be done only when you are fresh and rested. Doing it when you are fatigued will cause your body to produce less muscular power—exactly the opposite of what you are trying to accomplish.

Two of the benefits of plyometrics are greater strength and resiliency to injury in your feet and lower legs. Figure 12.9 shows what the height- or distance-bounding drill looks like. Start off doing the strides-plyometrics workouts with your nor-

Plyometric training consists of explosive bounding and jumping drills.

Plyometrics are most effective for improving running power and speed.

mal training shoes. After a few such sessions, do the workout with lightweight shoes such as racing flats. Eventually, after your feet and lower legs get stronger, you should be able to do all of the strides and plyometrics barefoot. Always do this workout on a fairly soft surface, such as grass. Before going barefoot, check to make sure there aren't any sharp objects or animal droppings on your run course. It's also best not to do them barefoot if you have a cut on your foot.

The bottom line here is never to stop doing the strides-plyometrics workout. It should be the most frequent workout of all your running sessions. It will improve your running speed by making you more economical. What you should *not* do is try to force your stride length to increase or your ground contact time to decrease. Doing so will only make you slower and less efficient. Be patient and allow the strides-plyometrics workouts to make the changes gradually. These changes will be imperceptible at first. Hang in there for the long term to realize the benefits.

If foul weather forces you to train indoors on a treadmill on a day when you were going to do strides, you can do the 20-second fast-form runs with the treadmill in the level setting. But doing plyometrics on a treadmill is not a good idea. Instead, jump rope. Double- and single-leg rope jumping is a simple form of plyometrics. It forces you to stay on the balls of your feet with a quick hopping motion.

STRENGTH TRAINING

Now let's move on to another way of improving your performance by further enhancing your neuromuscular system. In the last 20 years or so, strength training has become a common way for endurance athletes to train. A training program of only aerobic endurance exercise will improve your strength, but it has limits. The ceiling for strength development from such training is quite low compared with what it can be if you regularly focus on muscle development. Improving your strength a bit beyond what endurance training produces will increase your power and improve your efficiency. That means greater speed and less wasted energy. The usual way of doing this is with weight lifting.

Besides greater strength, there are several other reasons why lifting weights is beneficial for your race performance. The most critical is power. Power plays a key role in reaching a high performance level in endurance sports. Power is the product of force and speed:

Force × Speed = Power

Force results from neuromuscular strength and can be easily developed with weight training. Speed has to do with cadence. In this section, we will examine the strength component. The drills in Chapter 12 will improve your cadence.

Another reason for weight lifting is injury prevention. One scientific review of research studies on weight lifting with a total of 26,610 subjects found that it reduces the chance of injury by about half. What we normally think of as the best way to prevent injuries—stretching—was not found to prevent injuries at all. Soft-tissue breakdowns are the greatest impediment to consistent training. So by lifting weights you're not only becoming more powerful, you're also reducing the risk for lost training time.

Strength training has also been shown in recent research to reduce fatigue in the latter

Strength training will increase power and improve efficiency.

portions of a long endurance race. The combination of greater power and greater endurance helps you to finish a race strongly.

And finally, lifting weights increases bone density. This is an especially important benefit for older triathletes, who are typically at high risk for osteopenia and osteoporosis.

I've had endurance athletes in a wide variety of sports lift weights for more than 30 years and have found it to be the most effective form of training they can do aside from their primary sport training.

Weight Lifting Language

Before getting into the details of how to include weight lifting in your training program, it's important that you understand the language of strength building. The following are a few terms that will be used in the explanations of a proposed weight lifting program.

Free weights and machines. The illustrations for the program that follows show an athlete using free weights for many of the exercises, such as squats (Figure 13.1) and step-ups (Figure 13.4). Free weights must be held in your hands and balanced during the exercise. Balancing the load helps to improve small-muscle and core strength, but it's risky. You may fall or drop a weight. Some of the other exercises illustrated below show the athlete using strength machines, as for the leg press (Figure 13.6) and leg curl (Figure 13.7). Balance is not required with machines, so they are considerably safer. The downside, however, is that the small muscles that contribute to balance are not strengthened. If you are new to lifting weights, machines are probably the better way to go.

Sets and reps. A weight lifting workout is made up of several exercises to build strength. Each exercise consists of several repetitions. One of the strength building phases, for example, calls for doing 8 to 12 reps. That makes up 1 set. The following guidelines may call for 3 sets with a brief recovery break after each.

Load. This has to do with how heavy the weight is that you are lifting. Throughout each strength training phase, the loads are increased at the same time that the number of reps for each exercise is decreased. As the loads are slowly increased over several weeks, the body slowly adapts and grows stronger.

Repetition maximum (1RM). How great the load is for a given set of an exercise is typically based on how heavy the greatest load is that you can lift one time for that exercise. This is called *1RM*. The loads are then prescribed according to percentages of 1RM. For example, you may be instructed to use a load that is 80 percent of 1RM. The downside of this system is that you must challenge yourself to do one maximal effort periodically to find your 1RM. That's risky. You may become injured. If you are highly experienced in the weight room, then your risk is low. But if you're not an experienced weight lifter, I'd suggest a less risky method.

You can determine loads in the program that follows based on Table 13.1. To use this table, select a load you think you can lift only 4 to 10 times for a given exercise. Then see how many reps you can do with that load. Find your reps in the left-hand column and look to the right of it for your factor. To determine your predicted 1RM for that exercise, divide the load you lifted

Lifting weights increases bone density.

by the appropriate factor. Let's say you did 9 squats with a load of 80 pounds. The factor for 9 is 0.775. Dividing 80 by 0.775 predicts a 1RM of 103 pounds. This is a much less risky way of finding your 1RM for each exercise you do.

Another way to find your load for an exercise is merely to guess and see how many reps you can do. If you did more than is called for, then increase the load and try again. You'll soon determine the correct load for the exercise. From then on, you'll adjust the loads up and down based on how many reps you're supposed to do in a certain phase.

Recovery. Each of the phases in the following weight lifting program lists how many minutes you should spend recovering after each set. The purpose here is to make sure you have adequately recovered before doing the next set. If the recoveries are too short, you will not be able to lift as great a load as you are capable of lifting for the prescribed number of reps. The exercise then becomes an endurance workout. Because you are already doing plenty of endurance training outside the weight room, this is of little value. To build strength, and therefore power, you need to be able to challenge yourself with each set's load. That means starting each exercise well recovered.

Spotter. Some exercises, such as squats, involve the use of quite heavy loads with free weights. Your balance may be challenged, especially when you use heavy loads. It's wise to have a training partner—a "spotter"—who can assist you with balancing the load and guide you through the exercise. This reduces your risk for falling or dropping the weight.

TABLE 13.1 **Determining Your 1RM**

REPS	FACTOR
4	0.90
5	0.875
6	0.85
7	0.825
8	0.80
9	0.775
10	0.75

Find how many reps you can do for a given exercise. Divide your load for that exercise set by the corresponding factor to establish your 1RM for the exercise.

Concentric and eccentric contractions. Muscles always work in one of two ways—concentrically or eccentrically. In a concentric contraction, the muscle gets shorter as the load is lifted. This is like doing an arm curl with a hand-held weight; as you lift the weight up, the muscle shortens. In an eccentric contraction, the muscle gets longer as the weight is lowered. Imagine doing an arm curl in which you start with the weight near your shoulder, where it was when you finished the concentric lift. Now slowly lower the weight to waist height. As you do this, the muscle gets longer as the elbow joint opens up. The muscle is stretching as it tries to control the weight going down. Every strength exercise has a concentric and an eccentric component. You lift the weight (concentric), then you set it back down (eccentric).

You are capable of handling a much greater load when doing eccentric (lowering the weight) exercises. But eccentric exercises also place a great deal more strain on the muscle if the load is great enough. It's also usually a risky movement. So the weight must be set back down cautiously.

To build strength, start each exercise well recovered.

Speed of movement. Some of the exercises you will read about in the following program call for *ballistic* movement. These are often described as "explosive" lifts. In other words, the concentric portions are done very quickly—as fast as you can move the load. The loads are considerably lighter than those used for the more traditional slow movements, which are done with heavy weights. The ballistic loads are usually best as 50 percent or less of 1RM. This type of exercise is better at producing quick power, such as when you are running. The foot's ground contact must be very short if you are to run fast. It's *much* briefer than the time it takes to push the pedal on your bike through the entire downstroke, even at a very fast cadence. So, as you'll see shortly, I recommend ballistic movements with light loads for run-specific exercises and slow movements with heavy loads for bike-specific exercises. Research shows that both light ballistic and heavy slow exercises improve running power. There isn't much research on ballistic exercises, however.

When you are doing ballistic exercises, the concentric contraction (lifting the weight) is the movement that is done explosively; the eccentric portion (lowering the weight) is done slowly.

Replicating a sport's movements. There is little reason to do exercises that aren't similar to the sport in which you are trying to become stronger and more powerful. They can be a complete waste of your valuable training time when it comes to improving triathlon performance. For example, doing arm curls will not make you a faster cyclist. In the same way, knee extensions are certainly more similar than arm curls to what is done when you are pedaling a bike. But exercise can be improved in terms of sports speci-

ficity. Exercises such as squats, leg presses, and step-ups come much closer to replicating the movements used in pedaling a bike.

Multijoint exercises. The sports in triathlon involve the use of several joints that are driven by contracting muscles at the same time. Again, consider pedaling a bike. As you push down on the pedal, the knee doesn't extend in isolation from the hip and ankle. They all move at the same time. That's why knee extensions aren't as effective as squats or several other exercises I'll soon introduce in building pedaling-specific strength. When you are working on acquiring greater strength and power for a specific propulsive movement in a given sport, it's always best to do exercises involving all of the primary joints of that movement.

Balancing muscle strength. The exception to the multijoint exercise guideline presented above occurs when you are balancing muscle strength. Joint motion is controlled by two or more muscles. The working muscle for a joint is called the *agonist*. When the agonist is working, the other muscles for that joint are relaxing. They are the *antagonists*. For example, the elbow joint is controlled by a pair of muscles: the *biceps* and the *triceps*. When you are doing an arm curl, the biceps is the agonist and the triceps is the antagonist. But when you are doing a push-up, the triceps becomes the agonist and the biceps the antagonist.

There should be healthy ratio of strength between the two. If the agonist becomes too powerful, there is a risk for damage to the antagonist. So it's sometimes a good idea also to build strength in the antagonist to protect it from injury. The best example of this in triathlon is the quadriceps muscle of the thigh, which can become very strong when exercises such as squats are done. That presents some risk to the hamstrings, which are the antagonists when you are running or pedaling a bike. The antagonists may be strengthened by using a muscle-isolated exercise rather than a multijoint exercise. So you'll see leg curls in the following program to strengthen the hamstrings. Also, the loads and reps for the triathlon antagonist muscles are not the same in every phase as those for the agonists.

Other Weight Lifting Considerations

Weight lifting is no less complex than swimming, biking, and running. The following guidelines will help you avoid injury while you increase the potential for making significant strength and performance gains.

Workout spacing. Weight lifting sessions should be spaced as evenly as possible throughout the week. If you do two or three such workouts in a week, as is recommended for the early base period, and they are too closely spaced, there will be several back-to-back days with no strength sessions. That's all right when you are in a maintenance phase, but it's counterproductive when you are trying to build strength. Excessive spacing makes it difficult to make gains because strength is lost during those several days without weight lifting. Spacing sessions as evenly as possible throughout the week allows time for the muscles to adapt, which occurs during a couple of days of recovery, but not so much time away from strength work that excessive gains are lost. For example, two weekly sessions of weight lifting on Monday and Friday are preferable to

lifting on Monday and Tuesday. If you lift three times per week, sessions on Tuesday, Thursday, and Saturday are preferable to lifting on Tuesday, Wednesday, and Thursday.

Warm-up and cooldown. Just as before swimming, biking, and running workouts, there should be a warm-up before lifting weights. And as with the three sports, a cooldown afterward is beneficial. Let's start with the warm-up.

There are two steps in a strength training warm-up routine. The first is to increase blood flow slowly to the muscles that will soon be challenged by lifting heavy loads. As you'll see, most of the exercises in the following program involve the legs, and you can increase blood flow to the legs by riding a stationary bike or running on a treadmill, assuming you are at a facility such as a health club. It takes only 5 to 15 minutes of gradually increasing aerobic movement to accomplish this. Then you are *almost* ready to do the first strength building exercise.

The second stage of warm-up involves making the movement of the exercise by doing a few reps with a light load. For example, if you are about to do squats, start by doing a few with body weight only. Emphasize technique while doing these. Now you're ready to start the exercise. Do this second-stage warm-up before each subsequent exercise.

After a challenging strength session, cool down by spinning for a few minutes on a bike or walking on a treadmill (5 minutes is plenty). Of the two, I think the bike is the better option. You will most likely have done some heavy lifting for your legs, which has a tendency to alter your pedaling mechanics and cadence negatively. A few minutes spent spinning with good technique

Weight lifting sessions should be spaced evenly throughout the week.

After a challenging strength session, cool down by spinning for a few minutes on a bike or walking on a treadmill.

at a relatively high cadence will help to restore your neuromuscular firing sequence.

Exercise order. As you'll see later in this chapter, there is a preferred order for doing strength exercises. I recommend doing the exercises that involve the heaviest loads first. It's better (and safer) to lift heavy loads when you are fresh rather than fatigued. It's also safer to alternate muscle groups and movements. For example, you should avoid doing two exercises for hip-knee-ankle extension (such as squats and step-ups) back to back. It's best to insert another exercise with a different movement and muscle group between them.

Starting a new phase. When starting a new phase of strength training involving heavier loads than what you've been using, be conservative in selecting loads in the first session. While challenging yourself to lift heavier loads is a good idea at certain times in the season, the first session is not the time to do it. Save that for the subsequent workouts, when you are likely to have a better idea of how to challenge yourself.

New exercises. If unsure how to do an exercise, have someone who is experienced at weight lifting show you. Strength building is certainly a high-risk/high-reward form of training. The risk that you will injure yourself by doing the exercise incorrectly is quite high. Improper technique for many of the exercises, especially those involving heavy loads, is a sure way to get hurt. Ask for help. You might also have someone shoot a video of you doing the lifts and then search the Internet for examples of good technique to see how yours compares.

Do the exercises that involve the heaviest loads first.

Lifting to failure. You've probably heard of the practice of lifting until you can't lift the load again; it's a quite common practice among serious weight lifters. They often do reps of a given workout until they are unable to lift the weight one last time and need help setting it down. That may be all right for them, but I wouldn't recommend it for triathletes. The risk is much too great. Pay attention to how your muscles feel on each exercise and stop 1 or 2 reps short of failure. The strength benefits of going to failure instead of stopping short of it are insignificant, and your risk for injury is considerably higher.

Time available. The weight lifting program described below assumes you are like most triathletes and have limited time for training because of other responsibilities. That's why there are only a few exercises. These are the ones that are most likely to result in performance gains. Feel free to do more if you have the time, energy, and inclination.

Muscle mass. Some athletes, especially young males, are likely to bulk up when lifting weights. While that's good for strength, it can be counterproductive to triathlon performance. At some point, the increase in muscle size becomes detrimental to performance. That's a good reason to limit how much strength training you do and how many exercises you include in your weight lifting program. It's also why I suggest that the emphasis on serious weight lifting last only a handful of weeks. After those few weeks are over, strength training goes from strength building mode to maintenance mode.

Loads also play a role here. The program I recommend below builds up over a handful of weeks to heavier loads done with a few reps. There is research showing that lighter loads with a high number of reps done to exercise failure produces much the same muscle strength, but the high number of reps is also more likely to produce excessive muscle mass. Very few triathletes need to weigh more.

Food and strength. What and when you eat play a role in strength building. Body size and the difficulty of the workout have to do with how much you eat. Research suggests that eating 10 to 25 grams (0.35–0.875 ounces) of leucine-rich protein immediately after the session, but at least within 3 hours of lifting, enhances strength gains. This will help your body rebuild the tissues that have broken down as a result of the strain of lifting heavy loads.

The protein source doesn't have to be anything expensive, exotic, or designed by a scientist. Real food will do quite nicely. Common protein- and leucine-rich foods that can be stored in your refrigerator for a quick post-workout snack, and that provide about 10 grams (0.35 ounces) of protein and roughly 1,000 milligrams (0.035 ounces) of leucine, are boiled eggs (2 medium), cheddar cheese (1.5 ounces, or about 45 grams), and milk (10 ounces, or about 295 milliliters).

Special groups and weight lifting. Junior triathletes (those under the age of 18) should be especially cautious with weight lifting. The growth plates of the bones in young people may still be developing and are susceptible to damage from heavy loads. This is more likely to be an issue for juniors under age 16, but there are considerable differences in physical maturity at this age. That doesn't mean juniors shouldn't lift at all. For youngsters who show an interest, I'd recommend starting a weight training program at about age 12 with very light loads that focuses on developing and refining the techniques of common strength exercises. The youngsters may also benefit from doing ballistic exercises with very light loads. Like all exercise programs for youth, the program should be driven only by fun. At this stage of development, training schedules and strict routines are not recommended.

Triathletes over the age of 50 may reap the greatest benefits from weight lifting. Older endurance athletes' performances are often limited by their loss of muscle mass. They are also likely to experience a loss of bone density, making them susceptible to fractures. Strength training is likely to produce significant improvement in muscle power while rebuilding bones.

Young elite triathletes, both male and female, who have been training and racing for a long time probably don't need as much resistance training as age groupers. They are likely to reap a much smaller gain in performance, if any at all. Their youth is a factor in having a lot of natural power. And the mere fact that they are racing at an elite level says a lot about their innate physiology.

Those new to the sport are likely to benefit significantly from weight lifting. The most common issue for novices, however, is finding available time. They are typically going through a lifestyle change in their first year in the sport, and trying to fit swimming, biking, and running into their weekly routines is already a challenge. Wedging in yet another sport-related activity may not seem possible. Although weight lifting would definitely benefit their growth as triathletes, newbies will make rapid performance gains just by training in three sports. If you are a novice

Real food supplies plenty of protein. You don't need supplements.

in triathlon, I'd recommend omitting the maximum strength (MS) phase that is described later in this chapter. You will make great gains without it and keep your risk for injury low.

Strength Training Program

Here, I'm going to suggest the best strength building exercises by sport. After all three of the sports have been covered, I will lay out the phases and a suggested workout procedure. As in all forms of training, regardless of the sport, there are many ways to improve strength through weight lifting. If you have a program that has worked well for you in the past, stick with it. If you believe that sport-specific strength is a limiter for you, then strongly consider incorporating this program into your periodization plan, as suggested in Chapters 7, 8, and 9.

In the next few pages, I will describe strength training exercises by sport. The sports are listed in the order in which such training is most likely to be beneficial. That order is bike, run, then swim.

Bike

Heavy-load weight lifting has been shown by many research studies to be quite effective for cycling. If the bike leg of a triathlon is typically a limiter for you, then you are likely to make great gains from a strength building program as described here. How do you know if biking is a limiter? The most straightforward way is to see how you typically rank in your age-group race results for each leg of the triathlon—swim, bike, and run. For example, if you consistently rank in the top-10 split times for swimming and running, but well outside the top 10 on the bike, then cycling is limiting your performance. Weight lifting is likely to help you make great gains here.

The key to making significant gains is to build up to lifting heavy loads with a low number of reps by doing exercises that primarily work the extension of the hip, knee, and ankle joints at the same time. This extension imitates the primary movement that propels you when you are riding a bike. The power you produce results in part from how much muscular force you apply to the pedal in the downstroke. The more force you can generate without increasing your perceived effort, the faster you will become on the bike. You'll also climb better. Of course, muscular force isn't the only determiner of bike power. The other component is cadence. That's what Chapter 12 discussed. Here, we will look strictly at how to produce more force by strengthening the muscles that extend the hips, knees, and ankles.

There are six common weight lifting exercises that develop the muscles that drive these joints. While slightly different, they all benefit muscular force for pedaling. The exercises described in the following pages are the double-leg squat, single-leg squat, dead lift, step-up, lunge, and leg press. Choose one or two of these exercises that you will do in each weight lifting session. Or, you may opt to do several of them in the interest of variety over the course of the season. Note that the first five exercises use free weights; only the last one uses a machine. Many health clubs and gyms have machines that may be used for some of the first five should you decide to avoid the risks of free weights.

The leg curl is not a power-enhancing exercise for cycling. Its purpose is to balance the strength of the three hamstring muscles on the back of the thigh with that of the quadriceps muscle on the front of the thigh.

Double-Leg Squat

The *double-leg squat* (Figure 13.1) is perhaps the exercise for hip-knee-ankle extension that is most commonly used by experienced triathletes. The figure shows the athlete using a barbell, but the exercise can be done just as well with a dumbbell in each hand or even with a weight-loaded, heavy-duty backpack. The following instructions will help you learn the movement if you haven't done it before.

→ Consider wearing a weight belt to support your back, especially during the MS phase.

→ Stand with a barbell on your shoulders just above the scapulae (or a dumbbell in each hand) and with your feet apart about the same distance as your bike pedals. That's about 7 to 8 inches (18–20 centimeters) between your insteps. Your feet should be pointing straight ahead just as they are when you pedal your bike.

→ Stand with your back straight and head up.

→ Squat until your thighs are almost parallel to the floor—about the same knee bend as when your pedal is at the 2-o'clock position.

→ Keep your knees pointed straight ahead and over your feet as you squat.

→ Return to the start position with your back straight and eyes still looking straight ahead so that your head is up. Do *not* look down.

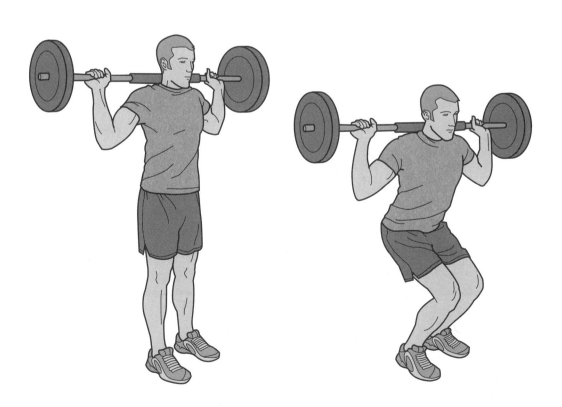

FIGURE 13.1 The double-leg squat

Single-Leg Squat

The advantage of doing the *single-leg squat* rather than the double-leg squat is that the load can be considerably lighter, reducing the risk for injury. The downside is that it requires good balance because you're standing on just one leg, with the other supported behind you as shown in Figure 13.2.

→ With a dumbbell in each hand (or with a barbell across your shoulders and just above the scapulae), stand about 2 feet (about 60 centimeters) from a bench or other approximately knee-high platform, facing away from it.

→ Reach back and place the top of one foot on the bench.

→ With your back straight and head up, squat on the forward leg until your thigh is almost parallel to the floor. The knee bend should be similar to what it is at the 2-o'clock pedaling position. You may need to adjust your distance from the bench to get the right knee bend.

→ With your back still straight and eyes looking forward, not down, return to the starting position.

→ Repeat the exercise in the same way for the other leg.

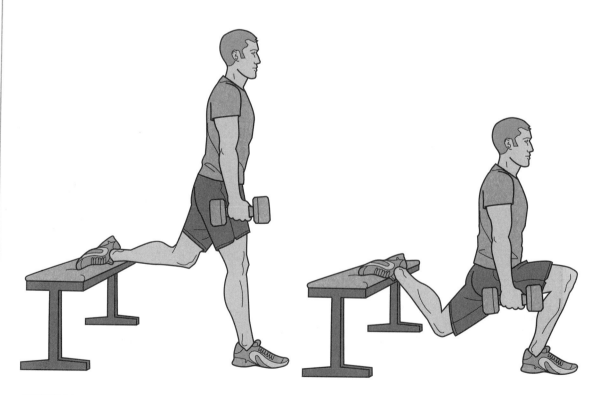

FIGURE 13.2 The single-leg squat

Dead Lift

The *dead lift* is an excellent exercise for building leg extension strength; however, it is perhaps a bit riskier than the squat exercises because those new to this exercise typically use their back muscles to do most of the lifting instead of their legs. This is one exercise in which you are likely to need some expert assistance to get it right. Another problem is that if you are using a fairly light load, as you should be when starting the season, the plates on the ends of the bar are small, requiring you to reach quite low with the knees considerably bent. Some gyms have floor racks or lightweight adaptors resembling large plates that may be put on the ends of the bar so that you start in a higher position. You can also do this exercise with dumbbells, which may be better for novices. Figure 13.3 illustrates how to do a dead lift.

→ Stand facing the barbell with your feet apart about the same distance as your bike pedals—approximately 7 to 8 inches (18–20 centimeters).

→ Start in a full squatting position with your knees bent so that your thighs are nearly parallel to the floor.

→ With your back straight, head up, and eyes looking forward (never down), reach down and grasp the bar with both hands slightly farther apart than your feet.

→ Stand up while using only your legs to do the heavy lifting—not your back.

→ Return to the starting position by using your legs while keeping your back straight, your head up, and your eyes looking forward.

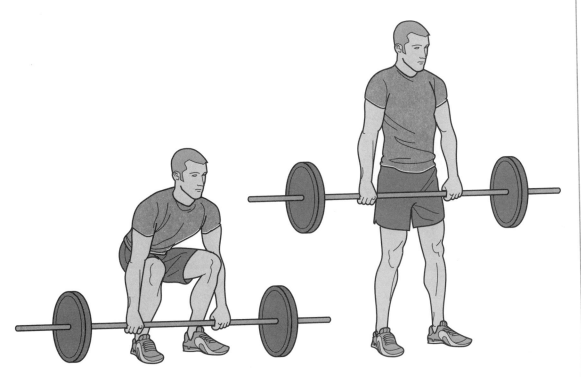

FIGURE 13.3 The dead lift

Step-Up

The *step-up* is a common exercise that you will also see later in the section on running (with a slight variation). Once again, for cycling this is an excellent exercise for building leg extension strength. Figure 13.4 shows how it's done. While this figure shows the athlete using a barbell, you can also do it with dumbbells, which is somewhat safer because the center of gravity is lower. For this exercise, it's very important that you get the height of the bench or other platform right. You're trying to replicate the position your legs have on the bike when one pedal is at the 6-o'clock position and the other is at the 12-o'clock position.

→ Stand facing a low bench or other platform that is about 13 to 15 inches (33–38 centimeters) high with a barbell across your shoulders and just above the scapulae (or with a dumbbell in each hand). Tall athletes will use a higher bench than short athletes.

→ Place one foot on the bench. Your raised knee should be slightly below your hip so that your thigh is almost parallel to the floor.

→ With your back straight, head up, and eyes looking straight ahead (not down), step up onto the bench so that both feet are on it.

→ Step back down with the same foot returning to the start position, then repeat the movement.

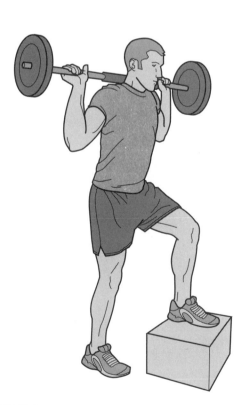
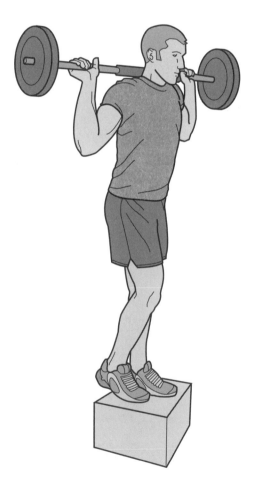

FIGURE 13.4 The step-up

Lunge

The *lunge* uses a lot of floor space because it involves taking long steps forward. It's a simple exercise but requires that you get the step distance right every time. Too short and you'll have a hard time getting low enough; too long and you place a great strain on the back leg's hip flexor. Figure 13.5 shows how it's done.

→ Stand tall with your feet together and a dumbbell in each hand (you can instead use a barbell across your shoulders).

→ Step forward placing your foot flat on the floor with your toes pointing straight ahead. Your knee should be directly over the forward foot and your weight mostly on that leg. The rear leg helps to maintain balance.

→ Lower your body until the forward thigh is almost parallel to the floor. The rear knee should come close to touching the floor.

→ Stand up and step forward with your back foot so that you return to the starting position.

→ Continue with a forward step with the other leg.

→ Keep your back straight and head up throughout the movement.

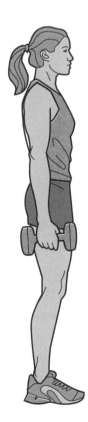
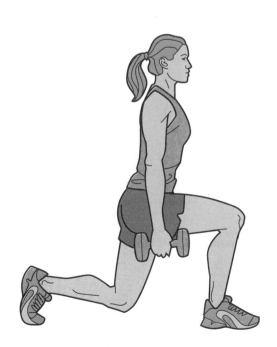

FIGURE 13.5 The lunge

Leg Press

The *leg press* is probably the safest of the leg extension exercises because it's done with a machine and doesn't require balancing heavy loads. But the loads here can be much heavier than with the other exercises, not only because there is no balancing but also because you're no longer lifting your body weight. So more external weight can be added to the machine. Figure 13.6 provides instructions.

→ Place your feet on the platform so they are about the same distance apart as your bike pedals—roughly 7 to 8 inches (18–20 centimeters). Your feet should point straight ahead—not flare outward.

→ With the platform in the low position, your knees should be at about the same bend as when you are pedaling with a foot at the 2-o'clock position. This means that the knee angle will be slightly greater than 90 degrees. Some machines have a handy locking mechanism that prevents the platform from going too low.

→ Press the platform up until your knees are almost straight and just short of locking out.

→ Lower the platform back to the start position.

→ Your knees should be in line with your feet throughout the movement—never turned outward or angled inward.

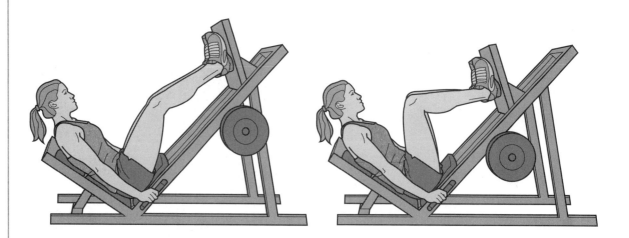

FIGURE 13.6 The leg press

Leg Curl

The purpose of doing leg curls is to help prevent hamstring strains due to an imbalance that is too great in favor of the quadriceps. The quad will always be stronger—perhaps twice as strong as the three hamstring muscles on the back of the thigh—and that kind of imbalance can lead to knee injuries. Some research suggests that women may have a greater need to strengthen their hamstrings because their quad-hamstrings imbalance may be even greater than men's. Focusing only on strengthening leg extension may compound the problem—thus the usefulness of this exercise to help balance things out.

Figure 13.7 shows a common hamstring exercise done on a machine. If you are doing your exercises in a home gym, you can use an elastic band, as shown in Figure 13.8.

→ Stand on the platform and bring one leg back to contact the lever.

→ Curl your leg to about a right angle at the knee. Return to starting position.

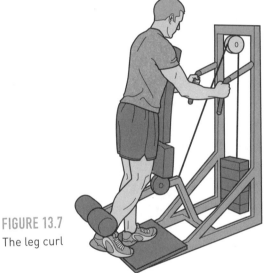
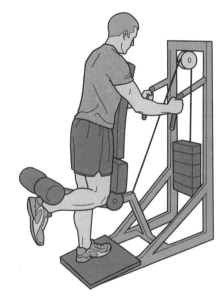

FIGURE 13.7
The leg curl

→ Put the loop of the elastic band around one ankle.

→ Lying prone, curl your leg to about a right angle at the knee. Return to starting position.

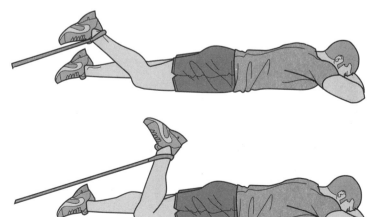

FIGURE 13.8 The alternative leg curl

Later in this chapter, you will read about how many sets and reps should be done at various times of the season for different exercises. Note that the leg curl exercise has smaller loads and more reps in some phases.

Run

While cycling seems to get the greater benefit from weight lifting, running power is also improved. If you do one or more of the above exercises for leg extension (along with leg curls), your running should improve. But I believe you can make even greater gains in running by doing ballistic weight lifting with lighter loads. So once again, you have an option here based on what you know about your race performance. If running is not a limiter, then doing more gym exercises for it may not prove beneficial. But if running is a limiter, I'd highly recommend incorporating one of the exercises that follow.

Recall from the section "Weight Lifting Language" that ballistic exercises are done very rapidly. The reason for this is to increase muscular power. In running, that pays off with a decrease in ground contact time. As you read in Chapter 12, a very brief footstrike is a hallmark of fast runners. So the following exercises, along with the plyometrics I suggested you do in the strides workout in Chapter 12, will help you shorten the time your foot is on the ground, thus increasing your speed.

Whenever you do ballistic weight lifting, the loads must be light. So for the following exercises, use loads of 50 percent of 1RM or less. Be aware that even though you are using light loads, explosive movements can still cause an injury due to poor technique or overuse. When doing these exercises, warm up with a very light load, perhaps only body weight, before progressing to somewhat heavier loads in the following sets.

There are two ballistic, power-building exercises I recommend for runners—the power step-up and the power clean. They are illustrated in Figures 13.9 and 13.10. Select one of these to do along with the cycling exercises described above if your weight lifting goal is to improve running.

Power Step-Up

The only differences between the step-up in Figure 13.4 and the *power step-up* described here are the lighter load and the speed of the movement. It's better to use handheld dumbbells rather than a barbell for the power step-ups to improve balance and to allow the arms to assist with the movement. Figure 13.9 shows how this exercise is done.

→ Stand facing a stable platform that is about 13 to 15 inches (33–38 centimeters) high with one foot resting on it and a light dumbbell in each hand.

→ Your back should be straight and your eyes looking straight ahead (not down).

→ Make a quick and explosive movement as you step up onto the platform by driving the back leg forward and up so that you finish with that knee in a nearly waist-high position.

→ Slowly return to the starting position and then repeat. Allow time for recovery between step-ups with your foot resting on the floor for approximately 5 seconds. Power development requires recovery.

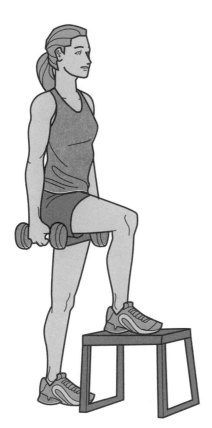
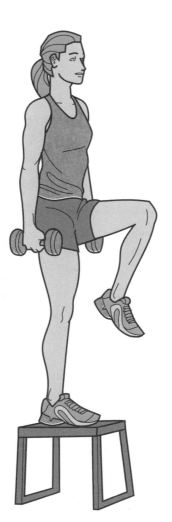

FIGURE 13.9 The power step-up

Power Clean

The *power clean* is an advanced power-building exercise that requires mastering a somewhat complex movement that is done explosively. This exercise is best learned initially by moving slowly and using a very light load. At first, that may be something as light as a broomstick. Eventually, you will progress to a bar only, and then perhaps to a bar with plates on it. The load is always less than 50 percent of 1RM. If you're unsure about what that load should be, err on the low side. Keep it light.

This exercise must be done with good technique to reduce the risk for injuring your back. If you are new to weight lifting, it's probably best to not attempt this exercise. The power step-up is probably the better choice for novices. Figure 13.10 shows how the power clean is done.

→ Start with the bar about halfway up your shins. Your knees should be bent, your head up, and your eyes looking forward (not down). Your butt is at about the same height as your knees.

→ Grasp the bar so that your palms are facing down with the knuckles forward of the bar.

→ In one continuous and explosive movement of the legs and arms, bring the bar to thigh height (your heels should come off the floor if it's truly explosive) and then continue moving the bar upward to shoulder height with your elbows flaring. Without pausing, rotate your arms so that the bar is resting on your hands with your elbows below the bar. Again, this must be a nonstop movement of the bar from the shin to the shoulders and done with primarily the legs used for lifting—not the back.

→ Set the weight down slowly by using your legs, not your back; rest for a few seconds, and then repeat. Recovery is necessary for building power.

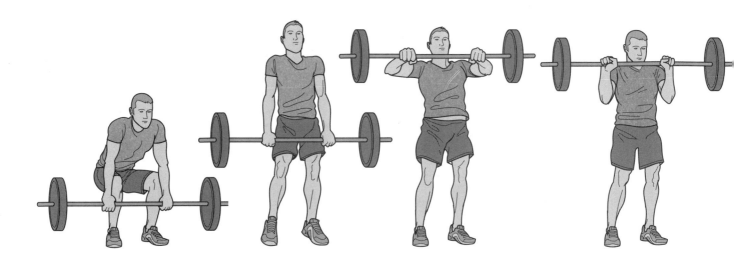

FIGURE 13.10 The power clean

Swim

Earlier in this chapter, I discussed the importance of replicating the movements of a sport when weight lifting. Building strength for movements that differ from what good technique in the sport calls for is largely a waste of time. You'll simply get stronger for a movement that's not used. Performance will not improve. This brings us to the challenge of improving strength for swimming. As mentioned at the start of this section, I'm describing strength exercises in the order of the sports that are most likely to benefit from such training. I've found that for most triathletes, swimming is the least likely to improve as a result of weight lifting.

The main reason for this is that the swim positions you must get into are very difficult to replicate in the gym. Recall from the PDLC swim technique described in Chapter 12 that the *L*

stands for length. Once you master this position, you'll find that you are rolled slightly to the side of your extended arm. Figure 13.11 illustrates this position. That is the "speedboat" position described in Chapter 12. It's very difficult to simulate this position in dryland training. But you can easily get into the "tugboat" position with no roll, which is to be avoided when swimming, for exercises such as lat pull-downs and push-ups. But all that means is that you are building strength for movement you shouldn't use and that will make you slower if you do.

There is one dryland exercise exception, but it doesn't require the use of weights or a weight machine. Just as in the alternative leg curl exercise shown earlier (Figure 13.8), you can use an elastic band to build strength while in the PDLC speedboat position. The exercise is called catch and pull.

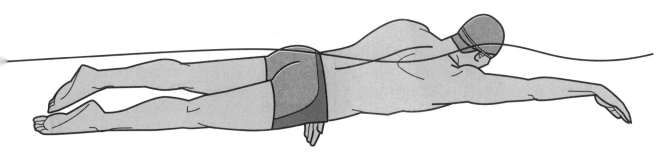

FIGURE 13.11 The long "speedboat" position of the freestyle stroke. Note the body roll.

Catch and Pull

I like this exercise because it improves your swimming strength while also reinforcing PDLC skill development. This is also a good way to warm up on race day when you can't get into the water before the start. Figure 13.12 shows how the catch and pull is done.

→ Stand facing the anchor point for an elastic band that is gripped with only one hand. Hold the band with the "catch" position— wrist bent and fingers pointing down.

→ Place the other hand on your hip.

→ Rotate your torso so that you are in a long, extended position with the torso slightly turned to the side of the extended arm.

→ Pull the extended arm backward and down as if catching the water with the fingers pointing at the floor (no death move!).

→ Continue pulling until your hand is at your waist. As your hand and arm move backward, rotate your shoulders until they are parallel to the floor.

→ To increase the load, stand farther away from the anchor point.

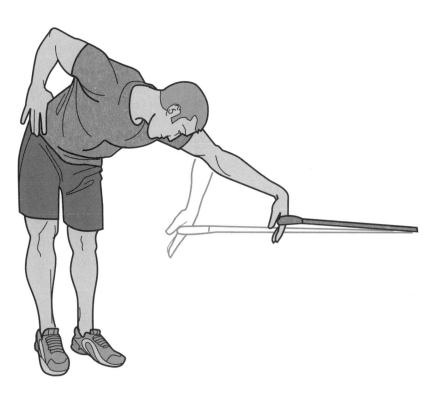

FIGURE 13.12 Catch and pull exercise

Sport-Specific Strength Training Alternatives

I've coached many athletes who didn't like going to the gym to lift weights. There have also been some who didn't have easy access to a gym or simply didn't have the time to devote to lifting.

How about you? Can you wedge a gym workout into your day? What if you have the time and would like to do some strength training, but don't have a handy gym? One option is to create a home gym by purchasing some dumbbells, a platform with adjustable height, a heavy-duty backpack that can be loaded with weights for hip-knee-ankle extension exercises, rubber tubing with handles, and a weight belt. If you shop around for low prices, a couple of hundred dollars will be enough for everything you need to turn a corner of your basement, garage, or some other room into a very handy gym. Problem solved.

What if you simply don't enjoy lifting weights and you'd much rather be swimming, biking, or running? Should you lift anyway? The answer comes down to why you do triathlons. If it's for fun, which I expect it is, then don't do things that aren't fun. That may mean not lifting. Don't do what isn't fun.

Of course, if you don't lift weights for any of these common reasons, you are less likely to achieve your potential for high performance as a triathlete. Strength training has many benefits, as you've already read in this chapter. If you aren't going to lift weights, wouldn't it be nice if you could reap much the same rewards without lifting weights? Well, you can—or at least some of the same benefits. There are swim, bike, and run workouts that you can do to develop strength without ever lifting a weight. They will make you stronger and more powerful, although they

aren't quite as effective as weight lifting. Let's take a look at how you can do that by examining the three sports in the order in which the benefit of such training is the greatest. It's the same order you read about above—biking, then running, and finally swimming.

While what I'm going to teach you here has significant strength rewards, there are also risks you need to be aware of. Just like weight lifting, these alternatives also require putting much bigger force loads on your muscles, tendons, and joints. There isn't any other way to build strength. This is quite obvious in the gym while you're lifting weights. It may not be quite so obvious when you're swimming, biking, and running. But the risk is still there. Doing one of these workouts could cause an injury and end your training in one or more of the sports for days, if not weeks. On the bike, you will be putting a great deal of stress on the knees. If you are prone to knee injuries, you should avoid the bike workout below. For runners, the primary areas of concern are the lower legs and feet. For swimmers, it's the shoulders.

You must be cautious and conservative when doing any of these exercises. Moderation is the key. The first time you do any of them, do only 2 or 3 reps and hold back on how much effort you put into each. In each subsequent session, you can slowly increase the reps and the effort as your body adapts to the loads. And of course be sure to warm up well before doing any of these workouts.

Biking

We're starting with biking because it's the sport where gains in strength performance are most likely to happen. I call this workout *force reps*. It's the most basic of the on-the-bike workouts for building strength. It involves using a small, steep hill and high gears. Having a power meter is very beneficial because it gives immediate feedback on the magnitude of each effort. You'll have to go by feel if you don't have a power meter, which is not a very precise method when it comes to determining if you are, for example, making progress over time. A heart rate monitor is of no use in this workout.

For the details of how to do force reps, go to Appendix C and look for "Muscular Force." The first workout listed there is "F1 Force Reps."

This workout calls for 3 sets of 3 reps each. Each set of this workout, with recoveries, takes 10 to 20 minutes. So doing 3 sets with a warm-up and cooldown requires at least 45 minutes and possibly as much as 90 minutes. Again, start conservatively with only 1 set and then gradually add more sets.

I'd advise you to do an easy workout the following day. The workout may not seem all that challenging while you are doing force reps, but fatigue often shows up the next day with very tired, and possibly very sore, muscles.

Running

Force reps for running are an alternative strength building workout for the triathlete who doesn't lift weights. Just like force reps on the bike, this run workout may be done along with weight lifting in the early base period. The combination of these two types of strength builders places great strain on the legs and so should be done with caution, if at all. I'll also describe an alternative version of force reps in which a weight vest is used; it will increase the reward in the form of greater force and therefore power, but it will also greatly increase the risk for injury. As with

the alternative cycling workout described above, when first doing this workout, you must be conservative with the number of reps, and also with the loads if you are using a weight vest. Start at low levels of both and over the course of a few sessions make cautious increases.

I've seen the force reps workout develop a great deal of running force, which, when combined with the strides workout in Chapter 12 and run training in general, ultimately produces more powerful and faster runners. Just as with the bike force reps, you need a steep hill. The hill can be quite short—about 10 to 15 yards/meters. It's best to do these on a grassy hill because the softer surface reduces some of the leg stress and therefore the risk for injury. If you decide to try the workout with a weight vest, wait until after you've done the workouts two or three times without it.

There are a few things to look for when purchasing a weight vest. The most obvious is fit. The vest should be rather snug so it doesn't bounce when you are running, yet not so tight as to restrict breathing. Look for one that has Velcro straps so the fit can be adjusted. Also look for a vest that allows you to adjust the amount of weight that can be carried. This usually involves small pockets into which weights can be placed. For the running force reps workout, you'll likely use about 5 to 10 percent of your body weight. However, the vest may also be used for weight lifting in a home gym, so you may want to have the option to greatly increase the load well above 10 percent of body weight. With a home gym, the vest replaces the possible need for a heavy-duty backpack for doing hip-knee-ankle extension exercises, such as squats and step-ups. For these gym exercises, you probably want a vest that can

Fatigue often shows up the next day with very tired muscles.

be adjusted to provide a much heavier load—30 to 50 pounds (14–23 kilograms).

For the details of this workout, turn to Appendix D and look under "Muscular Force" for workout MF1.

Again, I want to warn you to be very cautious with this workout. As with all such high-reward workouts, there is also a great risk. You must manage that risk. If at any time during this session you sense an unusual strain in a leg muscle, tendon, or joint, stop the workout immediately. No amount of running fitness is worth an injury. Be cautious and conservative with force reps, especially when using a weight vest.

Whether doing bike or run force reps, do this workout only one time per week for each sport. Within 6 weeks, you should be aware of feeling much stronger during this session. If you have a power meter on your bike, you'll be able to measure the improvement precisely as a max power increase. For running, if using the same hill and start point for each session, you should go farther up the hill in a given number of steps, indicating that you are getting stronger. This latter measurement method for gauging run progress also works on the bike if you don't have a power meter.

Swimming

There are also alternatives to lifting weights for the advanced triathlete who wants to build greater strength for swimming. I've already told you about using an elastic stretch cord to help you build swim strength while simulating the PDLC positions. Closely mimicking the swim postures and movements is key to developing effective strength on the deck. Of course, the best way to simulate swimming is to swim. So you may make greater neuromuscular gains by doing drills in the pool rather than by doing any dryland exercises.

When it comes to swimming, the most critical component of performance for most triathletes is technique. There is little reason to work on developing greater strength until you have refined the movements of swimming. If you are changing your movement pattern to the PDLC method described in Chapter 12, I'd recommend not doing any strength building until the changes have become well established. During these few weeks, concentrate your swim training on the fast-form 25s workout described in that chapter and listed in Appendix B under the heading "Speed Skills." Look for workout SS1.

Your new stroke technique is becoming well established when it happens without you concentrating on it. You can confirm this with head-on and side-view video recordings. When your movement patterns are well established, it's time to move on to building swim strength on the deck with an elastic cord, or in the pool with an alternative workout. You can find this in Appendix B under the "Muscular Force" category as workout MF1. You can read the details there. The quick summary is that it's the same workout as fast-form 25s, only with one change. When working on swim strength, you obviously can't use to hills to reap the positive benefits of overcoming gravity, as you can with cycling and running. The alternatives are to use hand paddles or wear a T-shirt while swimming. The paddles emphasize the catch portion of the stroke and simulate doing stretch cord pulls on the deck. Wearing a T-shirt increases the drag of swimming and causes you to work harder to overcome the resistance, so that you develop more swim-specific strength.

The most critical component of swimming performance is technique.

Wearing a T-shirt increases the drag of swimming and causes you to work harder.

Whether you choose to use paddles or a T-shirt, simply do the fast-form 25s just as before, only now with greater resistance. But be aware that just like the bike and run force reps, this workout has a certain amount of risk, especially to the shoulders if your length (*L* in PDLC) is too short, as when you are tugboat swimming. You must treat this drill with caution, and you must always include an adequate warm-up of 10 to 15 minutes in the pool, where you ratchet up the intensity followed by a few fast-form 25s *without* paddles or T-shirt. This portion of the workout is to reinforce good technique—especially length. After a few of these, it's time to do force reps.

To keep things simple, I recommend doing the force reps with 3 sets of 3 reps each and with long recoveries between reps and longer recoveries between sets (see workout SS1 in Appendix B for details). As with the bike and run force reps described above, start conservatively by doing only 1 set the first time. Over the course of a few weeks, increase the load gradually.

Some advanced triathletes may be able to do the MF1 swim workout two or three times a week as a part of another, longer session. Intermediate athletes (those in their second and third years in the sport) should probably limit this workout to once or perhaps twice per week. If in doubt, select the lower options. Novices should avoid this workout in their first year as triathletes and instead focus only on refining their swim technique.

Core Strength

You've probably heard a lot about core strength training and know the basic exercises. But I've found that most athletes really don't understand what the "core" is. Most seem to think it means strong abdominal muscles. It goes well beyond that. Core strength could also be called *torso strength*. It has to do with the small and big muscles from your armpits to your groin. These core muscles stabilize the spine, support the shoulders and hips, and transfer force between the arms and legs. Having a strong core ensures that you can effectively use any strength gains made in the arms and legs. Good core strength also reduces the likelihood of having lower back problems, which are all too common. Your core strength is very much akin to the foundation of a house. The more solid and sounder it is, the more stable the structure built onto it will be.

Poor core strength may show up in several ways. It's most obvious in running. Poor core strength is evidenced by a dropping hip on the side of a recovery leg, with the knee of the support leg collapsing slightly inward regardless of what the foot may be doing. Especially in running, injury is common when core strength is inadequate.

Poor core strength is less obvious in swimming and cycling, but it still affects technique. In swimming, it may result in "fishtailing"—the legs and hips wiggle from side to side as the catch is made. This is sometimes also due to faulty stroke mechanics, so it's hard to differentiate. In cycling, poor core strength may show up as a side-to-side rocking of the shoulders and spine when the pedal is pushed down, even when the saddle is the right height and the rider is not excessively mashing the pedals. This rocking is generally most evident when the rider is climbing while seated.

There is little doubt, even if it's not obvious in the athlete's movements, that poor core strength results in a loss of muscular force in all three sports. Having weak core muscles but strong arms and legs is like shooting a cannon out of a canoe.

How do you know if your core strength is adequate? One way is to have a physical therapist do an assessment. Find someone who works with endurance athletes and tell him or her that you would like a head-to-toe exam to pinpoint weaknesses and imbalances that could reduce performance or lead to injury. And find out what the therapist recommends to correct any shortcomings found. These fixes may be strengthening exercises, flexibility exercises, or postural improvement. This is perhaps the best way of finding out, but there is a cost. I have each of the athletes I coach examined by a physical therapist every winter. It provides a great start to the strength training program.

Another way to assess your core strength is to have someone make a video recording of you while running, then look for the dropping hip on the recovery side mentioned above. Run on a treadmill and shoot the video from the back. Tuck your shirt in so you can watch the waistband of your running shorts on the video to see if it dips from side to side when the recovery leg swings through. The waistband should remain stable with every stride. And check the knee of the support leg to see if it is buckling in slightly. You will probably have to view the video in slow motion several times to see the unwanted movements.

Now let's take a look at a few common exercises for building core strength. I'll show you only a few of the possibilities; there are many other similar exercises. You can easily fit these into your training no matter how you develop strength—with a weight lifting session or sport-specific alternative exercises. They can be also done as a stand-alone workout or included following a swim, bike, or run session.

The most basic of the core exercises is the front plank. The side plank engages and develops a different group of core muscles from those developed by the front plank. The front plank with rows is an advanced exercise that places a greater strain on the core muscles.

Core strength is akin to the foundation of a house.

Front Plank

The key to this exercise is forming a straight line from head to toes without sagging or raising your hips. You may need to have someone help you get into this position the first few times you try it.

→ Lie on the floor face-down with your weight supported on your toes, hips, and elbows. Your elbows should be shoulder-width apart and directly below your shoulders.

→ Your arms should point straight forward from your elbows or pointed in slightly.

→ Raise yourself onto your toes and elbows as shown in Figure 13.13. Your body should create a straight line from your head to your toes without a sag or hump at your hips.

→ Hold the pose for about 30 seconds. That's 1 rep.

→ Lower your hips and rest for a minute or so after each exercise, and then repeat.

→ Do 3 reps in each session.

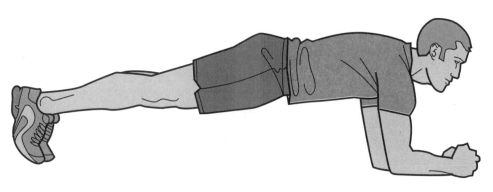

FIGURE 13.13 The front plank

Side Plank

The side plank is not a variation of the front plank because it targets a different set of core muscles. So don't substitute one exercise for the other; instead, do the front plank and the side plank in sequence.

→ Start on your side, with your hips on the floor, your feet stacked, and your upper body resting on your bent elbow.

→ Raise your hips up off the floor while balancing on the side of your lower foot and elbow, as shown in Figure 13.14.

→ Your legs, hips, shoulder, and head should form a straight line.

→ Your free hand may be held high, as shown in the figure, or placed on your hip.

→ Hold the position for 30 seconds. Rest for about a minute and repeat two more times.

→ Switch over to the other side and repeat.

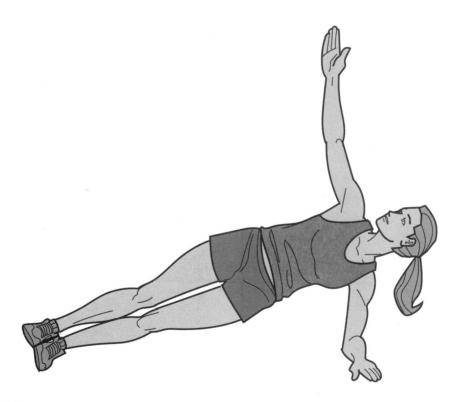

FIGURE 13.14 The side plank

Front Plank with Rows

This is a more difficult and advanced exercise than the front plank (Figure 13.13), so you need to master that one before attempting this one.

→ Assume the same basic starting position as the front plank, but instead of resting on your elbows, keep your arms straight with your weight on your hands while holding lightweight dumbbells.

→ Space your feet about the width of your hips.

→ While maintaining a straight-line posture from your head to your toes, slowly lift one of the weights straight up to your shoulder, as shown in Figure 13.15.

→ Slowly set the weight back down on the floor.

→ Do the same with the other arm. That makes 1 rep.

→ Do 5 reps in a set and then rest for a minute or so before repeating. Complete 3 sets in a session.

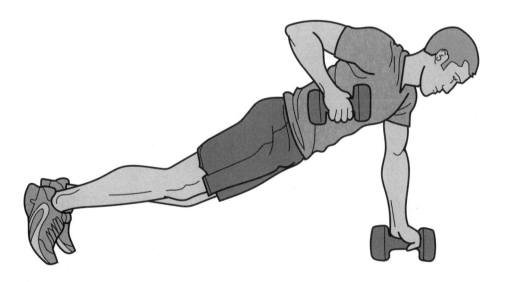

FIGURE 13.15 The front plank with rows

PERIODIZATION OF NEUROMUSCULAR TRAINING

Whether you do traditional weight lifting or an alternative strength building program with force reps while swimming, biking, and running, you need to ensure that it blends in with your other training. This takes us back to Chapters 7, 8, and 9, where you began laying out a plan for your season's training. Now it's time to merge your muscular force into that plan. As always, the key consideration in doing this is ensuring that you aren't doing so many stressful workouts back to back that you are chronically tired; that would reduce the quality and benefits of your training. That's why I strongly suggest having a periodization-based plan.

Periodization of Muscular Force

You've probably noticed that the number of weight lifting exercises is rather limited. I've recommended that you only do six or seven exercises in the gym—one or two hip-knee-ankle extension exercises, leg curls, one power exercise for running, the catch and pull for swimming, and two for core strength. This workout will probably take 45 minutes to an hour. The reason I suggest doing only a few strength exercises is that you probably have a very busy schedule with a lot going on and find it difficult to fit in gym time in addition to swimming, biking, and running (and that doesn't even take into consideration your family, career, and other commitments). The other reason for the small number of gym exercises is that I believe it's best to stay focused on what is likely to produce the most performance gains rather than doing a wide variety of strength exercises and hoping that something there works.

If you're an experienced triathlete, it's quite likely you already have a strength building program that works for you, not only in terms of the time commitment but also performance results. If that's the case, don't make any changes. Continue as you've been doing. If there's room for improvement and you believe that greater muscular force is the key, then consider the weight lifting or sport-specific alternative programs I've described above.

You may also pick and choose parts of them to blend into your current training based on your sport limiters. For example, if your cycling has lots of room for improvement but your swim and run are quite good, then you could focus on the hip-knee-ankle extension exercises, leg curls, and muscular force reps on the bike. That would considerably trim the amount of weekly training time devoted to strength while placing the emphasis on what will likely lift your race performance.

Whatever combination of weight lifting and sport-specific alternatives you decide to use to develop strength, it must be married to your other workouts in such a way as to keep fatigue manageable. Once again, that's why I emphasize using a periodization plan. This is the part of the muscular force program that hasn't been addressed so far. In Chapters 8 and 9, I mentioned including a strength program several times as you were developing an annual training plan. Those chapters offered suggestions on how to include it in your training throughout the season (see Figure 8.1 and Tables 8.1, 8.2, 8.6, 9.1, 9.2, 9.4, 9.5, and 9.8). Now it's time to get much more specific. This starts with understanding what you're trying to accomplish with neuromuscular

Limit your weight lifting to avoid excess fatigue.

TABLE 13.2 **The Weight Lifting Phases and Their Purposes**

WEIGHT LIFTING PHASE	PURPOSE
Anatomical adaptation (AA)	Becoming accustomed to the various exercises
Max transition (MT)	Gradually adapting to heavier loads
Max strength (MS)	Building strength
Strength maintenance (SM)	Maintaining the strength gains made in MS

training and when it needs to be accomplished. Let's examine the periodization of weight lifting and sport-specific alternatives, which are treated much the same when it comes to planning.

Periodization of Weight Lifting

Chapter 8 introduced the various weight lifting phases and showed you how to include them in your periodization plan for the season. Table 13.2 provides a summary of what you read about there.

Table 13.3 summarizes the program for the neuromuscular force–building exercises described earlier in this chapter under the heading "Strength Training Program." Note that this table includes the ballistic exercises described earlier in this chapter for running. It does not account for the core exercises. Core exercises may be included continually throughout the season with little concern for periodization.

For the best results, I'd suggest doing a weight lifting session immediately after a swim, bike, or run. If you can't lift then and must do it before another workout, you need to be very cautious because the muscle strain and fatigue can greatly affect the following workout. For example, when a swim session immediately follows weight lifting, technique is likely to be affected. This is counterproductive to mastering new swim skills. Should you lift before a run, the fatigue may also compromise technique and increase the risk for injury. If you must lift weights before another workout, it's probably best if that session is an

You can do core exercises continually without concern for periodization.

TABLE 13.3 **Details of the Weight Lifting Phases**

WEIGHT LIFTING PHASE	PERIOD	TOTAL SESSIONS	SESSIONS PER WEEK	LOAD (% 1RM)	SETS PER SESSION	REPS PER SET	RECOVERY (IN MINUTES)
Anatomical adaptation (AA)	Prep	4–6	2–3	40–60	3–5	15–20	1–1.5
Max transition (MT) and ballistic	Prep	4–6	2–3	70–80	3–5	8–12	2–3
Max strength (MS) and ballistic	Base 1	8–12	2–3	85–95	3–4	3–6	3–4
Strength maintenance (SM) and ballistic	Base 2 Base 3 Build 1 Build 2 Peak	Indefinite	1	60, 85	2	12, 6	1–2

TABLE 13.4 **Periodization of Force Reps for Swimming, Biking, and Running**

PERIOD	TOTAL SESSIONS	SESSIONS PER WEEK	SETS PER SESSION	REPS PER SET
Prep	4–6	2–3	1	3
Prep	4–6	2–3	2	3
Base 1 (may continue into early base 2)	8–12	2–3	3–4	3–6
Base 2 Base 3 Build 1 Build 2 Peak	Indefinite	1	1	3

easy recovery ride. The negative consequences are much less likely to affect bike performance or your wellness. The best way to address this matter of weight lifting before swimming, biking, or running is to separate the two sessions by several hours. For example, a weight lifting session early in the morning with swimming, biking, or running late in the day is likely to have only minor consequences, if any at all.

Periodization of Sport-Specific Alternatives

The force reps workouts done while swimming, biking, and running are intended to build neuromuscular strength similar to that resulting from weight lifting, only without any gym time. But these workouts are treated in much the same way as gym sessions when it comes to periodization. That's because the orthopedic stresses associated with such training are also rather great, so the training should be done at a time in the season when other training stresses are low—that is, in the prep and early base periods. Table 13.4 suggests a periodization pattern to use throughout the season. You'll notice that the only variables are how often these workouts are done and how many sets are included in a workout in the various periods.

As mentioned in the earlier discussion of force reps, these may be blended into a swim, bike, or run workout during which you are also working on other abilities. To reduce the risk for injury, however, the force reps portion should be done early in the workout immediately after you warm up. For example, if you are going for a ride in which the primary focus will be aerobic endurance, you could warm up for 15 to 30 minutes, do a force reps segment, then continue into the main set.

CONCURRENT TRAINING

Blending all neuromuscular training and endurance workouts together into a single plan is highly beneficial for endurance athletes, but also quite complex. Trying to fit in swim, bike, and run sessions along with plyometrics, weight lifting, and alternative strength workouts places quite a demand on your time and also on your

It's best to lift after a swim, bike, or run session, not before.

capacity for work. You probably can't do every-thing, so you will need to decide how much time and energy you have available for training, what your limiters and training limitations are, and what is therefore the most important of every-thing you *can* work on.

The solution to this conundrum comes down to your limiters, as explained in Chapter 6. The first consideration is which sport is your greatest limiter and how improved strength and plyomet-rics may benefit it. When it comes to limiters, your primary concern should be cycling because it accounts for about half of your total time in a race. So if you can't decide which one of two or three of the sports is your greatest limiter, the answer is simple: the bike.

If you are already a very strong cyclist, your focus should shift to swimming and running. Of these two, if you are unsure, you must focus on running because it likely accounts for a larger portion of your finishing time than swimming does and therefore may have a greater impact on overall performance.

So again, you don't have to do everything. If the bike is your primary limiter, then to improve race performance you may decide to lift weights or do alternative bike force reps. If running is where you need to focus your time and energy, then plyometrics or ballistic strength training, possibly along with force reps, should be con-sidered alongside running workouts. If it's swim-ming that is definitely holding you back, then the solution is likely to be improving your swim-ming efficiency. That takes you back to PDLC, described in Chapter 12. There is little reason to work on swim strength if your technique is poor. Once your skills improve, strength training may prove beneficial.

If you are pressed for time or simply unable to manage all of the training suggested in this and previous chapters, focus on your limiting sport and emphasize those things that are likely to pro-duce the greatest improvement for the time and energy invested. This may not be muscular force. The other ability options, described in Chapter 6, are aerobic endurance, speed skills, anaerobic endurance, and muscular endurance.

SUMMARY: MUSCULAR FORCE

Of the five abilities relevant to performance improvement in triathlon, the three most basic are aerobic endurance, speed skills, and muscu-lar force. This chapter examined the last of these three. It is commonly the first of the five abili-ties to be developed early in the season and then maintained with reduced workout frequency until the first A-priority race of the year.

Muscular force training is typically associ-ated only with weight lifting. But plyometrics and alternative strength exercises done during swimming, biking, and running can also be part of the plan. Plyometrics can have an especially great effect on running because the nervous sys-tem is trained to fire the muscles in such a way as to increase power. The alternative, sport-spe-cific strength building workouts, called muscular force reps, can take the place of weight lifting or complement it for the triathlete whose greatest limiter in a sport is muscular force.

Of these three strength building options, the one that has been most studied and supported by research as a way of improving muscular force is weight lifting. In order to produce positive results, weight lifting exercises must be done in such a way as to closely simulate the movements of the sport for which you are trying to increase strength. For the bike and run, leg extension exercises involving the hip, knee, and ankle are considered the most effective. Swimming is much more difficult to simulate with traditional weight lifting. Using an elastic band for resistance is a better approach than weights because it allows a more swimlike position to be assumed. For running, ballistic strength exercises are also a good alternative to heavy-load weight lifting.

The most common challenge facing triathletes is fitting muscular force workouts, regardless of type, into their available training time. The solution involves determining the most limiting sport of the three and how much insufficient muscular force contributes to that limiter. Most triathletes' race performances will benefit if they increase their neuromuscular strength in their weakest sport or sports. If they focus muscular force training on that sport, the necessary training time is kept in check. The other solution to the issue of restricted time involves placing the emphasis on neuromuscular training early in the season, especially the prep and base 1 periods, when swimming, biking, and running are not as demanding of your time.

Once you've developed muscular force early in the season by doing two or three weekly sessions, you can put strength training into a maintenance mode. This involves doing such workouts only once per week with a very brief session; you want to do it in such a way that it does not detract from your primary swimming, biking, and running workouts. But don't ignore it; for muscular force to be well maintained, you need to do this once-weekly workout consistently during the buildup to your next A-priority race.

THE TRAINING DIARY

THIS BOOK IS all about training, but of course the purpose of training is racing. Aside from swim, bike, run, and strength training, the most beneficial thing you can do to take your race performances to a higher level is to keep a detailed training diary. In your diary, you will draw up a plan for the season, record the details of workouts, add comments on how training is progressing, and summarize race results. At the end of the season, as you start thinking about the new season ahead, your training diary will provide answers to questions, including the most important one: What can I do to race better next year? The answer is in your diary. Without a diary, though, you're left to rely solely on memory, which isn't always clear or reliable.

The training diary is not an end in itself. If all you do is record workout data but never review it to consider how training is going, you will get little benefit from it. In that case, it's only a log, not a diary. The difference between a log and a diary is that a diary relies on your consideration of what's been recorded; it's a compilation of your reactions, thoughts, conclusions, questions, concerns, and more. A log is merely a bunch of numbers. A diary leads you on a journey of personal discovery. A log is only a record of what you did. A well-kept diary allows you to plan your training, recall the details of your past workouts and races, build self-confidence, and hold yourself accountable. What a diary does sounds surprisingly similar to what a good coach does. In fact, it's the best tool you have as a self-coached athlete.

The training diary comes in many formats. The most basic is on paper. A simple notebook will do. Or you can use an electronic, calendar-based diary stored on your computer. The third option is to use a web-based diary. There are several available for which you pay a small monthly fee. All of these variations are easy to find with a search of the Internet. Some provide advanced tools for planning and analysis that serve as your coach to help you make training decisions, and if you are truly serious about race performance, that's the way to go.

A diary doesn't have to be complex to be effective. In its simplest form, your diary is a list of your season's goals and training objectives, followed by a seasonal plan, weekly planned workouts, workout history, race results, and your thoughts on all of these. The diary can also serve as an early warning system to prevent injuries and other types of breakdowns (more on this below). It's for all of these reasons that I believe keeping a training diary is the single most important thing you can do aside from actually training.

PLANNING WITH A DIARY

Chapters 7, 8, and 9 described how I plan a season for an athlete. There, I introduced various periodization schemes to help you organize your season around key races. We looked at the volume of training, in which you used either weekly hours or training stress score (TSS), and how that volume would be distributed throughout the year. We also got into the details of designing an effective training week. All of this should be stored in your diary.

The diary is where you start to prepare for your next season. Once you find yourself thinking about what lies ahead, it's time to begin planning. Set aside an hour or so to make notes in your diary on what your goals and training objectives are (see Chapter 5 for details). Note the periodization system you're using (see Chapters 7 and 9), plug your A-priority races into the appropriate calendar weeks, note the volume to

be completed for every week of the buildup to your first race (see Tables 8.4 and 8.5), and create and record a weekly training routine that fits your schedule (see Chapter 8). This will take a lot of careful thinking the first time you do it, but it will pay off throughout the season. Once you are into your training year, when you come to each new week, the decisions about what you should do will already be made. All you have to do is follow the guidelines laid out in your diary. This will prove to be a great time-saver throughout the year while improving the focus of your training.

With a diary, planning your workouts for the coming week is a snap. At the end of the current week, open your diary to the coming week and plan the daily workouts by sport. Use the workout codes found in Appendixes B, C, D, and E to note the swim, bike, and run sessions. If you're also doing weight lifting, indicate the day or days and the type of workout (AA, MT, MS, or SM) as described in Chapter 13. Then indicate the planned workout durations or TSS for each session. All of this is illustrated in Figure 14.1 on a paper version from my book *The Triathlete's Training Diary*, which is available through Velo-Press (www.velopress.com). You've already done your long-range planning at the very start of the season, so planning for next week will take only a few minutes. Knowing exactly what you're going to do each day gives you a head start on the week and more productive workouts.

Having a plan builds confidence. You're training with a purpose, not by the seat of your pants. Certainly, the plan may change. In fact, it would be unusual if you made it all the way through the season with the same plan that you created at the start. In more than 30 years of coaching triathletes, I have never had anyone finish the season

The diary is where you start to prepare for your next season.

without changes in his or her plan. Something always comes up to force a change. And to be quite honest, it's not the plan that is important, but rather the planning. When it comes to success at anything in your life, planning how to get there, even if the plan changes, is the most important thing you can do.

WHAT TO RECORD

Once the plan is laid out for the season, you're ready to do the workouts and keep a record of what is most important. So what should you record? The answer varies considerably among athletes. Some really enjoy keeping detailed records and poring over the data. Others find it burdensome to keep any records at all and hate looking back at past workouts. If you are a serious triathlete with high goals, but detest record keeping, you should strongly consider hiring a coach to guide you. The coach will make sure you record only the most pertinent data and will take care of analysis.

If you are the other type of triathlete—one who really enjoys collecting and analyzing data—it's likely you'll record too much. You can get so bogged down in details that making decisions is difficult. Recording too much is just as bad as recording too little. You should strive to record only what you feel is vitally important and what you are likely to need in making future decisions about your training. The key is to make your diary simple and succinct.

The following are five categories designed to help you make decisions about training. Even though these suggestions are minimal, don't feel you have to record all of them. Customize your diary to fit your training perspective. Keep a record only of those things you are likely to consider later on.

Basic log entries. The most basic workout data includes the sport, date, time of day, planned workout, actual workout completed, course route or venue, distance and duration of the workout, and equipment used. When you look back at workout data several days, weeks, or months later, you will also want to know of anything that set the workout apart from the norm. Did it go particularly well or poorly? How did you account for that at the time? Was it cold, hot, windy, or rainy? Did the weather affect your workout that day? Did you have a training partner who caused you to work a little harder than usual, or not as hard? Who was it? Was there anything that happened out of the ordinary, such as a knee that didn't feel quite right or tires that were underinflated? Perhaps you tripped and fell during a run. Make a note of it. Even if you record only such basic workout information and you've never done that before, your training will improve.

Morning warnings. Chapter 11 introduced the idea of taking stock of your readiness to work out as you wake up each morning. Table 11.1 lists several indicators that I call *morning warnings*. Decide which of these are good indicators of unusual stress for you and that you also know you will measure and record regularly. Then assess and record them in your diary first thing in the morning when you wake up. You might use a simple "plus" or "minus" rating or a more detailed scale of 1 to 5. It may help to reread that section of Chapter 11 and decide how to keep tabs on your daily morning warnings.

If you have high goals but detest record keeping, you should hire a coach to guide you.

week beginning: _Feb 6, 2017_

Period: _Base 1b_   Planned Hours: _10_

MONDAY _2 / 6 / 17_

▢ sleep ▢ fatigue ▢ stress ▢ soreness

resting heart rate _____ weight _____

WORKOUT 1   S B R Ⓞ _weights_

planned workout _MS, 45 minutes_

route _____ dist. _____ time _____

avg. HR _____ avg. power _____

zone 1_____ 2_____ 3_____ 4_____ 5_____

WORKOUT 2   S B R 0 _____

planned workout _____

route _____ dist. _____ time _____

avg. HR _____ avg. power _____

zone 1_____ 2_____ 3_____ 4_____ 5_____

notes _____

nutrition _____

TUESDAY _2 / 7 / 17_

▢ sleep ▢ fatigue ▢ stress ▢ soreness

resting heart rate _____ weight _____

WORKOUT 1   Ⓢ B R 0 _____

planned workout _SS1, 45 minutes_

route _____ dist. _____ time _____

avg. HR _____ avg. power _____

zone 1_____ 2_____ 3_____ 4_____ 5_____

WORKOUT 2   S B Ⓡ 0 _____

planned workout _AE2, 1 hour_

route _____ dist. _____ time _____

avg. HR _____ avg. power _____

zone 1_____ 2_____ 3_____ 4_____ 5_____

notes _____

nutrition _____

FIGURE 14.1 Using a training diary to plan for the coming week

week goals: ■ *1) Improve swim catch, 2) Build aerobic endurance for bike and*
■ *run, 3) Develop mid-foot strike for running, 4) Increase loads used in gym.*
■

WEDNESDAY ___2___ / ___8___ / ___17___

■ sleep ■ fatigue ■ stress ■ soreness

resting heart rate _____ weight _____

WORKOUT 1   S Ⓑ R O _____

planned workout __*AE2, 1 hour*__

route _____ dist. _____ time _____

avg. HR _____ avg. power _____

zone 1_____ 2_____ 3_____ 4_____ 5_____

WORKOUT 2   S B R O _____

planned workout _____

route _____ dist. _____ time _____

avg. HR _____ avg. power _____

zone 1_____ 2_____ 3_____ 4_____ 5_____

notes _____

nutrition _____

THURSDAY ___2___ / ___9___ / ___17___

■ sleep ■ fatigue ■ stress ■ soreness

resting heart rate _____ weight _____

WORKOUT 1   S B Ⓡ O _____

planned workout __*SS1, 45 minutes*__

route _____ dist. _____ time _____

avg. HR _____ avg. power _____

zone 1_____ 2_____ 3_____ 4_____ 5_____

WORKOUT 2   Ⓢ B R O _____

planned workout __*SS1, 45 minutes*__

route _____ dist. _____ time _____

avg. HR _____ avg. power _____

zone 1_____ 2_____ 3_____ 4_____ 5_____

notes _____

nutrition _____

→

FRIDAY ___2_/_10_/_17___

▢ sleep ▢ fatigue ▢ stress ▢ soreness

resting heart rate _____ weight _____

WORKOUT 1 Ⓢ B R 0_____

planned workout _SS1, 30 minutes_

_____

_____

route _____ dist. _____ time _____

avg. HR _____ avg. power _____

zone 1_____ 2_____ 3_____ 4_____ 5_____

WORKOUT 2 S B R Ⓞ _weights_

planned workout _MS, 45 minutes_

_____

_____

route _____ dist. _____ time _____

avg. HR _____ avg. power _____

zone 1_____ 2_____ 3_____ 4_____ 5_____

notes _____

_____

_____

_____

_____

_____

_____

_____

_____

nutrition _____

_____

_____

_____

_____

SATURDAY ___2_/_11_/_17___

▢ sleep ▢ fatigue ▢ stress ▢ soreness

resting heart rate _____ weight _____

WORKOUT 1 S Ⓑ R 0_____

planned workout _AE2, 2 hours_

_____

_____

route _____ dist. _____ time _____

avg. HR _____ avg. power _____

zone 1_____ 2_____ 3_____ 4_____ 5_____

WORKOUT 2 S B Ⓡ 0 _____

planned workout _AE1, 30 minutes_

_____

_____

route _____ dist. _____ time _____

avg. HR _____ avg. power _____

zone 1_____ 2_____ 3_____ 4_____ 5_____

notes _____

_____

_____

_____

_____

_____

_____

_____

_____

nutrition _____

_____

_____

_____

_____

FIGURE 14.1 (continued)

→

SUNDAY   2 / 12 / 17

▨ sleep ▨ fatigue ▨ stress ▨ soreness

resting heart rate _____ weight _____

WORKOUT 1 (S) B R O _____

planned workout _SS1, 45 minutes_ _____

_____

route _____ dist. _____ time _____

avg. HR _____ avg. power _____

zone 1 _____ 2 _____ 3 _____ 4 _____ 5 _____

WORKOUT 2 S B (R) O _weights_

planned workout _AE1, 30 minutes_ _____

_____

route _____ dist. _____ time _____

avg. HR _____ avg. power _____

zone 1 _____ 2 _____ 3 _____ 4 _____ 5 _____

notes _____

_____
_____
_____
_____
_____
_____
_____

nutrition _____

_____
_____
_____

WEEKLY SUMMARY

	TIME	DISTANCE	YTD TIME	YTD DISTANCE
swim				
bike				
run				
strength				
other				
total				

notes

_____
_____
_____
_____
_____
_____
_____
_____

Physical notes. How did the workout go? Did you accomplish what you were intending? You may use a simple grading system of A to F, as if you were in school. Also keep track of workout details, such as time by heart rate, pace, or power zones. Chapter 4 discussed intensity distribution over the course of the season. Recording how much workout time you spent in each zone will help you to stay on the mark for how you plan to train as the season progresses. If you never pay attention to such data, you are likely to stray from the seasonal plan.

Mental notes. Some athletes view their feelings as unimportant, especially in comparison with the hard data that was recorded as physical notes. That's a big mistake. The best indicator of how you are progressing on a daily basis is most likely to be your emotions and impressions. Record how you felt about the workout. Are you satisfied with how it went? Do you feel as if you are making good progress? Do you have concerns? Make note of your thoughts and feelings after every workout. These notes may well provide a treasure trove of valuable information as you look back.

Miscellaneous notes. Other daily details you may include in your diary are anything unusual that might affect your workout: travel, environmental factors such as altitude and humidity, career-related stress such as working long hours, injuries and illnesses, and family activities that interrupt workouts. You may also note equipment changes made: new running shoes, a repositioned saddle, or new bike gears. Record changes made to your typical diet, especially what you eat before or during a race. And of course record the details of any races you do (more on this below).

> The best indicators of your daily progress are most likely your emotions and impressions.

TRAINING ANALYSIS

Triathlon training is a scientific experiment with only one subject—you. A scientific experiment has to do with changing controllable variables and then observing what happens. It's about hard evidence, not unfounded beliefs. The evidence will be found in your accumulating workout data. Recording workouts day after day for weeks, months, and years produces a tremendous reservoir of experimental data. What you're trying to discover from this data is the best way for *you* to train.

As an athlete, you are unique in many ways (remember the principle of *individualization* from Chapter 3?). You can't do exactly what your training partner does and expect the same results. By collecting and analyzing your workout data, you can learn what works for you and what doesn't. Using that information to make small training adjustments will help you stay on track to achieving your goals. You only need to know what data to collect and understand how to analyze it.

The starting place for analysis is asking yourself the most basic of training questions, such as these:

- Am I making progress toward my goals?
- Is my training too hard or too easy?
- Am I getting enough rest and recovery?
- Is my diet meeting my fueling needs?

You must always be honest in answering such questions. There's nothing to be gained by sugarcoating the answers. Early in the season, you probably can answer these without even keeping a diary. But as the season progresses and the sheer volume of workouts accumulates, it can be difficult to remember what you did last month, last week, and even yesterday. If you decide a training adjustment is needed, what will you change if you can't recall exactly how many intervals you've been doing, when in the season you started doing those intervals, the duration progression of your long workouts, how often you've included rest-and-recovery weeks, and what you've been eating after hard sessions? A daily written record of your training helps you to find the answers and therefore make informed training decisions.

The answers to the critical concerns about progress are found in your diary. It may take some searching, but the answers to questions such as How am I doing? are found there. The best indicator of future performance is past performance, especially if it is recent. If you are doing occasional B- and C-priority races, they will serve as the very best markers of progress toward your A-priority race. Other indicators come from periodic testing. Chapter 8 suggested that these be done at the end of rest-and-recovery weeks. Performance tests measure speed, pace, or power. These are the ultimate workout predictors for your A race. Occasionally measuring heart rate with testing will ensure that you have your zones right, but heart rate is not an indicator of performance. It tells you about effort, much the same as a rating of perceived exertion. Tests that combine heart rate and performance data, such as power for cycling and speed for running, however, are quite beneficial (see Appendixes C and D for "Aerobic Threshold" test workout examples).

RACE ANALYSIS

Good or bad, after every race—especially an A race—you need to assess how you did. If the race didn't go as planned and expected, it's criti-cal that you search for the reason why. It may be painfully obvious, such as a bike breaking down mechanically or going off course. Such matters can generally be corrected easily in the future. If everything else went well except for this, you know your training plan was effective.

If, on the other hand, you performed poorly in your race, you have a greater matter to consider. What exactly was the reason? It may be obvious, or it may take a lot of searching to find it. The best time to start the quest for an answer is generally the day after the race. The hours immediately following your finish are seldom the best time to give deep thought to the matter. Emotions are running high and will confuse your thinking. Your head won't be clear enough for you to draw good conclusions. It's best to wait until the next day and then begin the analysis. In the meantime, be reluctant to draw conclusions. You may think you know why immediately afterward, but give it a day.

The common reasons for a poor race performance have to do with race management. The most frequent cause of poor race management is incorrect pacing. What's the underlying cause? Uncontrolled emotions. This is most evident at the start of the bike leg of a triathlon. Most incorrectly paced races, and therefore poor race results, can be traced to the first quarter of the bike portion. Because emotional excitement is running high, the common tendency is to start harder than is realistic. I've seen Ironman athletes set new personal best times in the first 40 kilometers of the bike leg—and they still have 150 kilometers to go! You can't win the race in the first quarter, but you can certainly lose it. The first quarter of the bike leg is the time when you must have a conservative pacing strategy and rigidly stick to it. The goal

Good or bad, after every race—especially an A race—you need to assess how you did.

should be to do the second half of the bike leg at a slightly higher power output than the first half. That's called *negative splitting*. If you learn to do this, you come off the bike ready to have a fast run. The way to learn this skill is to rehearse it in training at least weekly in the last 12 weeks before the race.

Another common race management issue has to do with race-day conditions, especially heat. If it's a hot day, you need to make pacing adjustments. Go more slowly. I know that's hard to do, but if it's hot you'll either make such a decision or suffer the consequences of a really poor race performance. Every athlete in the race has to do this, so it's not as if you are the only one. This decision is often made on race day. But start considering it well in advance. Several weeks in advance, you should have a good idea of what the weather conditions have been for a particular race in past years and perhaps even an early indication of what might be expected this time. If it's going to be hot, you need to prepare well in advance by doing some heat adaptation. Wishing and hoping won't work. Prepare. Run frequently in the hottest part of the day in the last month or so before the race. If it's much cooler where you live than where the race will be held, you need to be creative. The bottom line is to be prepared for the conditions on race day.

But what if the race-day heat is totally unexpected? What then? It all comes back to race management and wise decisions. It's obvious that if it's a hot day and you aren't heat-adapted, you won't be able to go as fast as you had originally planned. You must be willing to change your pacing strategy by slowing down, especially coming out of T2. Failure to do so will without a doubt lead to poor performance.

> Race performance is highly predictable by analyzing how you've done in the past few weeks.

Unrealistic expectations are another common cause of poor race management. Your key workouts, tests, and B and C races in the last 6 weeks or so before your A race are strong indicators of what can be expected on race day. Just because you want to race fast doesn't mean you will. There is no magic on race day. You either have it or you don't. Race performance is highly predictable by simply analyzing how you've done in the past few weeks. Use that data to plan your race pacing strategy.

There are many, many other causes of a poor race performance. Experienced triathletes who have analyzed their races for several years have learned how to deal with the expected, such as heat, and with the unexpected, such as bike mechanicals. They can find the details in their training diaries of how they made adjustments in such situations and use those notes to be prepared for similar race circumstances in the future.

On the brighter side, what if you had a great race? Races in which everything went well deserve special attention. Did you do anything aside from the usual race preparation, especially in the week leading up to the race and on race day? Perhaps your workouts were unique in how they were arranged, or you rested more or less than usual, or maybe your lifestyle changed in some way, or your diet changed, or you paced the race perfectly. The possibilities are nearly endless. Give it considerable thought because there is something here you need to understand so you can do it again at the next race.

Figure 14.2 offers suggestions for analyzing your race. It will also help you keep a record of your race data as a reference for future races. Copy and complete this form after every race and store it in your training diary for future reference.

RACE EVALUATION FORM

race name _____ / / / _____ start time _____

location _____ type/distance _____

key competitors _____

weather_____ course conditions _____

race goal _____
_____

race strategy _____
_____
_____

pre-race meal _____
_____

warm-up description _____
_____

start line arousal: ▨ low   ▨ moderate   ▨ high

results (place, time, splits, etc.) _____
_____

what I did well _____
_____
_____

what I need to improve _____
_____

aches, pains, and problems before, during, or after _____
_____

comments on how the race went _____
_____
_____
_____

FIGURE 14.2 Race evaluation form

Or use it as a guide for race analysis with the comments noted in your diary. The information will prove to be of great value in preparing for future races, especially the same one next year.

SUMMARY: THE TRAINING DIARY

The training diary is your most valuable tool in preparing for a high-performance season. It holds the record of your season's goals so you see them every time you open your diary. They can be written on the cover, the first page, or a card that serves as a page marker. If you are using an electronic diary on your computer or on the Internet, you need to record your goals there and review them frequently. You can then use your diary to create seasonal and weekly plans for how you will achieve the goals while also gauging your progress toward achieving them.

Your overall seasonal plan may take an hour or so once each year to create, but once done, it will prove valuable to your goal achievement. The next weekly plan is created at the end of the current week and takes only a few minutes. This also will do wonders for your training if you've never done it before.

Your training diary helps you see not only the big picture of your season but also the details of what's happening along the way. Deciding what to record depends on your own perspective on training. This chapter suggests items to record, from the most basic to highly detailed. You should enter only what you are likely to look at

later when gauging your progress toward your goals. Recording too much data is as bad as recording too little.

As you test your athletic progress every few weeks, note these critical bits of information in your diary. The data here is even more valuable than your daily workout information and comments, so be sure to record all of what you think may be useful later when you look for trends. This may be in the form of field tests of performance (speed or power) or B- and C-priority race data. The results of field tests and races are your best markers of progress toward goals.

Periodically review your training diary while looking for trends. The best time to do this is every third or fourth week during a rest-and-recovery week. Review how your training went in the period you've just finished. Compare that with where your performance was during the previous rest-and-recovery week. Are you seeing progress toward your goals? If not, why not? If you are, what's working well?

After every race—good or bad—evaluate how you did. Poor race performances aren't fun to relive, but at the very least you should consider what you would do differently in preparation if you could do it all over again. That analysis may help you with the direction of your training before the next race. If the race went well, consider what you think was the underlying reason. Performance is directly related to training and racing management. Is your training effective and are you managing races in the best way? Your diary provides the answers.

The training diary is your most valuable tool in preparing for a high-performance season.

EPILOGUE

If you've made it this far, I'm sure you love triathlon as much as I do. Your love for the sport is undoubtedly fueled by your passion for seeking to achieve high goals. I hope you discovered a few things in *The Triathlete's Training Bible* that will help you with that undertaking. I wrote the book to introduce you to the latest training trends in sports science and my experience-based insights acquired during more than 30 years as a coach. I hope that the time you invested in reading it pays off with increased triathlon fitness and improved performance.

If you carefully studied a previous edition of *The Triathlete's Training Bible*, you surely discovered that many things have changed in this latest version. The commingled worlds of triathlon training and sports science are in a constant state of transformation. They are never stagnant. I continue to learn new ways of training from talking with athletes and other coaches, by observing how athletes respond to training, and through reading sports science research. Untried methods of training are not something to be avoided. They should be given careful consideration and even embraced as challenges that may help you achieve greater goals. Change is ultimately necessary for improving race performance.

With that in mind, I can guarantee you that the advanced triathlon-training methods described in this book will change over time. They are not now and never have been carved in stone. New ideas will continue to come along, and my own thoughts about what makes for effective training will evolve with them. The sport will move on. That's to be expected—and greatly desired.

Even though I researched and gave careful consideration to what I wrote here, *The Triathlete's Training Bible* should not be viewed as a set of immutable "rules" for training. Instead, think of it as a collection of proven guidelines to help you make smart decisions about the many factors that affect your training experience.

What all of this means is that you shouldn't now, after reading this book, expect to know how to train for as long as you continue in the sport. You must always seek better ways. Don't be afraid to experiment. Training is a research study with one subject—you. If you always train the same way, your performance will eventually plateau while other farsighted and creative triathletes go right on improving.

Training for triathlon is a malleable activity. If you are to continue to grow as a triathlete, you must be willing to consider new ways of preparing to race. You must always seek better results, regardless of what currently may be the accepted training procedures.

This book is not meant to be a fixed and rigid description of what athletes *must* do to race at a high level of performance. It is meant only as an introduction to becoming a more knowledgeable and wiser triathlete. Your creativity, curiosity, and desire to improve are, in the end, the keys to high performance.

APPENDIX A: ANNUAL TRAINING PLAN TEMPLATE

Athlete _____

Annual Volume _____

Year_____

WEEK	MON.	RACES	PRI.	PERIOD	VOLUME	WEIGHTS	SWIM							BIKE							RUN						
							AEROBIC ENDURANCE	MUSCULAR FORCE	SPEED SKILLS	MUSCULAR ENDURANCE	ANAEROBIC ENDURANCE	SPRINT POWER	TESTING	AEROBIC ENDURANCE	MUSCULAR FORCE	SPEED SKILLS	MUSCULAR ENDURANCE	ANAEROBIC ENDURANCE	SPRINT POWER	TESTING	AEROBIC ENDURANCE	MUSCULAR FORCE	SPEED SKILLS	MUSCULAR ENDURANCE	ANAEROBIC ENDURANCE	SPRINT POWER	TESTING
01	/																										
02	/																										
03	/																										
04	/																										
05	/																										
06	/																										
07	/																										
08	/																										
09	/																										
10	/																										
11	/																										
12	/																										
13	/																										
14	/																										
15	/																										
16	/																										
17	/																										
18	/																										
19	/																										
20	/																										
21	/																										
22	/																										
23	/																										
24	/																										
25	/																										
26	/																										

Season Goals

1. _____
2. _____
3. _____

Training Objectives

1. _____
2. _____
3. _____
4. _____

								SWIM							BIKE							RUN					
WEEK	MON.	RACES	PRI.	PERIOD	VOLUME	WEIGHTS	AEROBIC ENDURANCE	MUSCULAR FORCE	SPEED SKILLS	MUSCULAR ENDURANCE	ANAEROBIC ENDURANCE	SPRINT POWER	TESTING	AEROBIC ENDURANCE	MUSCULAR FORCE	SPEED SKILLS	MUSCULAR ENDURANCE	ANAEROBIC ENDURANCE	SPRINT POWER	TESTING	AEROBIC ENDURANCE	MUSCULAR FORCE	SPEED SKILLS	MUSCULAR ENDURANCE	ANAEROBIC ENDURANCE	SPRINT POWER	TESTING
27	/																										
28	/																										
29	/																										
30	/																										
31	/																										
32	/																										
33	/																										
34	/																										
35	/																										
36	/																										
37	/																										
38	/																										
39	/																										
40	/																										
41	/																										
42	/																										
43	/																										
44	/																										
45	/																										
46	/																										
47	/																										
48	/																										
49	/																										
50	/																										
51	/																										
52	/																										

APPENDIX B: SWIM WORKOUTS

The following are basic swim sets that you can combine in various ways into a single swim session. For example, following the warm-up, you may start the session with a speed skills set, followed by an anaerobic endurance set and then an aerobic endurance set, before the cooldown.

The typical order for ability sets within a single training session is aerobic endurance (AE) and/or speed skills (SS) as a warm-up, followed by muscular force (MF), anaerobic endurance (AnE), and muscular endurance (ME). The cooldown is commonly AE and/or SS. For example, if the main set (the portion that is neither warm-up nor cooldown) of the workout includes MF and ME, the order of all the sets within the session from warm-up through cooldown will be as follows:

1st set: SS
2nd set: MF
3rd set: ME
4th set: AE

A common exception is to insert an AE or SS set within the main set to allow a long recovery between high-effort sets.

The MF, ME, and AnE ability sets are always a part of the main set—the primary portions of the workout that are neither warm-up nor cooldown. They should always be preceded by a warm-up. Note that the more intense the main set of the workout, the longer the warm-up must be.

The intensities for most of the workouts below are based on pace; heart rate monitors are difficult to use while swimming. See Table 4.2 for swim-pace zones.

Aerobic Endurance Sets

AE1: Recovery

Swim steadily for 10 to 20 minutes or more in pace zone 1, concentrating on only one aspect of technique. You can use this as a recovery workout following a hard bike or run workout, or as a swim session cooldown.

AE2: Aerobic Threshold Intervals

Swim intervals in pace zone 2 at a distance that takes 6 to 12 minutes. Recover after each for 10 to 15 percent of the preceding work-interval time. Total work-interval distance may match the distance of the swim portion of your next A- or B-priority race. Build up to this set duration over a few sessions. A variation on this set is to recover between intervals with a 25- to 50-meter/yard drill. Example: 4 × 500 meters/yards in 7 minutes, 30 seconds, leaving every 8 minutes, 15 seconds. Or swim long and steady in pace zone 2, especially in open water.

AE3: Tempo Intervals

Swim 3 to 7 intervals, each taking about 3 to 5 minutes to complete. Intensity is pace zone 3. Recover after each for 5 to 10 percent of the preceding work-interval time. The total interval time for this session should be something in the range of 10 to 20 minutes. Example: 5 × 200 meters in 3:00, leaving on 3:15.

Muscular Force Sets

MF1: Muscular Force Reps

Note: Do not undertake this set until your SS are very well established because the risk for injury is high if your skills are poor.

Following an extensive warm-up including short, fast repeats (such as SS1), do 1 to 3 sets of 3 intervals of 25 meters/yards each. Wear a T-shirt or other such drag device, or use paddles for each interval. The purpose of using a drag device or paddles is to increase stress on the muscles and therefore generate greater force. Take a long (40–60 seconds), standing recovery at the wall after each. Between sets, swim easily as described for AE1 (above) for 25 to 50 meters/yards. The first time you do MF1, do only 1 set of 3 intervals. Gradually increase the number of sets. Stop this set at the first sign of shoulder discomfort, which is an indicator of poor swim skills. Instead of continuing, go to the SS1 set (below) to improve your technique before returning to the MF1 sets.

MF2: Open-Water-Current Intervals

Swim in a river, lake, or the ocean with alternating sets against and with the current. Swim each high-exertion set against the current at nearly maximal effort without breaking form, taking 8 to 10 strokes (each arm) in each set. Recover by swimming easily with the current for 60 to 90 seconds. Complete 3 to 8 of these sets. Do this only with a partner or group. Example: 5 × 8 strokes at nearly maximal effort into the current with 1-minute, easy-swim recoveries.

MF3: Paddles

Swim any set other than warm-up or cooldown while using paddles. When you first use paddles, start with small ones, use them only for AE sets (above), and do no more than 10 percent of the total workout distance with them. Over the course of several weeks, increase the size of the paddles. Don't do more than 50 percent of a workout with them, and never increase both paddle size and total distance within a workout at the same time. At the first sign of shoulder discomfort, discontinue using the paddles and return to an emphasis on SS training (below).

Speed Skills Sets

Remember that the term *speed skills* as used here doesn't mean high velocity but rather the ability to move the arms quickly, efficiently, and effectively. Revisit Chapter 12 for more details on SS training.

SS1: Fast-Form 25s

Start this set by swimming one length of the pool at a slow to moderate effort. Over the next several 25s, swim each subsequent length more briskly, but never all out. While swimming a length, focus your attention on the one PDLC skill you are trying to improve: posture, direction, length, or catch. Think of nothing else for each 25. Don't time these 25s; your focus must be on technique, not on increasing the effort.

When you finish a 25, stop and rest at the wall. Make each recovery long. Don't make the rest stops brief in order to improve your endurance.

The only focus is on skill. Let your mind wander while you rest at the wall. Think about anything except your swim performance. You should be breathing easily before starting the next 25.

When you are ready to swim the next length, bring your mental focus back to the PDLC skill you are concentrating on. Then swim another 25 focusing only on correctly making this movement. The number of 25s you do in a session can be just a few as a part of the warm-up or cooldown, or they can make up the entire swim session.

SS2: Toy Sets

Do any set wearing fins or keeping a pull buoy between your thighs. These "toys" are especially helpful during intervals within the main set for maintaining body position on top of the water while you focus on a single PDLC skill.

Muscular Endurance Sets

ME1: Long Cruise Intervals

This is a session with work intervals that take 6 minutes or longer. The recovery intervals are about 5 to 15 percent of the preceding work-interval duration. As fitness improves, reduce the duration of the recovery intervals. Intensity is pace zones 4 to 5a. The total work-interval distance for the set may gradually increase over a few weeks to equal the distance of your next A- or B-priority race. Example: 5 × 400 meters/yards in 6:00 leaving every 6:40.

ME2: Short Cruise Intervals

Swim intervals that take 3 to 5 minutes to complete. Intensity is pace zones 4 to 5a. Recover after each for about 5 to 10 percent of the preceding work-interval duration. Total work-interval time may be gradually increased to match the total distance of the swim portion of your next A- or B-priority race. Example: 8 × 200 meters in 3:00 leaving every 3:10.

ME3: Threshold

Swim steadily for 12 to 20 minutes in pace zone 3. Example: 1,200 meters/yards in 18:00.

Anaerobic Endurance Sets

AnE1: VO₂max Intervals

Complete 3 to 5 work intervals, each with a duration of 2 to 3 minutes and each with a recovery that is 10 to 25 percent of the work-interval time. Intensity is pace zone 5b. This session will gradually boost your aerobic capacity. Important: Do not allow technique to break down. Recovery intervals may be reduced to about 10 percent of the work interval during the build period as your fitness improves. Example: 5 × 200 meters/yards in 2:40 leaving every 3:00.

AnE2: Anaerobic Capacity Intervals

Swim 1 to 4 intervals with durations of 30 to 60 seconds at pace zone 5c and with long recoveries that have at least the same duration in order to fully recover before the next interval. The recovery intervals may get longer as the set progresses. Important: Focus on maintaining good posture, direction, length, and catch during each work interval. This set is particularly beneficial in the late build, peak, and race-week periods when you are preparing for a swim in which you anticipate starting the swim very fast. Total work-interval duration for 1 swim set is less than 4 minutes. Example: 3 × 50 meters/yards in 35 seconds leaving every 1:30.

Test Workouts

T1: Broken Kilometer

After your standard pretest warm-up, swim 10 × 100 meters/yards at a maximal but maintainable effort with exactly 10-second recovery intervals after each 100. Time the entire set, including recovery intervals, with a running clock from the start of the first 100 to the end of the 10th. Subtract 90 seconds (for recovery intervals) to produce a test "score." Perform this test at the end of a rest-and-recovery period. Record the time of this test set in your training diary to gauge progress over time.

T2: Functional Threshold Pace Test

Following your standard pretest warm-up, swim continuously for 1,000 meters/yards as if racing while concentrating on maintaining good technique. Record the time of this test set in your training diary to gauge progress over time. Use your finish time for this test to determine your swim-pace zones (see Table 4.2) for the next training period. You can do this test at the end of each rest-and-recovery break.

APPENDIX C: BIKE WORKOUTS

The following basic bike workouts for triathletes are categorized according to the five abilities described in Chapter 6: aerobic endurance (AE), muscular force (MF), speed skills (SS), muscular endurance (ME), and anaerobic endurance (AnE). By combining portions of the workouts that follow, you can create new workouts, including multiple-ability workouts, to match your specific needs. Merging multiple abilities into one workout is most commonly done in the build period of the season (see Chapters 7 and 8 for more on periodization of training).

The MF, ME, and AnE workouts listed below should be preceded by a warm-up. You should use these three ability categories only in the main set—the primary portion of the workout that is neither warm-up nor cooldown. Note that the more intense the main set of the workout, the longer your warm-up should be.

Workout intensities are described with power and heart rate. See Table 4.3 for bike heart rate zones and Table 4.5 for bike power zones. Note that heart rate and power zones don't always agree. You may want to reread "Zone Agreement" in Chapter 4, the section that discusses their relationship. If you have both devices, use the power meter to measure performance and the heart rate monitor to gauge effort. The power meter is the preferred intensity gauge for most workouts. There are some exceptions, which are described below.

Aerobic Endurance Workouts

AE1: Recovery

Do this workout in heart rate zone 1 while using the small chain ring on a flat course. Pedal with a comfortably high cadence. Alternatively, you can use an indoor trainer or rollers for these at any time of the year, especially if flat road courses are not available. Other options for recovery in the prep and early base periods include cross-training workouts, such as cross-country skiing on a relatively flat course, and various health club machines. Note that your heart rate zones for these activities are unlikely to be the same as those for the bike.

Although light exercise on a bike is quite beneficial for speeding recovery among advanced triathletes, novices benefit more by taking time off from exercise. Recovery workouts are not included in the annual training plan, but they are an integral part of training throughout the season.

AE2: Aerobic Threshold (AeT)

The AeT workout was briefly introduced in Chapter 4 in the section "Intensity Reference Points." An important purpose of this workout is to boost aerobic fitness by improving the body's capability for delivering and using oxygen to produce energy in muscle. Use a heart rate monitor to gauge the intensity of this workout. Your AeT heart rate is approximately 30 bpm below your anaerobic threshold heart rate (see "Setting Training Zones" in Chapter 4 for details).

Following a warm-up, ride at your AeT heart rate plus or minus 2 bpm on a flat to gently rolling course, or on an indoor trainer. The length of time you spend on the AeT portion of the workout depends on the length of your target race. For sprint and Olympic-distance triathlon training, the AeT portion is 1 to 1.5 hours long. If you are training for a half-Ironman, ride 2 to 2.5 hours. Ironman athletes should do an AeT portion of 3 to 4 hours. If you are also using a power meter, when the workout is over, divide the normalized power for the AeT portion by your average heart rate for the same portion to find your efficiency factor (EF) for this session. An increasing EF over time indicates that your AeT is improving. Note that it seldom rises linearly but instead "ratchets" up over several weeks as fitness improves.

You can also use the AeT workout as a test of AE (see "T1: Aerobic Threshold [AeT] Test" below). Do this workout year-round, initially to build and later on to maintain your AE. When you are using it to maintain AE, do this workout about half as frequently as when you were initially building aerobic fitness.

AE3: Intensive Endurance

This workout develops AE while also building ME. After a warm-up, ride for an hour or more on a course with small hills while staying mostly in heart rate zone 2, but with frequent, brief increases to zone 3. Remain seated on most hills. You can also do this workout on an indoor trainer by frequently shifting gears to increase the load and simulate hills. Accumulate several minutes of zone 3 in this manner within the ride. A common variation of this workout is to run 15 to 20 minutes immediately after the ride. The purpose of the workout is to boost your body's capacity for processing oxygen to produce energy.

Muscular Force Workouts

MF1: Force Reps

This is an interval workout involving 1 to 3 sets with 3 reps within each set. That means a total of 3 to 9 reps within the session. As with all such high-intensity workouts, warm up well before starting the reps. Do this workout no more than twice per week with at least 48 hours between workouts. Do not do this workout if you have knee problems. The workout is done as follows:

→ Find a short—about 30 to 50 yards or meters long—steep hill. The grade should be about 6 to 8 percent. There should be very little traffic.

→ For each rep, select a high gear, such as 53 × 16 or 50 × 15. The stronger you are, the higher and more challenging the gear can be. Your gear selection should be high enough that your highest cadence is less than 50 rpm by the end of a rep. The steepness of the hill will also play a role in gear selection, so you will need to experiment with gearing the first time you do this workout. Err on the low-gear (easy) side at first.

→ Coast back down to the base of the hill in that high (hard) gear and almost come to a complete stop while staying balanced.

→ As you start up the hill, stay seated. Do not stand. Drive the pedals down with a maximal effort for 5 to 10 revolutions. A revolution is 1 complete pedal stroke, so, for example, count your right foot driving the pedal down

8 times. Alternate the leg you count for subsequent reps because you are likely to push harder with the "counted" leg.

→ After a rep, shift to a low (easy) gear and pedal gently for 3 to 5 minutes to allow recovery. Do not shorten the recovery time between reps because this will reduce the workout benefit of strength development. Be sure your legs are recovered before doing the next rep.

→ Repeat the above steps 2 more times for a total of 3 reps. That's 1 set. If you are doing a second set (do only 1 set the first time you try this workout), pedal easily for 5 to 10 minutes after each set to ensure full recovery. Be aware of how your knees feel on each rep. This is a high-risk, high-reward workout. At the first sign of any tenderness, stop the workout. Do not continue, even if the tenderness in your knees is only slight.

→ Power, not heart rate, is the only gauge of intensity for this session. Strive to produce very high wattage on each rep.

MF2: Hilly Ride

Select a course that includes several moderately steep hills with a grade of up to about 6 percent that take 2 to 5 minutes to climb. *Stay seated* on all hills, pedaling from the hips. That means little or no rocking of the upper body. Cadence on the climbs is 60 rpm or higher. Increase power to zone 4 or 5 on each hill. Ride in power zones 1 and 2 on the latter portions of the course. Power is the preferred gauge of intensity for this workout, but if you are using only a heart rate monitor, stay below zone 5a on the hills. On an indoor trainer, you can simulate hills by placing a 5- to 7-inch riser under the front wheel and selecting high gears and a wheel-resistance setting that will produce a slow cadence. Do this workout no more than twice per week with at least 48 hours between workouts. Do not do this workout if you are prone to knee injury.

MF3: Hill Repeats

On a steep hill with a grade of about 6 to 8 percent that takes 30 to 60 seconds to climb, do 3 to 8 repeats with 2 to 4 minutes of recovery between them. Maintain power zone 5 for each uphill climb. Your heart rate may reach zone 5a or 5b by the top of the hill later in the workout, but it will be mostly in zones 3 and 4 early in the session, even though your power reading stays the same. To recover, coast while descending before starting the next rep. Climb in the saddle, holding the handlebar tops with minimal upper-body movement. Maintain a cadence of 70 rpm or lower on each rep. Stop the workout if you find your knees becoming sensitive. Do this workout no more than twice per week with at least 48 hours between workouts. Do not do this workout at all if you are prone to knee injury.

Speed Skills Workouts

SS1: Spin-Ups

On a flat or slightly downhill section of road, or on an indoor trainer set to light resistance and in a low (easy) gear, gradually increase cadence for 1 minute to your maximum. Maximum is the cadence you can maintain without bouncing on the saddle. As the cadence increases, allow your lower legs and feet to relax—especially your toes. Hold your maximum cadence for as long as possible, which will probably be only a few seconds. Recover for at least a minute. Repeat several times. This drill is best done with a handlebar computer that displays cadence. Heart rate and power ratings have no significance for this workout. The purpose is improvement of your pedaling efficiency, indicated by an increasing maximum cadence.

SS2: Isolated Leg

On a flat or slightly downhill section of road, do 90 percent of the work with one leg while the other rests. If you are performing this drill on an indoor trainer while using a light resistance, you can support your resting leg by placing your foot on a chair or stool. Spin with a high cadence. Change legs when fatigue begins to set in. Focus on eliminating the "dead" portions at the top and bottom of the stroke. Heart rate and power ratings have no significance for this workout.

Muscular Endurance Workouts

ME1: Tempo Intervals

After warming up, do 3 to 5 work intervals in zone 3 with brief recoveries. The work intervals may be 12 to 20 minutes long with recoveries that are about one-fourth as long. For example, following a 16-minute interval, recover for 4 minutes. This workout should be done on a mostly flat road course or an indoor trainer. Power is the preferred measure of intensity for this workout, but you can also use heart rate. If you are training only with a heart rate monitor, the work interval starts as soon as you begin pedaling hard—*not* when zone 3 is achieved. There will be a time lag during the interval as your heart rate catches up to your effort. During these times, use a perceived exertion of 5 to 6 on a scale of 0 to 10 (see Chapter 4 for details on rating of perceived exertion, or RPE). Avoid roads with heavy traffic and frequent stop signs. Stay in an aerodynamic position for each interval. Recover by using easy pedaling in zone 1. Tempo intervals are a foundational workout for long-course triathlon preparation.

ME2: Cruise Intervals

On a relatively flat course or an indoor trainer, complete 3 to 5 work intervals with a duration of 6 to 12 minutes. Each work interval is done in zone 4. Power is the preferred gauge of intensity for this workout, but heart rate may be used. If you are using heart rate, the timed interval begins as soon as the hard effort begins, *not* when the heart rate achieves zone 4. During this period of increasing heart rate, estimate intensity based on a perceived exertion of 7 on a scale of 0 to 10 (see Chapter 4 for details on RPE). Recover in zone 1 with easy pedaling for about one-fourth of the preceding interval. For example, after a 6-minute interval, recover for 90 seconds with easy pedaling in zone 1. During the first such workout of the new season, the duration of the work intervals should typically total 12 minutes or less (e.g., 2 × 6 minutes). Gradually, over a few weeks, increase the combined work-interval duration to 30 to 50 minutes (e.g., 5 × 6 minutes or 4 × 12 minutes). Stay relaxed and aerodynamic, and listen closely to your breathing. The work-interval intensity is very similar to that of an Olympic-distance triathlon. Pedal with a cadence similar to what you would use at such a race distance. An optional variation that challenges you to work harder is to shift occasionally between your "normal" gear for this intensity and a higher (harder) gear.

ME3: Hill Cruise Intervals

This session is the same as ME2 cruise intervals, except it is done on a hill with a long, low gradient, such as 2 to 4 percent, or into a strong head wind. Select a hill that has light traffic and no stop signs. As with ME2, a power meter is the preferred tool for measuring intensity while you are riding in zone 4, but a heart rate monitor may be used. If you are training only with a heart rate monitor, the work interval starts as soon as you begin pedaling hard—*not* when zone 4 is ultimately achieved. Note that you may not achieve heart rate zone 4 during the first or perhaps even the second interval. That's common. During these periods of slowly increasing heart rate, use a perceived exertion of 7 on a scale of 0 to 10 to gauge intensity (see Chapter 4 for details on RPE). Stay in the aero position for each climb, and work on a smooth stroke with minimal upper-body motion. Recover after each climb by turning around and returning to the bottom of the hill in zone 1. This descent means that the recovery intervals will be longer than when you are doing ME2 intervals, but with a somewhat increased intensity for each interval and a slightly greater benefit for MF. A variation on this workout is to shift between your "normal" gear for such a climb and a higher (harder) gear every 30 seconds or so. Be sure to stay in zone 4 when doing this.

ME4: Crisscross Intervals

This workout is very similar to ME2 but somewhat more challenging. On a mostly flat course with little traffic and no stop signs, or on an indoor trainer, do 3 to 5 intervals with durations of 4 to 8 minutes in power zone 4 or heart rate zones 4 and 5a. After each interval, recover for one-fourth of the duration of the preceding interval. The combined total of the work intervals in a single session may be 12 to 25 minutes (for example, 3 × 4 minutes or 5 × 5 minutes). During each work interval, shift to a higher (harder) gear or increase your cadence to build gradually to the top of zone 4 (power) or 5a (heart rate), taking 1 to 2 minutes to do so. Then gradually reduce the intensity by shifting to a lower (easier) gear or by reducing cadence so that you slowly drop back to the bottom of zone 4, taking 1 or 2 minutes to do so. Continue this pattern throughout each interval. Power is the preferred tool for gauging intensity for this workout, but a heart rate monitor may be used. If you are training only with a heart rate monitor, the work interval starts as soon as you begin pedaling hard—*not* when zone 4 is finally achieved. You may not achieve heart rate zone 4 during the first two intervals. That's common. During these periods of slowly increasing heart rate, use a perceived exertion of 6 to 8 on a scale of 0 to 10 to gauge intensity (see Chapter 4 for details on RPE).

This is an advanced workout that shouldn't be attempted until you have done 30 minutes or more of combined work-interval time with workout ME2. The first of these workouts in a season should include short intervals (e.g., 4 minutes) with a low total combined interval time (e.g., 12 minutes).

ME5: Threshold Ride

On a mostly flat course, ride 20 to 40 minutes nonstop in power zone 4 (preferred) or heart rate zone 4. Stay focused on steady pacing while listening to your breathing throughout. Don't attempt a threshold ride until you've completed at least 4 ME interval workouts.

Anaerobic Endurance Workouts

AnE1: Group Ride

Ride with a group of triathletes that includes some who are somewhat stronger riders than you. There is no structure to this ride. Push yourself to stay with the faster riders for as long as you can. If you are unable to ride at the front with them, sit in by drafting at the back of the group or break off and ride alone. The intensity goal is to achieve zone 5 (power) or zone 5b (heart rate) for a few minutes several times during the ride. Be cautious with this workout, not only in terms of how intense it may become, but also in regard to road safety; pay attention to traffic and to other riders who may not be skilled at riding in groups. Power is the preferred metric for this workout; because of lag, heart rate is not indicative of the work being accomplished.

AnE2: VO₂max Intervals

After a long warm-up, on a mostly flat course with no stop signs and light traffic, do several work intervals, each with a duration of 30 seconds to 4 minutes. Recover with easy pedaling in zone 1 for as long as the previous interval. As your fitness improves, reduce the recovery time by half. Start with about 5 minutes of total interval time within a workout (e.g., 10×30 seconds) and gradually, over several sessions, build to about 15 minutes in a session (e.g., 5×3 minutes). A power meter is the preferred tool for measuring intensity here. Heart rate lag makes heart rate monitors ineffective for gauging intensity. The goal intensity is power zone 5. If you don't have a power meter, use a rating of perceived exertion of 9 on a scale of 0 to 10 for each interval (see Chapter 4 for details on RPE). Cadence for these intervals is at the high end of your comfort range.

AnE3: Pyramid Intervals

This workout is the same as the AnE2 session, except the work-interval progression is 1, 2, 3, 4, 3, 2, and 1 minutes in power zone 5. The recovery after each interval is equal to the preceding work interval. After having done a few of these or the AnE2 workouts, reduce the recovery durations by half. For example, following a 2-minute work interval, recover for 1 minute in zone 1. Heart rate is an ineffective gauge of intensity because of heart rate lag and the shortness of these intervals. If you don't have a power meter, use an RPE of 9 on a scale of 0 to 10 for each interval (see Chapter 4 for details on RPE). Cadence for these intervals is at the high end of your comfort range.

AnE4: Hill Intervals

Find a relatively steep hill with a gradient of 6 to 8 percent, light traffic, and no stop signs that takes 2 to 3 minutes to climb. Following a thorough warm-up, do 5 to 7 climbs in power zone 5 for a total of 10 to 15 minutes of workout climbing time (e.g., 7×2 minutes or 5×3 minutes). Sit upright with your hands on the handlebar tops while staying on the saddle with a cadence at 60 rpm or higher. Recover by coasting down the hill. Start a new interval every 2 to 3 minutes (e.g., following a 2-minute climb recover for 2 minutes). This is a very hard workout that is best done only once in a week and followed by at least 48 hours of recovery.

Test Workouts

T1: Aerobic Threshold (AeT) Test

This test of your aerobic fitness is best done after 3 to 5 days of greatly reduced training to allow rest and recovery. Follow the instructions for workout AE2 above. Although you may also be doing the AE2 workout during a "normal" training week, your results after a short rest-and-recovery break from hard training are a better indicator of your progress because fatigue is unlikely to be a mitigating factor. As with the AE2 workout above, following the session, divide your normalized power for the AeT portion by your average heart rate for the same portion to determine your current EF. Your EF value will increase over time as your aerobic fitness improves. During a period of greatly reduced training, such as at the end of the season, you should expect your EF to decrease, indicating a loss of aerobic fitness. That is normal and to be expected because fitness must decline at certain times of the year. This test should be done year-round at least every 6 to 8 weeks. If possible, use the same course every time.

T2: Functional Threshold Test

The purpose of this test is to determine your functional threshold power (FTPo) and functional threshold heart rate (FTHR). Do this test following 3 to 5 days of active rest and recovery. Find a stretch of road with a wide bike lane, light traffic, no stop signs, and few intersections and corners that is flat to slightly uphill (grade of less than 3 percent). You will probably need 5 to 10 miles depending on how fast you are. A safe course is critical. (You may also do this on an indoor trainer.) Throughout the test, keep your head up so you can see ahead. Ride as if you are in a race that lasts 20 minutes. Hold back slightly in the first 5 minutes (most athletes start much too fast). Every 5 minutes, decide whether you should go slightly faster or more slowly for the next 5 minutes. After the workout, find your average heart rate for the 20-minute test. Subtract 5 percent and you have a good estimate of your bike FTHR. Then use Table 4.3 to compute your training zones. To determine FTPo from the same test, subtract 5 percent from your average power (not "normalized" power) and you have a good estimate of FTPo. You can then use Table 4.5 to set your power training zones.

T3: Functional Aerobic Capacity Test

This test is done to determine your functional aerobic capacity (VO_2max) power. It requires a power meter. It may be done in place of a costly clinical test of VO_2max. This test is best done following reduced training for 3 to 5 days. The course you use for the test should be safe. That means light traffic, no stop signs, few intersections, no turns, and a wide bike lane. For safety, you should look straight ahead throughout the test. Do *not* ride with your head down. The selected test course should also be a flat to slightly uphill (grade of less than 3 percent) section of road that you can use every time you do this test. (You may also do this on an indoor trainer.) Warm up thoroughly and then do a steady, all-out effort for 5 minutes. Your average power for the 5-minute test portion is a good predictor of your power at aerobic capacity.

T4: Time Trial

After a thorough 15- to 30-minute warm-up, complete a 10-km time trial on a flat course. The section of road you choose should be safe, with light traffic, few intersections, no stop signs, and a wide bike lane. Keep your head up throughout the test so you can see traffic and possible road obstacles, such as potholes. The course should be flat to very slightly uphill (grade of less than 2 percent). Mark your start point and finish point for later reference, or note landmarks so you can test on the same course every time. (You may also do this on an indoor trainer.) Expect faster times as your AnE and ME improve. In addition to your time, note your average heart rate and normalized power for the test portion in your training diary. You can use any gear combination, and you may shift during the test. Treat this test like a race.

APPENDIX D: RUN WORKOUTS

Below are basic run workouts for triathlon grouped according to the five abilities described in Chapter 6: aerobic endurance (AE), muscular force (MF), speed skills (SS), muscular endurance (ME), and anaerobic endurance (AnE). These workouts may be considered modules that can be paired with others to create unique sessions. Combining multiple abilities into one workout is most commonly done in the build period of the season (see Chapters 7 and 8 for more on periodization of training).

The MF, ME, and AnE workouts listed below should be preceded by a warm-up. You should perform these three ability categories only in the main set—the primary portion of the workout that is neither warm-up nor cooldown. Note that the more intense the main set of the workout, the longer your warm-up should be. AE and SS workouts may also be in the main sets and are commonly part of the warm-up and cooldown.

Workout intensities are described here with pace and heart rate. See Table 4.4 for run heart rate zones and Table 4.6 for run pace zones determined by using a GPS device, a measured course, or a track. As explained in the section "Zone Agreement" in Chapter 4, heart rate and pace zones don't always align. If you have both a heart rate monitor and a GPS device, pace is used to evaluate performance, while heart rate expresses your effort. Pace (or speed) is the preferred metric for most workouts because the goal of training is to improve performance measurably. Although not reflective of workout accomplishment, heart rate may also be used as an indirect way of expressing intensity. Some workouts rely heavily on heart rate. For very brief intervals, as in MF and AnE sessions, and for SS workouts, heart rate is of limited value.

Aerobic Endurance Workouts

AE1: Recovery

This workout is done in zone 1, preferably on a flat, soft surface such as a park or golf course. You can instead use a treadmill for these at any time of the year, especially if flat courses are not available. The purpose is active recovery following a hard workout in the past day or so. Most age-group triathletes will be better off swimming or cycling for recovery because of the risk for an injury resulting from running on tired legs. Novices generally recover faster by taking time off from exercise. Cross-training in other sports may also be beneficial for recovery, especially in the prep and base periods. Recovery workouts are not scheduled in the annual training plan but are an integral part of training throughout the season. The duration or TSS for this workout should be the lowest in a given week of training.

AE2: Aerobic Threshold (AeT)

AeT is explained in Chapter 4 under the heading "Intensity Reference Points." A primary reason for doing this workout is to improve aerobic fitness by increasing your physical capacity for delivering and using oxygen to produce energy in muscle.

Use a heart rate monitor to gauge intensity. Your AeT heart rate is approximately 30 bpm below your anaerobic threshold heart rate (see "Setting Training Zones" in Chapter 4 for details). Following a warm-up, run from 30 minutes to 2 hours at your AeT heart rate plus or minus 2 bpm on a flat to gently rolling course or indoor trainer. The longer your intended race, the longer the AeT portion of the workout should be. For sprint- and Olympic-distance triathlon training, the AeT portion is 30 to 45 minutes. If you are training for a half-Ironman, run about 1 to 1.5 hours at AeT heart rate. Ironman athletes should do AeT portions of 1.5 to 2 hours. Build to these durations over several weeks with weekly AeT workouts. If you are also using a GPS device, when the workout is over, divide the normalized graded pace (NGP) for the AeT portion by your average heart rate for the same portion to find your efficiency factor (EF) for this session. An increasing EF over time indicates that your aerobic fitness is improving. Note that EF rises and falls over several sessions, but the trend should show an increase if your training is going well. You can also use the AeT workout as a test of aerobic endurance following a rest-and-recovery period (see "T1: Aerobic Threshold [AeT] Test" below). This workout should be done year-round, initially for building and later on for maintaining AE. To maintain AE, do this workout about half as frequently as when you were initially building your aerobic fitness.

AE3: Intensive Endurance

This workout develops AE while also contributing to improved ME. After a warm-up, run for 20 to 90 minutes or more on a course with small hills while staying mostly in heart rate zone 2, but with frequent, brief increases into zone 3. You can also use an indoor trainer by frequently changing the grade or speed to increase the workload. The purpose of this workout is to boost your body's capacity for processing oxygen to produce energy.

Muscular Force Workouts

MF1: Force Reps

This is a very challenging repeated-segment workout composed of 1 to 3 sets of 3 repetitions each, yielding a total of 3 to 9 reps within a workout. As with all such high-intensity workouts, warm up well before starting the reps. The purpose is to build greater force by strengthening your running muscles. Combining the greater force produced from doing this workout with the increased cadence of SS training results in improved running power. This workout has the potential for high reward, but it also involves high risk. Avoid this workout if you are prone to foot, Achilles tendon, calf, or knee injuries. If your legs are fully capable of handling the stress, you may increase the workload by wearing a weight vest equal to 5 to 10 percent of your body weight. Force reps are done as follows:

→ Find a short, steep (grade of 6 to 8 percent) hill that you can run to as a warm-up. Grass or dirt is the preferred surface. The hill should be at least 10 yards/meters from base to peak.

→ After warming up thoroughly, walk to the base of the hill and come to a complete stop. Then quickly run up the hill with great effort on each push-off.

→ Your stride length is determined by the steepness of the hill and by whether or not you are wearing a weight vest.

→ Keep your head up in a neutral posture as you run up the hill. Do *not* look at your feet.

→ Produce a total of 10 to 20 maximal-effort steps on each brief hill repeat. A "step" is a footstrike with either foot. The fewer steps you take in one ascent of the hill, the greater the effort should be.

→ After each hill rep, *walk* slowly back down the hill and fully recover for 2 to 3 minutes. Don't run during the recoveries or try to make the recoveries briefer. Doing so will only increase the risk and decrease the potential reward. The purpose of this workout is to increase maximum muscular strength, not to build endurance. Allow your muscles to recover before doing the next rep.

→ Repeat the above steps 2 more times for a total of 3 reps comprising 1 set. If you are doing a second or third set (it's best to do only 1 set of 3 reps the first time you do this workout), walk and run slowly for 3 to 5 minutes after each set to ensure full recovery. Again, this is a high-risk workout. Be very aware of your legs and feet on each rep. Stop the workout at the first sign of any tenderness. Do not continue even if the tenderness is only slight. No amount of fitness is worth an injury.

MF2: Hilly Run

Select a course that includes several moderately steep hills with grades of about 4 to 6 percent, each taking 2 to 5 minutes to run up. Or run on a treadmill, changing the gradient to create "hills." On the uphill portions, run at a rating of perceived exertion (RPE) of 7 or 8 on a scale of 0 to 10 (see Table 4.1 for RPE zones). Maintain a "proud" posture—head up and tall—while going up the hills.

On the flatter portions of the course, run in pace zones 1 and 2. RPE and pace are the preferred gauges of intensity for this workout, but if you are using a heart rate monitor, stay below zone 5a on the hills. Although you are working hard, you may only achieve heart rate zone 3 on hills in the early portion of this workout. Do this workout no more than once per week. Do not do this workout if you are prone to knee, foot, or lower-leg injury.

MF3: Hill Repeats

On a steep hill with a grade of about 6 to 8 percent that takes 30 to 60 seconds to climb, do 3 to 8 repeats with 2 to 4 minutes of recovery between them. Maintain an RPE in zone 7 or 8 on a scale of 0 to 10 for each uphill run (see Table 4.1 for RPE zones). Heart rate may reach zone 5a by the time you are at the top of the hill later in the workout but will be mostly in zones 3 and 4 early in the session, even though RPE is appropriately high. Maintain a "proud" posture—head up and tall—while going up the hills. To recover, slowly jog or walk back down the hill before starting the next rep. If you are wearing a weight vest, only walk down the hill to help prevent an injury to the knees. Stop the workout if your legs show signs of excessive stress, such as soreness and extreme fatigue. Do this workout no more than once per week. Do not do this workout at all if you are prone to any running injuries.

Speed Skills Workouts

SS1: Strides

The purpose of this workout is to refine your running skills. Run fast down a very slight hill (grade of 1 percent) with a soft surface such as grass or dirt for 20 seconds (RPE of 9 on a scale of 0 to 10). Do this 4 to 8 times. Focus on one aspect of your technique on each stride. This could be, for example, cadence. Count your right footstrikes for the 20 seconds with a goal of 28 to 32. A variation is to run these barefoot, but only if the grass is free of sharp objects and there are no breaks in the skin on your feet. Heart rate has no significance for this workout.

SS2: Pickups

Within an endurance run such as AE3 above, randomly insert several 20-second accelerations to a speed faster than 5-km race pace (heart rate is not a good indicator of intensity for these). The primary focus should be on your technique, such as working on a flat footstrike. Other goals may be maintaining a relaxed posture or a high cadence. Recover for several minutes between these pick-ups by returning to zone 2 steady running.

Muscular Endurance Workouts

ME1: Tempo

Warm up thoroughly. Then, on a mostly flat course or on a treadmill, run at pace zone 3 (preferred) or heart rate zone 3 for an extended time without recovery. Start with about 10 to 15 minutes of zone 3 and build to 30 to 45 minutes or more by adding 5 minutes or so each week to the tempo portion of this workout. You can do this workout once or twice weekly.

ME2: Cruise Intervals

Warm up thoroughly before doing this main set. On a relatively flat course or a treadmill, complete 3 to 5 work intervals, each with a duration of 6 to 12 minutes. Build to pace zone 4 (preferred) or heart rate zone 4 on each work inter-

val. If you are training with a heart rate monitor, the work interval starts as soon as you begin running with high effort—not when zone 4 is finally achieved. During this heart rate lag period, run at an RPE of about 7 on a scale of 0 to 10 (see Chapter 4 for details on RPE). Between intervals, recover in zone 1 by walking or jogging for one-fourth the duration of the previous interval. A variation is to run cruise intervals on a track with 1- to 2-mile work intervals in pace zone 4. Stay relaxed with a tall posture and a quick cadence while closely monitoring your breathing.

ME3: Hill Cruise Intervals

This workout is the same as ME2 cruise intervals above, except it is done on a hill with a long, low gradient (2 to 4 percent). Maintain a tall posture and quick cadence. The recovery between intervals will be longer than in ME2 because you must return to the bottom of the hill. Do this by walking and jogging slowly.

ME4: Crisscross Intervals

Complete at least 2 cruise-interval workouts before doing this workout, and warm up thoroughly before doing this main set. On a mostly flat course, run 10 to 20 minutes in pace zones 4 and 5a (preferred) or heart rate zones 4 and 5a. Once zone 4 is attained, gradually build to the top of zone 5a, taking 1 or 2 minutes to do so. Then gradually back off and slowly come to the bottom of zone 4, again taking 1 or 2 minutes. Continue this pattern throughout the run.

ME5: Threshold Run

Warm up thoroughly before starting. On a mostly flat course, run 10 to 20 minutes nonstop in pace zone 4 (preferred) or heart rate zone 4. Maintain good technique while listening to your breathing throughout. Don't attempt a threshold run until you've completed at least four of the other ME interval workouts.

Anaerobic Endurance Workouts

AnE1: Group Run

This is an unstructured workout. After a thorough warm-up, run fast with other triathletes of similar ability. Gradually increase speed until you are running in pace or heart rate zones 4 and 5a (pace preferred) with periodic surges or hill climbs in which you achieve zone 5b. This may be on mixed terrain, especially something similar to what you anticipate for your short-course race. The duration of the fast portion may vary based on your race goals and current level of fitness.

AnE2: VO$_2$max Intervals

After a long warm-up, move to a mostly flat road course, treadmill, or track. Do several work intervals with a duration of 30 seconds to 4 minutes, each in pace zone 5b. Recover after each with easy jogging and walking in zone 1 for as long as the previous interval. As your fitness improves, reduce the recovery time by half. Start with about 5 minutes of total interval time within a workout (e.g., 10 × 30 seconds) and gradually, over several sessions, build to about 15 minutes in a session (e.g., 5 × 3 minutes). A GPS device is the preferred tool for measuring intensity during this workout. Heart rate lag makes heart rate monitors ineffective for gauging intensity for such short intervals. If you don't have a GPS device, run at an RPE of 9 on a scale of 0 to 10 for each interval (see Chapter 4 for details on RPE). Concentrate on good running technique.

AnE3: Hill Intervals

Find a relatively steep (grade of 6 to 8 percent) hill that takes 2 to 3 minutes to run up. Following a thorough warm-up, do 5 to 7 climbs at a perceived exertion of 9 on a scale of 0 to 10 (see Chapter 4 for details on RPE) for a total of 10 to 15 minutes of total workout climbing time (e.g., 7 × 2 minutes or 5 × 3 minutes). (Heart rate lag makes heart rate monitors ineffective for this workout.) Recover by slowly jogging and walking down the hill, then start a new interval when you reach the base. This is a very hard workout that is best done only once in a week and followed by at least 48 hours of recovery. Complete at least 2 AnE2 and 2 MF workouts before doing this one.

Test Workouts

T1: Aerobic Threshold (AeT) Test

This test of your aerobic fitness is best done after 3 to 5 days of greatly reduced training to allow rest and recovery. Follow the instructions for workout AE2 above. While you may also be doing the AE2 workout during a "normal," non-recovery training week, your results after a short rest-and-recovery break from hard training are a better indicator of your progress because fatigue is unlikely to be a mitigating factor. As with the AE2 workout above, following the session, divide your NGP for the AeT portion by your average heart rate for the same portion to determine your current EF. As your aerobic fitness improves over time, your EF value will trend upward. During a period of greatly reduced training, such as at the end of the season, you should expect your EF to decline steadily, indicating a loss of aerobic fitness. That is normal and to be expected because fitness must subside at certain times of the year.

TABLE D.1 Estimation of VO₂max from a 1.5-Mile Run Test

TIME FOR 1.5 MILES (MIN:SEC)	ESTIMATED VO₂MAX (ML/KG/MIN)
7:30 and faster	75
7:31–8:00	72
8:01–8:30	67
8:31–9:00	62
9:01–9:30	58
9:31–10:00	55
10:01–10:30	52
10:31–11:00	49
11:01–11:30	46
11:31–12:00	44
12:01–12:30	41
12:31–13:00	39
13:01–13:30	37
13:31–14:00	36
14:01–14:30	34
14:31–15:00	33
15:01–15:30	31
15:31–16:00	30
16:01–16:30	28
16:31–17:00	27
17:01–17:30	26
17:31–18:00	25

This test should be done year-round at least every 6 to 8 weeks. If possible, use the same course every time and keep other conditions (e.g., shoes, warm-up, time of day, and before-workout meals) the same from one test to the next.

T2: Functional Threshold Test

The purpose of this test is to determine your functional threshold pace (FTPa) and functional threshold heart rate (FTHR) for running in order to set your training zones. Do this test following 3 to 5 days of active rest and recovery. A road course should be relatively flat for this test, or do it on a track (preferred). Use the same course every time. (Most treadmills can't be calibrated closely enough to attain the accuracy required for this test.) Run as if you are in a race that lasts 20 minutes. Hold back slightly in the first 5 minutes (most athletes start much too fast). Every 5 minutes, decide whether you should go slightly faster or more slowly for the next 5 minutes. Cool down afterward with easy jogging and walking. Following the workout, find your average heart rate for the 20-minute test. *Subtract* 5 percent and you have a good estimate of your run FTHR. Then use Table 4.4 to compute your heart rate training zones. If you are using a GPS device on a road course, *add* 5 percent to your NGP to determine FTPa. If you performed the test on a track, use the track measurements to determine pace and also *add* 5 percent for an estimate of FTPa. Table 4.6 may then be used to set your pace training zones.

T3: Functional Aerobic Capacity Test

Use this test to determine your functional aerobic capacity (VO₂max) pace. A GPS device is required if the test is done on the road. If you are on a track, use its measurements to determine pace. (Most treadmills can't be calibrated closely enough to attain the accuracy required for this test.) This test is best done following reduced training for 3 to 5 days. Warm up thoroughly and then run a steady, all-out effort for 5 minutes. Your NGP from a road test or the actual pace from a track-based test for the 5-minute test portion is a good predictor of your pace at aerobic capacity. This test may be done in place of a costly clinical test of VO₂max.

T4: VO$_2$max Estimation Time Trial

The following test may be used as a predictor of your VO$_2$max (milliliters of O$_2$ per kilogram per minute) in place of a costly clinical test. After a thorough 10- to 20-minute warm-up, complete a 1.5-mile, maximum-effort time trial on a track or a flat and precisely measured road course. (Most treadmills can't be calibrated closely enough to attain the accuracy required for this test.) Record the time for the time trial in your training diary to compare with future time trials. In addition to time, record your average and peak heart rates. Keep the conditions the same from one time trial to the next. You can estimate your VO$_2$max from your time in this 1.5-mile time trial as shown in Table D.1.

APPENDIX E: COMBINED BIKE-RUN ("BRICK") WORKOUTS

These basic combined bike-run workouts are categorized into the five abilities presented in Chapter 6: aerobic endurance (AE), muscular force (MF), speed skills (SS), muscular endurance (ME), and anaerobic endurance (AnE). Combined bike-run workouts are commonly called *bricks* by triathletes. There are many other possible brick workouts that are variations on these, including multiple-ability workouts that may have two abilities within the bike and run portions or a different ability focus in each of the two sports. For example, the bike or run portion could include both AE and ME. Another variation could focus on AE for the bike portion and ME for the run. The possibilities are many. You can vary the bricks you create to fit your specific needs relative to the anticipated demands of your targeted race. The only limit is your creativity in designing workouts. The merging of two or more abilities into a single brick workout is most commonly done in the build period of the season (see Chapters 7 and 8 for more on periodization of training).

The order of sports within a brick is typically bike followed by run. But duathletes often do run-bike-run workouts because that's their common race design. You can also do bricks with several alternating stages of the two sports, such as bike-run-bike-run. Such workouts are often done at a running track with a stationary trainer set up nearby for the bike portions. Swim-to-bike bricks are rare, but there is certainly merit in rehearsing the first transition. You will see an example of this below in the SS workouts.

When you transition from the bike to the run in one of these brick workouts, it's recommended that you follow the same procedure you intend to use in your targeted race; doing so will serve as practice for your transition in your race. Lay out your transition area to be as similar as possible to the way it will be on race day. As you end the bike ride, quickly and efficiently change shoes and put on any other run clothing while also grabbing whatever food or equipment that you will need.

How long should the run portion of a brick be? It depends, of course, on the type of race you are targeting. But it's often best to keep the run portions short because running on legs that are tired from a long bike ride increases your risk for an injury. Even for long-course races, a 15-minute run following a long bike ride is beneficial for learning to cope with the strange sensation of running on bike-weary legs. For short-course races, a brick that has about the same duration that you expect the combined bike and run portions of the race to have is common. For long-course racing, however, bricks that are equal in duration to the anticipated combined bike and run portions of the race are not recommended because the recovery afterward takes too long.

When the bike portion of a brick calls for ME or AnE, the workout should be preceded by a warm-up. (MF workouts are best *not* done as bricks.) These two ability categories are used only in the brick's main set—the primary portion of the workout that is neither warm-up nor cooldown. Note that the more intense the main set of the workout, the longer your warm-up should be. In a brick, the bike portion always serves as a warm-up for the following run.

Aerobic Endurance Workouts

AE1: Aerobic Threshold (AeT) Brick

Complete a long ride on a rolling course while staying primarily in heart rate zone 2. Then transition to a run on a mostly flat course, also in heart rate zone 2. The total time for this brick may vary from 90 minutes to 5 hours depending on the distance of the race you are preparing for and your periodization. You can emphasize the run portion one week and the bike the next week.

AE2: Intensive Endurance Brick

Following a warm-up, ride on a rolling course with more than half of the time in power zones 2 and 3 (preferred) or heart rate zones 2 and 3, accumulating as much zone 3 time as possible. Then transition to a run, also primarily in pace (preferred) or heart rate zones 2 and 3. You can vary emphasizing the bike and run portion durations from week to week by alternately doing a long bike ride followed by a short run and then reversing the durations the following week. This is an especially good workout when you are preparing for a long-course race.

Muscular Force Workouts

MF workouts are best done in isolation as stand-alone bike or run sessions. Combining them greatly increases the risk for injury.

Speed Skills Workouts

SS1: Transition 1 (T1) Practice

At the pool or other swimming venue, set up your bike on a trainer. Swim several race-pace sets and then transition to the bike for 5 minutes at race intensity. The transition involves putting on cycling shoes and helmet, and possibly removing a wet suit (the latter should be rehearsed if you are doing a race with a wet suit swim). Repeat this 3 to 5 times. Emphasis should be placed on making T1 as efficient and quick as possible.

SS2: Transition 2 (T2) Practice

At the running track or other handy venue, set up your bike on a trainer. After a warm-up, ride 5 minutes at race pace and then transition by changing into run shoes and putting on a cap or any other materials you will use during the run in your race. Following the transition, run for 3 to 5 minutes at T2-exit, goal-race pace. Repeat the bike-to-run workout 3 to 5 times. Emphasis should be placed on making T2 as efficient and quick as possible.

Muscular Endurance Workouts

ME1: Tempo Brick

Depending on the length of your next race, bike for 60 to 90 minutes including a 10- (sprint), 20- (Olympic), 30- (half-Ironman), or 40-km (Ironman) effort at racelike intensity on a course similar to that of your next A- or B-priority race. Ride the measured portion at an intensity similar to or slightly greater than that planned for your next important race. Then transition to a 10-

(sprint), 20- (Olympic), 30- (half-Ironman), or 40-minute (Ironman) run at your goal-race pace.

ME2: Hilly Brick

In preparation for a hilly race, design a brick course that closely simulates the race course. This can be a hilly bike and flat run or a flat bike and hilly run, or both the bike and run may be hilly. The emphasis of the workout is on the hilly portions, where you should rehearse proper pacing on the climbs. The bike and run courses should be considerably shorter than those in the race, at about one-half of the race distance or less. On the flat portions, ride and run steadily at an intensity (power, pace, heart rate, or RPE) similar to what you will do in the race. On the uphill portions, increase the power, run speed, or heart rate by *no more than* two zones. This intensity variation is recommended for the race so that the workout can be a rehearsal.

Anaerobic Endurance Workouts

AnE1: Bike-Intervals Brick

This workout is recommended for short-course triathletes only. Ride 45 to 90 minutes on a flat to rolling course. After warming up on the bike, do 3 to 5 work intervals, each with a duration of 2 to 4 minutes. The interval intensity should be above your functional threshold power (FTPo). Power is the preferred measurement, but if you are using a heart rate monitor, you are unlikely to achieve heart rates above zone 4 because of heart rate lag. In this case, use a rating of perceived exertion

(RPE) of 8 to 9 on a scale of 0 to 10. Recover after each work interval for a time equal to half of the preceding work-interval time. For example, after a 4-minute work interval, recover for 2 minutes. Accumulate up to about 15 minutes of total work-interval time on the bike. Transition to a run with a duration about half the duration of the preceding bike portion (e.g., if you rode for 60 minutes, run for 30 minutes). During the run and immediately following the transition, include 10 to 20 minutes of steady state in pace zone 4 (preferred) or heart rate zone 4.

AnE2: Run-Intervals Brick

Take your indoor bike trainer to a running track. Run for 10 to 20 minutes in pace (preferred) or heart rate zones 1 to 3 for warm up. Then, on the bike trainer, ride for 5 to 10 minutes while achieving power (preferred) or heart rate zone 4 in the last minute or so. Transition to running shoes and complete 2 to 4 work intervals that last 2 to 4 minutes, with intensity rising into pace (preferred) zone 5b on each. You may also do these work intervals with intensity based on an RPE of 8 to 9 on a scale of 0 to 10. Heart rate is ineffective because of the shortness of the intervals. Recovery intervals are half the duration of the previous work interval and done in zone 1. Return to the bike and again ride 5 minutes, building to zone 4. Repeat this alternating bike-run pattern 1 to 3 more times before cooling down for 10 minutes or so on the bike. Aim for a total of about 20 minutes or 3 miles of work intervals for running.

GLOSSARY

Ability. In the context of this book, a category of workouts focusing on an intended physical adaptation in preparation for racing. See *adaptation, aerobic endurance, muscular force, speed skills , muscular endurance, anaerobic endurance,* and *sprint power.*

Active recovery. Low-intensity exercise intended to allow recovery. See *passive recovery.*

Adaptation. The body's physiological adjustment to a physical-training stress placed on it over a period of time. The purpose is to improve an element of fitness. Adaptation requires that the training ability be stressed repeatedly over many weeks. See *ability* and *fitness.*

Aerobic. Occurring in the presence of oxygen; aerobic metabolism uses primarily oxygen to produce energy. Also refers to any exercise intensity below the anaerobic threshold.

Aerobic capacity (AeC). The maximal volume of oxygen an athlete can process to produce energy during a maximal and prolonged exertion. Also known as VO_2max. Aerobic capacity is determined in a graded exercise test by measuring oxygen uptake (in milliliters), dividing it by the athlete's body weight (in kilograms), then dividing the quotient by the duration of exercise (in minutes) at maximal intensity: $VO_2max = O_2$ uptake (mL)/body weight (kg)/duration at maximal intensity (min). See VO_2max.

Aerobic endurance. In the context of this book, a category of workouts done at or near the aerobic threshold and intended to improve an athlete's aerobic ability.

Aerobic threshold (AeT). The exercise intensity at which blood lactate begins to rise above the resting level. Exercise is fully aerobic at this intensity, with fuel supplied primarily by stored body fat. In terms of heart rate, the aerobic threshold is about 20 to 40 bpm below the anaerobic or lactate threshold.

Agonist muscles. The primary movement muscles, which contract with the purpose of propelling the body for activities such as swimming, cycling, and running. See *antagonist muscles.*

Anaerobic. Literally, "without oxygen." Describes very high-intensity exercise during which the demand for oxygen is greater than can be met. The primary fuel during anaerobic exercise is carbohydrate. Also used to describe the intensity of exercise performed above the anaerobic or lactate threshold.

Anaerobic endurance. In the context of this book, a category of workouts done to improve an athlete's ability to maintain a high level of intensity above the anaerobic threshold for an extended period of time.

Anaerobic threshold (AnT). A high level of intensity that occurs immediately before exercise becomes anaerobic. Above this level, energy production becomes anaerobic, with energy supplied by stored carbohydrate. Intensities above the AnT can be maintained continuously for a few minutes up to about an hour, depending on how high the level of intensity.

Antagonist muscles. Muscles that oppose the contraction of agonist muscles. For example, the triceps is an antagonist muscle for the biceps because the biceps flexes the elbow and the triceps extends it. See *agonist muscles*.

Base period. In seasonal periodization, the training period during which the workouts are "general," meaning not exactly like the demands of the targeted event. The purpose of training in this period is to prepare the body for the training stresses of the build period. See *prep period*, *build period*, *peak period*, *race period*, and *transition period*.

Beats per minute (bpm). The number of heartbeats per minute during exercise.

Bonk. A state of extreme exhaustion during a very long endurance session related to the depletion of glycogen. See *glycogen*.

Breakthrough (BT). A challenging workout intended to cause a significant, positive, adaptive response. These workouts generally

must be followed by 36 or more hours of active rest for adequate recovery.

Brick. A combined and continuous bike-run workout commonly done by triathletes.

Build period. In seasonal periodization, the training period during which the workouts are "specific," meaning very much like the demands of the targeted event. The purpose of training in this period is to prepare the body for the training stresses of racing. See *prep period*, *base period*, *peak period*, *race period*, and *transition period*.

Cadence. Revolutions per minute of the swim stroke, pedal stroke, or running stride.

Capillaries. Small blood vessels located between arteries and veins in which the exchange of oxygen and fuel between tissue (e.g., muscle) and blood occurs. Generally, several capillaries at a given site form a capillary bed. As aerobic fitness improves in a given muscle, the capillary beds for that muscle are enlarged.

Carbohydrate loading. A dietary procedure intended to elevate muscle and liver glycogen stores by emphasizing carbohydrate consumption for a few days prior to a race.

Cardiorespiratory system. The system comprising the heart, blood vessels, and lungs, which interact to supply fuel and oxygen to the working muscles during exercise.

Catch. In freestyle swimming, the portion of the stroke during which the arm is fully extended in front of the athlete's body and the fingers are pointed toward the bottom of the pool. The catch phase of the stroke starts as the fingers enter the water and lasts until the hand exits the water. This is the primary propulsive movement of swimming and is critical to performance.

Central nervous system. The brain and spinal cord.

Circuit training. Selected exercises or activities performed rapidly and in sequence. A term often used in weight training.

Compound exercise. In weight lifting, an exercise that uses multiple joints, usually in the same manner in which they are recruited during swimming, cycling, and running. For example, the squat is a compound exercise involving the hips, knees, and ankles and is somewhat similar to the lower body's movement in pedaling a bicycle.

Concentric contraction. Muscular contraction during which the muscle shortens, as when the biceps muscle is used in an arm-curling exercise. During bicycle pedaling, the quadriceps muscle is used concentrically. See *eccentric contraction*.

Cooldown. Low-intensity exercise at the end of a training session intended to return the body gradually to a resting state.

Cranks. On a bicycle, the levers to which the pedals are attached.

Crosstraining. Workouts that involve activities not usually part of an athlete's primary sport. For example, weight lifting and cross-country skiing are crosstraining activities for a triathlete.

Direction. In freestyle swimming, placement of the extended hand and arm in front of the athlete's body before the hand enters the water. The hand and arm must point in the direction of the intended path of movement.

Drafting. Swimming, biking, or running closely behind another athlete in order to reduce effort.

Drops. The lower portion of turned-down handlebars, commonly seen on road bicycles.

Duration. The length of time of a given workout.

Eccentric contraction. Muscular contraction during which the muscle lengthens as it contracts, as, for example, when the biceps muscle is used to slowly lower a weight that was lifted during an arm curl. In running, the quadriceps muscle is used eccentrically. See *concentric contraction*.

Economy. The physiological cost of swimming, biking, or running. Economy is commonly expressed as liters of oxygen consumed for a given duration or distance. As an athlete becomes more economical, the amount of oxygen that is consumed at any given pace or power decreases. See *fitness*.

Efficiency factor (EF). In the context of this book, the normalized power divided by the average heart rate for a steady, aerobic workout or segment thereof, such as an aerobic interval. An increasing EF over time suggests improving aerobic fitness. See *normalized power*.

Endurance. The ability to persist or to resist fatigue for a relatively long duration.

Ergogenic aid. A substance, device, or phenomenon that can improve athletic performance. For example, caffeine is often considered an ergogenic aid for endurance sports. Some ergogenic aids are banned from triathlon.

Fartlek. A Swedish term meaning speed play. An unstructured, interval-type workout in which the intensity and duration of the intervals and recovery times between them are completely subjective and spur-of-the-moment decisions.

Fast-twitch (FT) fiber. A muscle fiber characterized by a fast contraction time, high anaerobic capacity, and low aerobic capacity, all making the fiber suited for high-power activities such as sprints. See *slow-twitch fiber*.

Fatigue. In sport, the long-term accumulation of tiredness resulting from training.

Fitness. In endurance sport, the combined product of an athlete's aerobic capacity, anaerobic threshold (as a percentage of aerobic capacity), and economy. See *aerobic capacity*, *anaerobic threshold*, and *economy*.

Foot strike. The brief moment when the foot makes initial contact with the ground during running.

Force. The muscular work done to overcome a resistance. For example, pushing down on a bicycle pedal exerts force. See *torque*.

Form. An athlete's readiness to race. Specifically, on race day the athlete should have a relatively high level of fitness and be fresh, without fatigue.

Free weights. Weights, such as barbells and dumbbells, that are not part of an exercise machine.

Frequency. The number of times per week that an athlete trains.

Functional threshold (FT, FTPa, FTPo). The term *functional threshold pace* (FTPa) is used in swimming and running, while the term *functional threshold power* (FTPo) is used in cycling. Both terms refer to an intensity level that is similar to the anaerobic threshold or lactate threshold. The intensity level is determined through a field test, instead of in a clinic by measuring oxygen expenditure or lactate accumulation. The most common test duration is 20 minutes. FTPa is determined by subtracting 5 percent of the average speed in swimming and running; FTPo is determined by subtracting 5 percent of the average power in cycling. See *anaerobic threshold* and *lactate threshold*.

Gear, high and low. On a bicycle, one crank revolution in a high gear results in the bike going a greater distance than one revolution in a low gear. During bicycle riding, greater force is required to turn the cranks in a high gear than in a low gear.

Glycogen. A source of fuel for exercise derived primarily from dietary carbohydrate. Glycogen is the body's storage form of sugar.

GPS device. An electronic mechanism worn by an athlete, usually on the wrist, or installed on the handlebars of a bicycle. It determines position and is used to measure distance and speed with the U.S. navigational Global Positioning System. Data from the device may be downloaded to a computer following the session for analysis.

Hammer. A slang term used to describe a fast, sustained, nearly maximal effort.

Hamstring. Muscle on the back of the thigh that flexes the knee and extends the hip.

Heart rate monitor. An electronic device that measures and displays an athlete's pulse and may be downloaded to a computer for analysis following a training session.

Hoods. On drop handlebars, the rubber covers over the brake lever mechanisms.

Human growth hormone. A hormone secreted by the anterior lobe of the pituitary gland that stimulates physical growth and development.

Individuality, principle of. The theory that any training program must consider the specific needs and abilities of the individual for whom it is designed, as individual athletes often vary considerably in their responses to training.

Intensity. The qualitative element of training referring to effort, speed, velocity, pace, force, and power.

Intensity factor (IF). A power metric that quantifies workout intensity. IF is determined by dividing the workout's normalized power by the rider's functional threshold power (IF = NP ÷ FTP). See *intensity*, *normalized power*, and *functional threshold power*.

Intervals. A system of generally high-intensity work marked by short but regularly repeated periods of hard exercise interspersed with periods of recovery. See *work interval* and *recovery interval*.

Isolated leg training (ILT). Pedaling a bicycle with one leg in order to focus on improving technique. Generally done on an indoor trainer.

Kickboard. A flat, floating device held in a swimmer's hands during kicking drills.

Kilojoule (kJ). In training with a power meter, the unit used to express how much energy is expended throughout a workout or portion of a workout. The cumulative training load for a given period of time, such as a week, may also be measured in kilojoules. A kilojoule is the average power (in watts) multiplied by the number of seconds within a workout or selected portion of a workout; this product is then divided by 1,000. See *workload*.

Lactate. A chemical formed in the body that enters the bloodstream following the production of lactic acid in the muscles. See *lactic acid*.

Lactate threshold (LT). The intensity during exercise at which blood lactate begins to accumulate because of the body's inability to process it, resulting in labored breathing. The LT is similar to the anaerobic threshold

(AnT), but LT is determined by sampling blood lactate, whereas AnT is measured by sampling inhaled and expired oxygen. See *anaerobic threshold*.

Lactic acid. A by-product of the incomplete breakdown of glucose (sugar) during the production of energy in the muscles. Lactic acid is produced during both rest and exercise. See *lactate*.

Length, pool. Often referred to as a *lap* in swimming.

Long-course triathlon. A race distance equal to that of a half-Ironman (70.3 miles/113 km) or an Ironman (140.6 miles/226 km) race. See *short-course triathlon*.

Long, slow distance (LSD). A form of continuous training in which an athlete performs at a relatively low intensity, usually below the aerobic threshold, for a long duration.

Macrocycle. In training periodization, a period of training that includes several mesocycles. Usually refers to an entire season but may also refer to the preparation period for a single race. See *mesocycle* and *microcycle*.

Main set. The primary portion of a workout session that is focused on a specific training ability. This typically follows the warm-up and precedes the cooldown.

Mash. To push a high gear on a bicycle at a slow cadence.

Mesocycle. In training periodization, a period of training generally 2 to 6 weeks long. See *macrocycle* and *microcycle*.

Microcycle. In training periodization, a period of training of approximately 1 week. See *macrocycle* and *mesocycle*.

Muscular endurance. In the context of this book, a category of workouts done to improve the ability of a muscle or muscle group to perform repeated contractions for a long period of time while overcoming resistance.

Muscular force. In the context of this book, a category of workouts done as brief repeats at a maximal intensity with long recoveries between repeats for the purpose of increasing an athlete's ability for sport-specific strength.

Negative splits. Producing a faster time or pace, or a greater power output, in the second half of a workout, race, or interval. See *pacing*.

Normalized graded pace (NGP). In running, the adjusted pace at which an athlete runs with consideration for hills. Effort expended is represented more closely by NGP than by average pace. A GPS device and software are necessary to measure NGP. See *GPS*.

Normalized power (NP). A measurement of performance derived from an algorithm that computes the average power attained during cycling and assigns greater numerical weight to surges. The NP for a workout is typically somewhat higher than the workout's average power. A power meter and software are necessary to measure NP. See *power meter* and *surging*.

Open water. A term used to refer to swim venues that are not pool-based, such as lakes, rivers, and the ocean.

Overload, principle of. A training load that challenges the body's current level of fitness and causes adaptation. See *adaptation* and *fitness*.

Overreaching. Training above the workload that will produce overtraining if such a training load is continued long enough.

Overtraining. A physical and mental condition marked by extreme fatigue and caused by training for an excessive period of time at a workload higher than that to which the body can readily adapt. It's the result of an imbalance between training stress and rest.

Pace. A measurement of the intensity of a swim or run workout based on the relationship between time and distance.

Pacing. The act of carefully managing the expenditure of energy during a workout, race, or interval to produce a steady speed or power, thus leading to the best possible performance. Unsteady pacing wastes energy. See *negative splits* and *surging*.

Passive recovery. A day or group of days with no workouts, the goal of which is complete rest. See *active recovery*.

Peak period. In seasonal periodization, the training period during which workouts are "specific," meaning very much like the demands of the targeted event, and workout durations are decreased while intensity remains high. The peak period typically follows the build period and precedes the race period. The purpose of this period is to produce form gradually by allowing the body to recover from the previous period of hard training while steadily becoming race-ready. See *form, base period, prep period, build period, race period,* and *transition period.*

Periodization. A seasonal planning method of structuring training into periods based on training volume and intensity, with each period focused on a specific training objective. See *intensity, volume, macrocycle, mesocycle,* and *microcycle.*

Posture. In freestyle swimming, a hydrodynamic body position requiring the athlete's head, spine, and hips to be in alignment and nearly parallel to the water surface.

Power meter. An electronic device that measures cadence and either torque (cycling) or force (running), thus providing a wattage reading as an indicator of intensity. The data may be downloaded to a computer for analysis following the session.

Preparation (prep) period. In seasonal periodization, the training period during which the workouts are very "general," meaning not exactly the same as the demands of the targeted event. The purpose of training in this period is to return gradually to a structured training program following a break from focused training during the preceding transition period. See *base period, build period, peak period, race period,* and *transition period.*

Progression, principle of. The theory that an athlete's training workload must be gradually increased over time, accompanied by intermittent periods of recovery.

Pull buoy. A floating device placed between the thighs and used by swimmers during some types of drills in order to allow concentration on the upper body's movements. A pull buoy may also be used to reduce the intensity of a workout, as during swimming for recovery only.

Quadriceps. The large muscle at the front of the thigh that extends the lower leg and flexes the hip.

Race period. In seasonal periodization, the training period during which the workouts are "specific," meaning very much like the demands of the targeted event, and workout durations are very brief while intensity remains high. This period typically follows the peak period and culminates with the targeted race. The purpose of this period is to recover completely from the previous periods of hard training and become race-ready. See *prep period, base period, build period, peak period,* and *transition period.*

Rating of perceived exertion (RPE). A subjective assessment of how hard one is working that generally uses a scale of 0 (low) to 10 (high).

Recovery interval. The relief period between work intervals within an interval workout. The recovery interval is defined by its duration and intensity, which is usually quite low. See *work interval.*

Repetition maximum (RM). In weight lifting, the maximum load that an athlete can lift in one attempt. Also called *1-repetition maximum* (1RM).

Repetitions (reps). The number of times a task, such as a work interval or lifting a weight, is repeated. See *set.*

Rest-and-recovery (R&R) period. In periodization, a period of moderate training that follows a block of hard training. During R&R, passive recovery and active recovery are emphasized. R&R is typically included in training after about 2 or 3 weeks of focused training in the base and build periods.

Sculling. A swimming drill in which only the arms and hands are used to propel the body while it is in a prone or supine position. The arms and hands make a figure-eight movement, similar to the movement made when one is treading water, in order to move the body through the water.

Session. A single workout or race.

Set. A group of repetitions. See *repetitions.*

Short-course triathlon. Sprint- and Olympic-distance ("standard") races (16 miles/25.75 km and 47.93 miles/51.5 km, respectively). See *long-course triathlon.*

Sighting. To stay on course while swimming in open water, an athlete occasionally glances above the water line to see course buoys or landmarks on the shore.

Slow-twitch (ST) fiber. A muscle fiber characterized by a slow contraction time, low anaerobic capacity, and high aerobic capacity, all making the fiber suited for low-power, long-duration activities.

Specificity, principle of. The theory that training must stress the specialized systems critical for optimal performance in order to achieve the desired training adaptations.

Speed skills. Within the context of this book, a category of workouts focused on improving the ability to move the body efficiently in order to produce optimal performance—for example, the ability to run efficiently with a high cadence.

Sprint power. In the context of this book, a category of workouts done at a maximal effort for a very brief time and typically at a very high cadence with long recovery periods between high efforts. This workout is intended to improve sprinting ability. Sprint-power workouts are common in some sports, such as bicycle road racing, but are not recommended for triathletes who do nondrafting workouts.

Surging. Swimming, cycling, or running unsteadily with a great deal of unnecessary energy expenditure during brief accelerations. Surging wastes energy in a triathlon. See *pacing* and *negative splits*.

Tapering. A training method initiated a few days or weeks prior to an important race in which training volume is gradually reduced in order for an athlete to come into form on race day. See *form*.

Tempo. Maintaining moderately hard intensity between the aerobic and anaerobic thresholds.

Torque. In pedaling a bicycle, the rotational force applied to the pedals. See *force*.

Training. A comprehensive program or portions thereof intended to prepare an athlete for competition.

Training stress score (TSS). The numerical value assigned to a session by using an algorithm based on session duration and intensity. A power meter, heart rate monitor, GPS, or other device is required for accurately measuring intensity. Because it involves both duration and intensity, cumulative TSS may be used to create a training seasonal plan. See *power meter*, *GPS device*, *heart rate monitor*, *periodization*, *duration*, *intensity*, and *workload*.

Training zones. Consecutive categories of intensity based on heart rate, pace, or power that are unique to an athlete's physical capacity. Training zones are typically based on percentages of an athlete's unique physiological marker, such as anaerobic threshold, lactate threshold, or functional threshold. Typically used to predetermine how intense a workout or portion of a workout will be. See *anaerobic threshold*, *lactate threshold*, and *functional threshold*.

Transition. The enclosed area at a triathlon where each athlete has an assigned stall and where swim, bike, and run gear are stored. Here, the athlete makes equipment changes from swim to bike (transition 1, or T1) and from bike to run (transition 2, or T2).

Transition (tran) period. In seasonal periodization, the training period during which workouts are quite easy, allowing full recovery in the days immediately following a targeted race. The purpose of this period is to recover completely from the stresses of recent training and racing. See *prep period*, *base period*, *build period*, *peak period*, and *race period*.

Variability index (VI). An indicator of how steadily (or nonsteadily) paced a workout, race, or interval is when a bicycle power meter is used. It is determined by dividing normalized power by average power. A resulting quotient of 1.05 or less is an indicator of steady pacing. A VI rising above 1.05 indicates progressively nonsteady riding marked by surging. See *pacing*, *negative splits*, and *surging*.

Ventilatory threshold (VT). The moment during steadily increasing exertion at which breathing first becomes labored. The VT closely corresponds to the lactate and anaerobic thresholds.

VO$_2$max. An athlete's physical capacity for oxygen consumption during a maximal endurance exertion. Also known as *aerobic capacity* and *maximal oxygen consumption*. VO$_2$max is numerically expressed as milliliters of oxygen consumed per kilogram of body weight per minute (mL/kg/min). VO$_2$max is closely related to endurance fitness. See *aerobic capacity* and *fitness*.

Volume. A quantitative element of training that expresses how much training is done in a given time frame, such as a week. Volume is commonly based on the cumulative training stress score (TSS), on total miles or kilometers, or on collective hours of training. Volume results from the combination of individual workout durations and their frequency. See *training stress score*, *duration*, and *frequency*.

Warm-up. The period of gradually increasing the intensity of exercise at the start of a training session, with the intent of readying the body for the physical stress of the main set. See *main set*.

Work interval. High-intensity efforts within an interval workout separated by recovery intervals. Work intervals are commonly defined by their durations and intensities. See *intervals* and *recovery interval*.

Workload. The measured stress applied in training through the combination of frequency, intensity, and duration for a given period of time, such as a week. This expresses both the quantitative and qualitative aspects of training in a single number. Common measurements are cumulative training stress score (TSS) and kilojoules (kJ) for the designated time frame. See *training stress score* and *kilojoules*.

Workout. A complete training session that is focused on a specific outcome and typically includes a warm-up, main set, and cooldown. See *warm-up*, *main set*, and *cooldown*.

BIBLIOGRAPHY

Chapter 1: Mental Fitness

Blanchfield, A. W., J. Hardy, H. M. De Morree, W. Staiano, and S. M. Marcora. "Talking Yourself Out of Exhaustion: The Effects of Self-Talk on Endurance Performance." *Medicine and Science in Sports and Exercise* (2014) 46 (5): 998–1007.

Casey, B. J., L. H. Somerville, I. H. Gotlib, O. Ayduk, N. T. Franklin, M. K. Askren, J. Jonides, M. G. Berman, N. L. Wilson, T. Teslovich, G. Glover, V. Zayas, W. Mischel, and Y. Shoda. "Behavioral and Neural Correlates of Delay of Gratification 40 Years Later." *Proceedings of the National Academy of Sciences of the United States of America* (2011) 108 (36): 14998–15003.

Jones, G. "How the Best of the Best Get Better and Better." *Harvard Business Review* (2008) 86 (6): 123–127, 142.

Zadow, E. K., N. Gordon, C. R. Abbiss, and J. J. Peiffer. "Pacing, the Missing Piece of the Puzzle to High-Intensity Interval Training." *International Journal of Sports Medicine* (2015) 36 (3): 215–219.

Chapter 2: Physical Fitness

Bouchard, C., M. A. Sarzynski, T. K. Rice, W. E. Kraus, T. S. Church, Y. J. Sung, D. C. Rao, and T. Rankinen. "Genomic Predictors of Maximal Oxygen Uptake Response to Standardized Exercise Training Programs." *Journal of Applied Physiology* (2010) 110 (5): 1160–1170.

Ericsson, K. A. "Training History, Deliberate Practice and Elite Sports Performance: An Analysis in Response to Tucker and Collins Review—What Makes Champions?" *British Journal of Sports Medicine* (2013) 47 (9): 533–535.

Lehmann, M. J., W. Lormes, A. Opitz-Gress, J. M. Steinacker, N. Netzer, C. Foster, and U. Gastman. "Training and Overtraining: An Overview and Experimental Results in Endurance Sports." *Journal of Sports Medicine and Physical Fitness* (1997) 37 (1): 7–17.

Meeusen, R., D. Martine, C. Foster, A. Fry, M. Gleeson, D. Nieman, J. Raglin, G. Rietjens, J. Steinacker, A. Urhausen, European College of Sport Science, and American College of Sports Medicine. "Prevention, Diagnosis and Treatment of the Overtraining Syndrome: Joint Consensus Statement of the European College of Sport Science (ECSS) and the American College of Sports Medicine (ACSM)." *European Journal of Sport Science* (2013) 13 (1): 1–24.

Chapter 3: Basic Training Concepts

Bangsbo, J., T. P. Gunnarsson, J. Wendell, L. Nybo, and M. Thomassen. "Reduced Volume and Increased Training Intensity Elevate Muscle Na+/K+ {alpha}2-Subunit Expression as Well as Short- and Long-term Work Capacity in Humans." *Journal of Applied Physiology* (2009) 107 (6): 1771–1780.

Bannister, E. W., R. H. Morton, and J. Fitz-Clarke. "Dose/Response Effects of Exercises Modeled from Training: Physical and Biochemical Measures." *Annals of Physiology and Anthropology* (1992) 11 (3): 345–356.

Borg, G. "Perceived Exertion as an Indicator of Somatic Stress." *Scandinavian Journal of Rehabilitation Medicine* (1970) 2 (2): 92–98.

Brisswalter, J., P. Legros, and M. Durand. "Running Economy, Preferred Step Length Correlated to Body Dimensions in Elite Middle Distance Runners." *Journal of Sports Medicine and Physical Fitness* (1996) 36 (1): 7–15.

Busso, T., R. Candan, and J. R. Lacour. "Fatigue and Fitness Modelled from the Effects of Training on Performance." *European Journal of Applied Physiology and Occupational Physiology* (1994) 69 (1): 50–54.

Costill, D. L., R. Thomas, R. A. Robergs, D. D. Pascoe, C. P. Lambert, S. I. Barr, and W. J. Fink. "Adaptations to Swimming Training: Influence of Training Volume." *Medicine and Science in Sports and Exercise* (1991) 23 (3): 371–377.

Ekblom, B., and A. N. Golobarg. "The Influence of Physical Training and Other Factors on the Subjective Rating of Perceived Exertion." *Acta Physiologica Scandinavica* (1971) 83 (3): 399–406.

Fitz-Clarke, J. R., R. H. Morton, and E. W. Banister. "Optimizing Athletic Performance by Influence Curves." *Journal of Applied Physiology* (1991) 71 (3): 1151–1158.

Helgerud, J., K. Hoydal, E. Wang, T. Karlsen, P. Berg, M. Bjerkaas, T. Simonsen, C. Helgesen, N. Hjorth, R. Bach, and J. Hoff. "Aerobic High-Intensity Intervals Improve VO$_2$max More Than Moderate Training." *Medicine and Science in Sports and Exercise* (2007) 39 (4): 665–671.

Kubukeli, Z. N., T. D. Noakes, and S. C. Dennis. "Training Techniques to Improve Endurance Exercise Performances." *Sports Medicine* (2002) 32 (8):489–509.

Laursen, P. B., and D. G. Jenkins. "The Scientific Basis for High-Intensity Interval Training: Optimizing Training Programmes and Maximising Performance in Highly Trained Endurance Athletes." *Sports Medicine* (2002) 32 (1): 53–73.

Lehmann, M., H. Mann, V. Gastmann, J. Keul, D. Vetter, J. M. Steinacker, and D. Haussinger. "Unaccustomed High-Mileage vs Intensity Training-Related Changes in Performance and Serum Amino Acid Levels." *International Journal of Sports Medicine* (1996) 17 (3): 187–192.

Lindsay, F. H., J. A. Hawley, K. H. Myburgh, H. H. Schomer, T. D. Noakes, and S. C. Dennis. "Improved Athletic Performance in Highly Trained Cyclists After Interval Training." *Medicine and Science in Sports and Exercise* (1996) 28 (11):1427–1434.

Midgley, A. W., L. R. McNaughton, and N. M. Wilkinson. "Is There an Optimal Training Intensity for Enhancing the Maximal Oxygen Uptake of Distance Runners?: Empirical Research Findings, Current Opinions, Physiological Rationale and Practical Recommendations." *Sports Medicine* (2006) 36 (2): 117–132.

Millet, G. P., A. Lambert, B. Barbier, J. D. Rouillon, and R. B. Candan. "Modelling the Relationships Between Training, Anxiety, and Fatigue in Elite Athletes." *International Journal of Sports Medicine* (2005) 26 (6): 492–498.

Morton, R. H. "Modeling Training and Overtraining." *Journal of Sports Sciences* (1997) 15 (3): 335–340.

Morton, R. H., J. R. Fitz-Clarke, and E. W. Banister. "Modeling Human Performance in Running." *Journal of Applied Physiology* (1990) 69 (3): 1171–1177.

Neal, C. M., A. M. Hunter, L. Brennan, A. O'Sullivan, D. L. Hamilton, G. DeVito, and S. D. Galloway. "Six Weeks of a Polarized Training Intensity Distribution Leads to Greater Physiological and Performance Adaptations Than a Threshold Model in Trained Cyclists." *Journal of Applied Physiology* (2013) 114 (4): 461–471.

Taha, T., and S. G. Thomas. "Systems Modelling of the Relationship Between Training and Performance." *Sports Medicine* (2003) 33 (14): 1061–1073.

Tanaka, H. "Effects of Cross-Training. Transfer of Training Effects on VO$_2$max Between Cycling, Running and Swimming." *Sports Medicine* (1994) 18 (5): 330–339.

Westgarth-Taylor, C., J. A. Hawley, S. Rickard, K.H. Myburgh, T. D. Noakes, and S. C. Dennis. "Metabolic and Performance Adaptations to Interval Training in Endurance-Trained Cyclists." *European Journal of Applied Physiology and Occupational Physiology* (1997) 75 (4): 298–304.

Chapter 4: Training Intensity

Bendke, R., R. M. Leithauser, and Q. Ochentel. "Blood Lactate Diagnostics in Exercise Testing and Training." *International Journal of Sports Physiology and Performance* 6 (1) (2011): 8–24.

Estave-Lanao, J., C. Foster, S. Seiler, and A. Lucia. "Impact of Training Intensity Distribution on Performance in Endurance Athletes." *Journal of Strength and Conditioning Research* 21 (3) (2007): 943–949.

Estave-Lanao, J., A. F. San Juan, C. P. Earnest, C. Foster, and A. Lucia. "How Do Endurance Runners Actually Train? Relationship with Competition Performance." *Medicine and Science in Sports and Exercise* (2005) 37 (3): 496–504.

Fiskerstrand, A., and S. Seiler. "Training and Performance Characteristics Among Norwegian International Rowers 1970-2001." *Scandinavian Journal of Medicine & Science in Sports* (2004) 14 (5): 303–310.

Gaskill, S. E., R. C. Serfass, D. W. Bacharach, and J. M. Kelly. "Responses to Training in Cross-Country Skiers." *Medicine and Science in Sports and Exercise* (1999) 31 (8): 1211–1217.

Helgerud, J., K. Hoydal, E. Wang, T. Karlsen, P. Berg, M. Bjerkaas, T. Simonsen, C. Helgesen, N. Hjorth, R. Bach, and J. Hoff. "Aerobic High-Intensity Intervals Improve VO$_2$max More Than Moderate Training." *Medicine and Science in Sports and Exercise* (2007) 39 (4): 665–671.

Impellizzeri, F., A. Sassi, M. Rodriguez-Alonso, P. Mognoni, and S. Marcora. "Exercise Intensity During Off-Road Cycling Competitions." *Medicine and Science in Sports and Exercise* (2002) 34 (11): 1808–1813.

Ingham, S. A., H. Carter, G. P. Whyte, and J. H. Doust. "Physiological and Performance Effects of Low- Versus Mixed-Intensity Rowing Training." *Medicine and Science in Sports and Exercise* (2008) 40 (3): 579–584.

Ingham, S. A., B. W. Fudge, and J. S. Pringle. "Training Distribution, Physiological Profile, and Performance for a Male International 1500-M Runner." *International Journal of Sports Physiology and Performance* (2012) 7 (2): 193–195.

Jacobs, I. "Blood Lactate: Implications for Training and Sports Performance." *Sports Medicine* (1986) 3 (1): 10–25.

Laursen, P. B., and D. G. Jenkins. "The Scientific Basis for High-Intensity Interval Training: Optimizing Training Programmes and Maximising Performance in Highly Trained Endurance Athletes." *Sports Medicine* (2002) 32 (1): 53–73.

Lehmann, M., H. Mann, V. Gastmann, J. Keul, D. Vetter, J. M. Stewacker, and D. Haussinger. "Unaccustomed High-Mileage vs. Intensity Training-Related Changes in Performance and Serum Amino Acid Levels." *International Journal of Sports Medicine* (1996) 17 (3): 187–192.

Loftin, M., and B. Warren. "Comparison of a Simulated 16.1-km Time Trial, VO$_2$max and

Related Factors in Cyclists with Different Ventilatory Thresholds." *International Journal of Sports Medicine* (1994) 15 (8): 498–503.

Midgley, A. W., L. R. McNaughton, and N. M. Wilkinson. "Is There an Optimal Training Intensity for Enhancing the Maximal Oxygen Uptake of Distance Runners?: Empirical Research Findings, Current Opinions, Physiological Rationale and Practical Recommendations." *Sports Medicine* (2006) 36 (2): 117–132.

Mujika, I., J. C. Chatard, T. Busso, A. Geyssant, F. Barale, and L. Lacoste. "Effects of Training on Performance in Competitive Swimming." *Canadian Journal of Applied Physiology* (1995) 20 (4): 395–406.

Munoz, I., S. Seiler, J. Bautista, J. Espana, E. Larumbe, and J. Esteve-Lanao. "Does Polarized Training Improve Performance in Recreational Runners?" *International Journal of Sports Physiology and Performance* (2013) 9 (2): 265–272.

Neal, C. M., A. M. Hunter, L. Brennan, A. O'Sullivan, D. L. Hamilton, G. DeVito, and S. D. Galloway. "Six Weeks of a Polarized Training Intensity Distribution Leads to Greater Physiological and Performance Adaptations Than a Threshold Model in Trained Cyclists." *Journal of Applied Physiology* (2013) 114 (4): 461–471.

Ready, E. A., and H. A. Quinney. "Alterations in Anaerobic Threshold as the Result of Endurance Training and Detraining." *Medicine and Science in Sports and Exercise* (1982) 14 (4): 292–296.

Seiler, S. "What Is Best Practice for Training Intensity and Duration Distribution in Endurance Athletes?" *International Journal of Sports Physiology and Performance* (2010) 5 (3): 276–291.

Seiler, S., and G. Kjerland. "Quantifying Training Intensity Distribution in Elite Endurance Athletes: Is There Evidence for an 'Optimal' Distribution?" *Scandinavian Journal of Medicine & Science in Sports* (2006) 16 (1): 49–56.

Seiler, S., and E. Tonnessen. "Intervals, Thresholds, and Long Slow Distance: The Role of Intensity and Duration in Endurance Training." *Sportscience* (2009) 13: 32–53.

Skinner, J., and T. McLellan. "The Transition from Aerobic to Anaerobic Metabolism." *Research Quarterly for Exercise and Sport* (1980) 51 (1): 234–248.

Swensen, T. C., C. R. Harnish, L. Beltman, and B. A. Keller. "Noninvasive Estimation of the Maximal Lactate Steady State in Trained Cyclists." *Medicine and Science in Sports and Exercise* (1999) 31 (5): 742–746.

Chapter 5: Getting Started

Jones, G. "How the Best of the Best Get Better and Better." *Harvard Business Review* (2008) 86 (6): 123–127, 142.

McGehee, J. C., C. J. Tanner, and J. A. Houmard. "A Comparison of Methods for Estimating the Lactate Threshold." *Journal of Strength and Conditioning Research* (2005) 19 (3): 553–558.

Millet, G. P., V. E. Vleck, and D. J. Bentley. "Physiological Differences Between Cycling and Running: Lessons from Triathletes." *Sports Medicine* (2009) 39 (3): 179–206.

O'Toole, M. L., and P. S. Douglas. "Applied Physiology of Triathlon." *Sports Medicine* (1995) 19 (4): 251–267.

Chapter 6: Building Fitness

Bendke, R., R. M. Leithauser, and Q. Ochentel. "Blood Lactate Diagnostics in Exercise Testing and Training." *International Journal of Sports Physiology and Performance* (2011) 6 (1): 8–24.

Cairns, S. P. "Lactic Acid and Exercise Performance: Culprit or Friend?" *Sports Medicine* (2006) 36 (4): 279–291.

Coyle, E. F. "Integration of the Physiological Factors Determining Endurance Performance Ability." *Exercise, Sport, and Science Review* (1995) 23: 25–63.

Coyle, F. F., M. E. Feltner, S. A. Kantz, M. T. Hamilton, S. J. Montain, A. M. Baylor, L. D. Abraham, and G. W. Petrek. "Physiological and Biomechanical Factors Associated with Elite Endurance Cycling Performance." *Medicine and Science in Sports and Exercise* (1991) 23 (1): 93–107.

Gleim, G. W., N. S. Stachenfield, and J. A. Nicholas. "The Influence of Flexibility on the Economy of Walking and Jogging." *Journal of Orthopedic Research* (1990) 8 (6): 814–823.

Grossl, T., R. Dantas De Lucas, K. Mendes De Souza, and G. A. Guglielmol. "Maximal Lactate Steady-State and Anaerobic Thresholds from Different Methods in Cyclists." *European Journal of Sport Science* (2012) 12 (2): 161–167.

Hunter, G. R., K. Katsoulis, J. P. McCarthy, W. K. Ogard, M. M. Bamman, D. S. Wood, J. A. DenHollander, T. E. Blandeau, and B. R. Newcomer. "Tendon Length and Joint Flexibility Are Related to Running Economy." *Medicine and Science in Sports and Exercise* (2011) 43 (8): 1492–1499.

Larsen, H. B. "Kenyan Dominance in Distance Running." *Comparative Biochemistry and Physiology Part A: Molecular & Integrative Physiology* (2003) 136 (1): 161–170.

Lucia, A., J. Hoyos, M. Perez, A. Santalla, and J. L. Chicharro. "Inverse Relationship Between VO$_2$max and Economy/Efficiency in World-Class Cyclists." *Medicine and Science in Sports and Exercise* (2002) 34 (12): 2079–2084.

McGehee, J., C. Tanner, and J. Houmard. "A Comparison of Methods for Estimating the Lactate Threshold." *Journal of Strength and Conditioning Research* (2005) 19 (3): 553–558.

Midgley, A. W., and L. R. Naughton. "Time at or Near VO$_2$max During Continuous and Intermittent Running. A Review with Special Reference to Considerations for the Optimisation of Training Protocols to Elicit the Longest Time at or Near VO$_2$max." *Journal of Sports Medicine and Physical Fitness* (2006) 46 (1): 1–14.

Midgley, A. W., L. R. Naughton, and M. Wilkinson. "Is There an Optimal Training Intensity for Enhancing the Maximal Oxygen Uptake of Distance Runners?: Empirical Research Findings, Current Opinions, Physiological Rationale and Practical Recommendations." *Sports Medicine* (2006) 36 (2): 117–132.

Millet, G. P., V. E. Vleck, and D. J. Bentley. "Physiological Differences Between Cycling and Running: Lessons from Triathletes." *Sports Medicine* (2009) 39 (3): 179–206.

Myers, J., and E. Ashley. "Dangerous Curves. A Perspective on Exercise, Lactate, and the Anaerobic Threshold." *Chest* (1997) 111 (3): 787–795.

Nicholls, J. F., S. L. Phares, and M.J. Buono. "Relationship Between Blood Lactate Response to Exercise and Endurance Performance in Competitive Female Master Cyclists." *International Journal of Sports Medicine* (1997) 18 (6): 458–463.

Pate, R. R., and J. D. Branch. "Training for Endurance Sport." *Medicine and Science in Sports and Exercise* (1992) 24 (9): S340–S343.

Saunders, P. U., D. B. Pyne, R. D. Telford, and J. A. Hawley. "Factors Affecting Running Economy in Trained Distance Runners." *Sports Medicine* (2004) 34 (7): 465–485.

Saunders, P. U., R. D. Telford, D. B. Pyne, E. M. Peltola, R. B. Cunningham, C. J. Gore, and J. A. Hawley. "Short-Term Plyometric Training Improves Running Economy in Highly Trained Middle and Long Distance Runners." *Journal of Strength and Conditioning Research* (2006) 20 (4): 947–954.

Slawinski, J., A. DeMarle, J. P. Koralsztein, and V. Billat. "Effect of Supra-Lactate Threshold Training on the Relationship Between Mechanical Stride Descriptors and Aerobic Energy Cost in Trained Runners." *Archives of Physiology and Biochemistry* (2001) 109 (2): 110–116.

Stendel-Numbers, K. L., T. D. Weaver, and C. M. Wall-Scheffler. "The Evolution of Human Running: Effects of Changes in Lower-Limb Length on Locomotor Economy." *Journal of Human Evolution* (2007) 53 (2): 191–196.

Swensen, T. C., C. R. Harnish, L. Beltman, and B. A. Keller. "Noninvasive Estimation of the Maximal Lactate Steady State in Trained Cyclists." *Medicine and Science in Sports and Exercise* (1999) 31 (5): 742–746.

Turner, A. M., M. Owings, and J. A. Schwane. "Improvement in Running Economy After 6 Weeks of Plyometric Training." *Journal of Strength and Conditioning Research* (2003) 17 (1): 60–67.

Chapter 7: Planning a Season

Fry, R. W., A. R. Morton, and D. Keast. "Periodisation of Training Stress—A Review." *Canadian Journal of Sport Sciences* (1992) 17 (3): 234–240.

Gaskill, S. E., R. C. Serfass, D. W. Bacharach, and J. M. Kelly. "Responses to Training in Cross-Country Skiers." *Medicine and Science in Sports and Exercise* (1999) 31 (8): 1211–1217.

Hagberg, J. M., R. C. Hickson, A. A. Ehsani, and J. O. Holloszy. "Faster Adjustment to and Recovery from Submaximal Exercise in the Trained State." *Journal of Applied Physiology* (1980) 48 (2): 218–224.

Hautala A. J., A. M. Kiviniemi, T. H. Makikallio, H. Kinnunen, S. Nissila, H. V. Huikuri, and M. P. Tulppo. "Individual Differences in the Responses to Endurance and Resistance Training." *European Journal of Applied Physiology* (2006) 96 (5): 535–542.

Morton, R. H. "Modeling Training and Overtraining." *Journal of Sports Sciences* (1997) 15 (3): 335–340.

Paton, C. D., and W. G. Hopkins. "Seasonal Changes in Power of Competitive Cyclists: Implications for Monitoring Performance." *Journal of Science and Medicine in Sport* (2005) 8 (4): 375–381.

Chapter 8: Planning a Week

Banister, E. W., R. H. Morton, and J. Fitz-Clarke. "Dose/Response Effects of Exercise Modeled from Training: Physical and Biochemical Measures." *Annals of Physiology and Anthropology* (1992) 11 (3): 345–356.

Busso, T., R. Candau, and J. R. Lacour. "Fatigue and Fitness Modelled from the Effects of Training on Performance." *European Journal of Applied Physiology and Occupational Physiology* (1994) 69 (1): 50–54.

Costill, D. L., R. Thomas, R. A. Robergs, D. Pascoe, C. Lambert, S. Barr, and W.J. Fink. "Adaptations to Swimming Training: Influence of Training Volume." *Medicine and Science in Sports and Exercise* (1991) 23 (3): 371–377.

Esteve-Lanao, J., C. Foster, S. Seiler, and A. Lucia. "Impact of Training Intensity Distribution on Performance in Endurance Athletes." *Journal of Strength and Conditioning Research* (2007) 21 (3): 943–949.

Esteve-Lanao, J., A. F. San Juan, C. P. Earnest, C. Foster, and A. Lucia. "How Do Endurance Runners Actually Train? Relationship with Competition Performance." *Medicine and Science in Sports and Exercise* (2005) 37 (3): 496–504.

Fitz-Clarke J. R., R. H. Morton, and E. W. Banister. "Optimizing Athletic Performance by Influence Curves." *Journal of Applied Physiology* (1991) 71 (3): 1151–1158.

Gaskill, S. E., R. C. Serfass, D. W. Bacharach, and J. M. Kelly. "Responses to Training in Cross-Country Skiers." *Medicine and Science in Sports and Exercise* (1999) 31 (8): 1211–1217.

Gomes, P. S., and Y. Bhambhani. "Time Course Changes and Dissociation in VO_2max at Maximum and Submaximum Exercise Levels as a Result of Training in Males." *Medicine and Science in Sports and Exercise* (1996) 28 (5): S81.

Hautala, A. J., A. M. Kiviniemi, T. H. Mäkikallio, H. Kinnunen, S. Nissilä, H. V. Huikuri, and M. P. Tulppo. "Individual Differences in the Responses to Endurance and Resistance Training." *European Journal of Applied Physiology* (2006) 96 (5): 535–542.

Helgerud J., K. Høydal, E. Wang, T. Karlsen, P. Berg, M. Bjerkaas, T. Simonsen, C. Helgesen, N. Hjorth, R. Bach, and J. Hoff. "Aerobic High-Intensity Intervals Improve VO_2max More Than Moderate Training." *Medicine and Science in Sports and Exercise* (2007) 39 (4): 665–671.

Hellard P., M. Avalos, C. Hausswirth, D. Pyne, J. F. Toussaint, and I. Mujika. "Identifying Optimal Overload and Taper in Elite Swimmers Over Time." *Journal of Sports Science and Medicine* (2013) 12 (4): 668–678.

Houmard, J. A. "Impact of Reduced Training on Performance in Endurance Athletes." *Sports Medicine* (1991) 12 (6): 380–393.

Laursen, P. B. "Training for Intense Exercise Performance: High-Intensity or High-Volume Training?" *Scandinavian Journal of Medicine & Science in Sports* (2010) 20 (supplement 2): 1–10.

Laursen, P. B., and D. G. Jenkins. "The Scientific Basis for High-Intensity Interval Training: Optimising Training Programmes and Maximising Performance in Highly Trained Endurance Athletes." *Sports Medicine* (2002) 32 (1): 53–73.

Midgley, A. W., L. R. McNaughton, and M. Wilkinson. "Is There an Optimal Training Intensity for Enhancing the Maximal Oxygen Uptake of Distance Runners?: Empirical Research Findings, Current Opinions, Physiological Rationale and Practical Recommendations." *Sports Medicine* (2006) 36 (2): 117–132.

Millet, G. P., A. Groslambert, B. Barbier, J. D. Rouillon, and R. B. Cantan. "Modeling the Relationships Between Training, Anxiety, and Fatigue in Elite Athletes." *International Journal of Sports Medicine* (2005) 26 (6): 492–498.

Morton, R. H. "Modeling Training and Overtraining." *Journal of Sports Sciences* (1997) 15 (3): 335–340.

Morton, R. H., J. R. Fitz-Clarke, and E. W. Banister. "Modeling Human Performance in Running." *Journal of Applied Physiology* (1990) 69 (3): 1171–1177.

Mujika I., J. C. Chatard, T. Busso, A. Geyssant, F. Barale, and L. Lacoste. "Effects of Training on Performance in Competitive Swimming." *Canadian Journal of Applied Physiology* (1995) 20 (4): 395–406.

Mujika, I., A. Goya, S. Padilla, A. Grijalba, E. Gorostiaga, and J. Ibañez. "Physiological Responses to a 6-d Taper in Middle-Distance Runners: Influence of Training Intensity and Volume." *Medicine and Science in Sports and Exercise* (2000) 32 (2): 511–517.

Seiler, S., and E. Tonnessen. "Intervals, Thresholds, and Long Slow Distance: The Role of Intensity and Duration in Endurance Training." *Sportscience* (2009) 13: 32–53.

Shepley, B., J. D. MacDougall, N. Cipriano, J. R. Sutton, M. A. Tarnopolsky, and G. Coates. "Physiological Effects of Tapering in Highly Trained Athletes." *Journal of Applied Physiology* (1992) 72 (2): 706–711.

Taha, T., and S. G. Thomas. "Systems Modelling of the Relationship Between Training and Performance." *Sports Medicine* (2003) 33 (14): 1061–1073.

Thomas, L., I. Mujika, and T. Busso. "Computer Simulations Assessing the Potential Performance Benefit of a Final Increase in Training During Pre-Event Taper." *Journal of Strength and Conditioning Research* (2009) 23 (6): 1729–1736.

Chapter 9: Planning Alternatives

Bosquet, L., J. Montpetit, D. Arvisais, and I. Mujika. "Effects of Tapering on Performance: A Meta-Analysis." *Medicine and Science in Sports and Exercise* (2007) 39 (8): 1358–1365.

Breil, F. S., S. N. Weber, S. Koller, H. Hoppeler, and M. Vogt. "Block Training Periodization in Alpine Skiing: Effects off 11-Day HIT on VO_2max and Performance." *European Journal of Applied Physiology* (2010) 109 (6): 1077–1086.

Buchheit M., and P. B. Laursen. "High-Intensity Interval Training, Solutions to the Programming Puzzle. Part II: Anaerobic Energy, Neuromuscular Load and Practical Applications." *Sports Medicine* (2013) 43 (10): 927–954.

Fleck, S. J. "Non-linear Periodization for General Fitness & Athletes." *Journal of Human Kinetics* (2011) 29A: 41–45.

García-Pallarés, J., M. García-Fernández, L. Sánchez-Medina, and M. Izquierdo. "Performance Changes in World-Class Kayakers Following Two Different Training Periodization Models." *European Journal of Applied Physiology* (2010) 110 (1): 99–107.

García-Pallarés, J., L. Sánchez-Medina, L. Carrasco, A. Diaz, and M. Izquierdo. "Endurance and Neuromuscular Changes in World-Class Level Kayakers During a Periodized Training Cycle." *European Journal of Applied Physiology* (2009) 106 (4): 629–638.

Hartmann, H., K. Wirth, M. Keiner, C. Mickel, A. Sander, and E. Szilvas. "Short-Term Periodization Models: Effects on Strength and Speed-Strength Performance." *Sports Medicine* (2015) 45 (10): 1373–1386.

Issurin, V. B. "Block Periodization Versus Traditional Training Theory: A Review." *Journal of Sports Medicine and Physical Fitness* (2008) 48 (1): 65–75.

Issurin, V. B. "New Horizons for the Methodology and Physiology of Training Periodization." *Sports Medicine* (2010) 40 (3): 189–206.

Issurin, V. B. "Training Transfer: Scientific Background and Insights for Practical Application." *Sports Medicine* (2013) 43 (8): 675–694.

Jeukendrup, A. E., M. K. Hesselink, A. C. Snyder, H. Kuipers, and H. A. Keizer. "Physiological Changes in Male Competitive Cyclists After Two Weeks of Intensified Training." *International Journal of Sports Medicine* (1992) 13 (7): 534–541.

Kibler, W. B., and T. J. Chandler. "Sport-Specific Conditioning." *American Journal of Sports Medicine* (1994) 22 (3): 424–432.

Kiely, J. "Periodization Paradigms in the 21st Century: Evidence-Led or Tradition-Driven?" *International Journal of Sports Physiology and Performance* (2012) 7 (3): 242–250.

Kirwan, J. P., D. L. Costill, M. G. Flynn, J. B. Mitchell, W. J. Fink, P. D. Neufer, and J. A. Houmard. "Physiological Responses to Successive Days of Intense Training in Competitive Swimmers." *Medicine and Science in Sports and Exercise* (1988) 20 (3): 255–259.

Lehmann, M., P. Baumgartl, C. Wiesenack, A. Seidel, H. Baumann, S. Fischer, U. Spöri, G. Gendrisch, R. Kaminski, and J. Keul. "Training-Overtraining: Influence of a Defined Increase in Training Volume vs Training Intensity on Performance, Catecholamines and Some Metabolic Parameters in Experienced Middle- and Long-Distance Runners." *European Journal of Applied Physiology and Occupational Physiology* (1992) 64 (2): 169–177.

Lehmann, M., H. Wieland, and U. Gastmann. "Influence of an Unaccustomed Increase in Training Volume vs Intensity on Performance, Hematological and Blood-Chemical Parameters in Distance Runners." *Journal of Sports Medicine and Physical Fitness* (1997) 37 (2): 110–116.

Muñoz, I., R. Cejuela, S. Seiler, E. Larumbe, and J. Esteve-Lanao. "Training-Intensity Distribution During an Ironman Season: Relationship with Competition Performance." *International Journal of Sports Physiology and Performance* (2014) 9 (2): 332–339.

Rhea, M. R., S. D. Ball, W.T. Phillips, and L. N. Burkett. "A Comparison of Linear and Daily Undulating Periodized Programs with Equated Volume and Intensity for Strength." *Journal of Strength and Conditioning Research* (2002) 16 (2): 250–255.

Rhea, M. R., W. T. Phillips, L. N. Burkett, W. J. Stone, S. D. Ball, B. A. Alvar, and A. B. Thomas. "A Comparison of Linear and Daily Undulating Periodized Programs with Equated Volume and Intensity for Local Muscular Endurance." *Journal of Strength and Conditioning Research* (2003) 17 (1): 82–87.

Rønnestad, B. R., S. Ellefsen, H. Nygaard, E. E. Zacharoff, O. Vikmoen, J. Hansen, and J. Hallén. "Effects of 12 Weeks of Block Periodization on Performance and Performance Indices in Well-Trained Cyclists." *Scandinavian Journal of Medicine & Science in Sports* (2014) 24 (2): 327–335.

Rønnestad, B. R., J. Hansen, and S. Ellefsen. "Block Periodization of High-Intensity Aerobic Intervals Provides Superior Training Effects in Trained Cyclists." *Scandinavian Journal of Medicine & Science in Sports* (2014) 24 (1): 34–42.

Rønnestad, B. R., J. Hansen, V. Thyli, T. A. Bakken, and Ø. Sandbakk. "5-Week Block Periodization Increases Aerobic Power in Elite Cross-Country Skiers." *Scandinavian Journal of Medicine & Science in Sports* (2016) 26 (2): 140–146.

Szabo, S., Y. Tache, and A. Somogyi. "The Legacy of Hans Selye and the Origins of Stress Research: A Retrospective 75 Years After His Landmark Brief 'Letter' to the Editor of Nature." *Stress* (2012) 15 (5): 472–478.

Tønnessen, E., Ø. Sylta, T. A. Haugen, E. Hem, I. S. Svendsen, and S. Seiler. "The Road to Gold: Training and Peaking Characteristics in the Year Prior to a Gold Medal Endurance Performance." *PLoS One* (2014) 9 (7): e101796.

Chapter 10: Training Stress

Aubry, A., C. Hausswirth, J. Louis, A. J. Coutts, and Y. Le Meur. "Functional Overreaching: The Key to Peak Performance During the Taper?" *Medicine and Science in Sports and Exercise* (2014) 46 (9): 1769–1777.

Hausswirth, C., J. Louis, A. Aubry, G. Bonnet, R. Duffield, and Y. Le Meur. "Evidence of Disturbed Sleep and Increased Illness in Overreached Endurance Athletes." *Medicine and Science in Sports and Exercise* (2014) 46 (5): 1036–1045.

Lehmann, M., U. Gastmann, K.G. Peterson, N. Bachl, A. Seidel, A. N. Khalaf, S. Fischer, and J. Keul. "Training-Overtraining: Performance, and Hormone Levels, After a Defined Increase in Training Volume Versus Intensity in Experienced Middle- and Long-Distance Runners." *British Journal of Sports Medicine* (1992) 26 (4): 233–242.

Lehmann, M., H. Wieland, and U. Gastmann. "Influence of an Unaccustomed Increase in Training Volume vs Intensity on Performance, Hematological and Blood-Chemical Parameters in Distance Runners." *Journal of Sports Medicine and Physical Fitness* (1997) 37 (2): 110–116.

Le Meur, Y., A. Pichon, K. Schaal, L. Schmitt, J. Louis, J. Gueneron, P.P. Vidal, and C. Hausswirth. "Evidence of Parasympathetic Hyperactivity in Functionally Overreached Athletes." *Medicine and Science in Sports and Exercise* (2013) 45 (11): 2061–2071.

Meeusen, R., M. Duclos, C. Foster, A. Fry, M. Gleeson, D. Nieman, J. Raglin, G. Rietjens, J. Steinacker, and A. Urhausen. "Prevention, Diagnosis, and Treatment of the Overtraining Syndrome: Joint Consensus Statement of the European College of Sport Science and the American College of Sports Medicine." *Medicine and Science in Sports and Exercise* (2013) 45 (1): 186–205.

Vesterinen, V., K. Häkkinen, T. Laine, E. Hynynen, J. Mikkola, and A. Nummela. "Predictors of Individual Adaptation to High-Volume or High-Intensity Endurance Training in Recreational Endurance Runners." *Scandinavian Journal of Medicine & Science in Sports* (2016) 26 (8): 885–893.

Chapter 11: Rest and Recovery

Ali, A., M. P. Caine, and B. G. Snow. "Graduated Compression Stockings: Physiological and Perceptual Responses During and After Exercise." *Journal of Sports Sciences* (2007) 25 (4): 413–419.

Ali, A., R. H. Creasy, and J. A. Edge. "Physiological Effects of Wearing Graduated Compression Stockings During Running." *European Journal of Applied Physiology* (2010) 109 (6): 1017–1025.

Ali, A., R. H. Creasy, and J. A. Edge. "The Effect of Graduated Compression Stockings on Running Performance." *Journal of Strength and Conditioning Research* (2011) 25 (5): 1385–1392.

Areta, J. L., L. M. Burke, M. L. Ross, D. M. Camera, D. W. West, E. M. Broad, N. A. Jeacocke, D. R. Moore, T. Stellingwerff, S. M. Phillips, J. A. Hawley, and V. G. Coffey. "Timing and Distribution of Protein Ingestion During Prolonged Recovery from Resistance Exercise Alters Myofibrillar Protein Synthesis." *Journal of Physiology* (2013) 591 (9): 2319–2331.

Berardi, J. M., T. B. Price, E. E. Noreen, and P. W. Lemon. "Postexercise Muscle Glycogen Recovery Enhanced with a Carbohydrate-

Protein Supplement." *Medicine and Science in Sports and Exercise* (2006) 38 (6): 1106–1113.

Berry, M. J., and R. G. McMurray. "Effects of Graduated Compression Stockings on Blood Lactate Following an Exhaustive Bout of Exercise." *American Journal of Physical Medicine* (1987) 66 (3): 121–132.

Bossingham, M. J., N. S. Carnell, and W. W. Campbell. "Water Balance, Hydration Status, and Fat-Free Mass Hydration in Younger and Older Adults." *American Journal of Clinical Nutrition* (2005) 81 (6): 1342–1350.

Breen, L., A. Philip, O. C. Witard, S. R. Jackman, A. Selby, K. Smith, K. Barr, and K. D. Tipton. "The Influence of Carbohydrate-Protein Co-ingestion Following Endurance Exercise on Myofibrillar and Mitochondrial Protein Synthesis." *Journal of Physiology* (2011) 589 (16): 4011–4025.

Chatard, J. C., D. Atlaoui, J. Farjanel, F. Louisy, D. Rastel, and C. Y. Guezennec. "Elastic Stockings, Performance and Leg Pain Recovery in 63-Year-Old Sportsmen." *European Journal of Applied Physiology* (2004) 93 (3): 347–352.

Crispim, C. A., I. Z. Zimberg, B. G. dos Reis, R. M. Diniz, S. Tufik, and M. T. de Mello. "Relationship Between Food Intake and Sleep Pattern in Healthy Individuals." *Journal of Clinical Sleep and Medicine* (2011) 7 (6): 659–664.

Davies, D. J., K. S. Graham, and C. M. Chow. "The Effect of Prior Endurance Training on Nap Sleep Patterns." *International Journal of Sports Physiology and Performance* (2010) 5 (1): 87–97.

Davies, V., K. G. Thompson, and S. M. Cooper. "The Effects of Compression Garments on Recovery." *Journal of Strength and Conditioning Research* (2009) 23 (6): 1786–1794.

De Pauw, K., B. De Geus, B. Roelands, F. Lauwens, J. Verschueren, E. Heyman, and R.R. Meeusen. "Effect of Five Different Recovery Methods on Repeated Cycle Performance." *Medicine and Science in Sports and Exercise* (2011) 43 (5): 890–897.

Duffield, R., J. Cannon, and M. King. "The Effects of Compression Garments on Recovery of Muscle Performance Following High-Intensity Sprint and Plyometric Exercise." *Journal of Science and Medicine in Sport* (2010) 13 (1): 136–140.

Duffield, R., J. Edge, R. Merrells, E. Hawke, M. Barnes, D. Simcock, and N. Gill. "The Effects of Compression Garments on Intermittent Exercise Performance and Recovery on Consecutive Days." *International Journal of Sports Physiology and Performance* (2008) 3 (4): 454–468.

Ebrahim, I. O., C.M. Shapiro, A. J. Williams, and P. B. Fenwick. "Alcohol and Sleep I: Effects on Normal Sleep." *Alcoholism, Clinical and Experimental Research* (2013) 37 (4): 539–549.

Eliakim, M., E. Bodner, Y. Meckel, D. Nemet, and A. Eliakim. "Effect of Rhythm on the Recovery from Intense Exercise." *Journal of Strength and Conditioning Research* (2012) 27 (4): 1019–1024.

French, D. N., K. G. Thompson, S. W. Garland, C. A. Barnes, M. D. Portas, P. E. Hood, and G. Wilkes. "The Effects of Contrast Bathing and Compression Therapy on Muscular Performance." *Medicine and Science in Sports and Exercise* (2008) 40 (7): 1297–1306.

Fudge, B. W., C. Easton, D. Kingsmore, F. K. Kiplamai, V. O. Onywera, K. R. Westerterp, B. Kayser, T. D. Noakes, and Y. P. Pitsiladis. "Elite Kenyan Endurance Runners Are Hydrated Day-to-Day with Ad Libitum Fluid Intake." *Medicine and Science in Sports and Exercise* (2008) 40 (6): 1171–1179.

Garrido, M., D. González-Gómez, M. Lozano, C. Barriga, S. D. Paredes, and A. B. Rodríguez. "A Jerte Valley Cherry Product Provides Beneficial Effects on Sleep Quality. Influence on Aging." *Journal of Nutrition, Health & Aging* (2013) 17 (6): 553–560.

Goh, S. S., P. B. Laursen, B. Dascombe, and K. Nosaka. "Effect of Lower Body Compression Garments on Submaximal Running Performance in Cold (10° C) and Hot (32° C) Environments." *European Journal of Applied Physiology* (2011) 111 (5): 819–826.

Goulet, E. D. "Effect of Exercise-Induced Dehydration on Time-Trial Exercise Performance: A Meta-Analysis." *British Journal of Sports Medicine* (2011) 45 (14): 1149–1156.

Hagberg, J. M., R. C. Hickson, A. A. Ehsani, and J. O. Holloszy. "Faster Adjustment to and Recovery from Submaximal Exercise in the Trained State." *Journal of Applied Physiology* (1980) 48 (2): 218–224.

Halson, S. L. "Does the Time Frame Between Exercises Influence the Effectiveness of Hydrotherapy for Recovery?" *International Journal of Sports Physiology and Performance* (2011) 6 (2): 147–159.

Halson, S. L., M. W. Bridge, R. Meeusen, B. Busschaert, M. Gleeson, D. A. Jones, and A. E. Jeukendrup. "Time Course of Performance Changes and Fatigue Markers During Intensified Training in Trained Cyclists." *Journal of Applied Physiology* (2002) 93 (3): 947–956.

Halson, S. L., G. I. Lancaster, J. Achten, M. Gleeson, and A. E. Jeukendrup. "Effects of Carbohydrate Supplementation on Performance and Carbohydrate Oxidation After Intensified Cycling Training." *Journal of Applied Physiology* (2004) 97 (4): 1245–1253.

Hemmings, B., M. Smith, J. Graydon, and R. Dyson. "Effects of Massage on Physiological Restoration, Perceived Recovery, and Repeated Sports Performance." *British Journal of Sports Medicine* (2000) 34 (2): 109–114.

Higgins, T., G. A. Naughton, and D. Burgess. "Effects of Wearing Compression Garments on Physiological and Performance Measures in a Simulated Game-Specific Circuit for Netball." *Journal of Science and Medicine in Sport* (2009) 12 (1): 223–226.

Hill, D. W., D. O. Borden, K. M. Darnaby, and D. N. Hendricks. "Aerobic and Anaerobic Contributions to Exhaustive High-Intensity Exercise After Sleep Deprivation." *Journal of Sports Sciences* (1994) 12 (5): 455–461.

Howatson, G., P. G. Bell, J. Tallent, B. Middleton, M. P. McHugh, and J. Ellis. "Effect of Tart Cherry Juice (Prunus cerasus) on Melatonin Levels and Enhanced Sleep Quality." *European Journal of Nutrition* (2012) 51 (8): 909–916.

Ingram, J., B. Dawson, C. Goodman, K. Wallman, and L. Beilby. "Effect of Water Immersion Methods on Post-Exercise Recovery from Simulated Team Sport Exercise." *Journal of Science and Medicine in Sport* (2009) 12 (3): 417–421.

Ivy, J. L. "Dietary Strategies to Promote Glycogen Synthesis After Exercise." *Canadian Journal of Applied Physiology* (2001) 26 (Supplement): S236–S245.

Ivy, J. L., H. W. Goforth Jr., B. M. Damon, T. R. McCauley, E. C. Parsons, and T. B. Price. "Early Postexercise Muscle Glycogen Recovery Is Enhanced with a Carbohydrate-Protein Supplement." *Journal of Applied Physiology* (2002) 3 (4): 1337–1344.

Jakeman, J. R., C. Byrne, and R. G. Eston. "Lower Limb Compression Garment Improves Recovery from Exercise-Induced Muscle

Damage in Young, Active Females." *European Journal of Applied Physiology* (2010) 109 (6): 1137–1144.

Jentjens, R., and A. Jeukendrup. "Determinants of Post-Exercise Glycogen Synthesis During Short-Term Recovery." *Sports Medicine* (2003) 33 (2): 117–144.

Kaikkonen, P., E. Hynynen, T. Mann, H. Rusko, and A. Nummela. "Heart Rate Variability Is Related to Training Load Variables in Interval Running Exercises." *European Journal of Applied Physiology* (2012) 112 (3): 829–838.

Kemmler, W., S. Von Stengel, C. Kockritz, J. Mayhew, A. Wassermann, and J. Zapf. "Effect of Compression Stockings on Running Performance in Men Runners." *Journal of Strength and Conditioning Research* (2009) 23 (1): 101–105.

Kenney, W. L., and Chiu P. "Influence of Age on Thirst and Fluid Intake." *Medicine and Science in Sports and Exercise* (2001) 33 (9): 1524–1532.

Kenney, W. L., C. G. Tankersley, D. L. Newswanger, D. E. Hyde, S. M. Puhl, and N. L. Turner. "Age and Hypohydration Independently Influence the Peripheral Vascular Response to Heat Stress." *Journal of Applied Physiology* (1990) 68 (5): 1902–1908.

Kephart, W. C., C. B. Mobley, C. D. Fox, D. D. Pascoe, J. M. Sefton, T. J. Wilson, M. D. Goodlett, A. N. Kavazis, M. D. Roberts, and J. S. Martin. "A Single Bout of Whole-Leg, Peristaltic Pulse External Pneumatic Compression Upregulates PGC-1α mRNA and Endothelial Nitric Oxide Synthase Protein in Human Skeletal Muscle Tissue." *Experimental Physiology* (2015) 100 (7): 852–864.

Killer, S. C., I. S. Svendsen, A. E. Jeukendrup, and M. Gleeson. "Evidence of Disturbed Sleep and Mood State in Well-Trained Athletes During Short-Term Intensified Training with and Without a High Carbohydrate Nutritional Intervention." *Journal of Sports Sciences* (2015): 1–9. [Epub ahead of print]

Kovacs, E. M., J. M. Senden, and F. Brouns. "Urine Color, Osmolality and Specific Electrical Conductance Are Not Accurate Measures of Hydration Status During Postexercise Rehydration." *Journal of Sports Medicine and Physical Fitness* (1999) 39 (1): 47–53.

Kraemer, W. J., S. D. Flanagan, B. A. Comstock, M. S. Fragala, J. E. Earp, C. Dunn-Lewis, J. Y. Ho, G. A. Thomas, G. Solomon-Hill, Z. R. Penwell, M. D. Powell, M. R. Wolf, J. S. Volek, C. R. Denegar, and C. M. Maresh. "Effects of a Whole Body Compression Garment on Markers of Recovery After a Heavy Resistance Workout in Men and Women." *Journal of Strength and Conditioning Research* (2010) 24 (3): 804–814.

Lamberts, R. P., J. Swart, B. Capostagno, T. D. Noakes, and M. I. Lambert. "Heart Rate Recovery as a Guide to Monitor Fatigue and Predict Changes in Performance Parameters." *Scandinavian Journal of Medicine & Science in Sports* (2010) 20 (3): 449–457.

Le Meur, Y., A. Pichon, K. Schaal, L. Schmitt, J. Louis, J. Gueneron, P. P. Vidal, and C. Hausswirth. "Evidence of Parasympathetic Hyperactivity in Functionally Overreached Athletes." *Medicine and Science in Sports and Exercise* (2013) 4 (11): 2061–2071.

Levenhagen, D. K., C. Carr, M. G. Carlson, D. J. Maron, M. J. Borel, and P. J. Flakoll. "Postexercise Protein Intake Enhances Whole-Body and Leg Protein Accretion in Humans." *Medicine and Science in Sports and Exercise* (2002) 34 (5): 828–837.

Lindseth, G., P. Lindseth, and M. Thompson. "Nutritional Effects on Sleep." *Western Journal of Nursing Research* (2013) 35 (4): 497–513.

MacRae, B. A., J. D. Cotter, and R. M. Laing. "Compression Garments and Exercise: Garment Considerations, Physiology and Performance." *Sports Medicine* (2011) 41 (10): 815–843.

MacRae, B. A., R. M. Laing, B. E. Niven, and J. D. Cotter. "Pressure and Coverage Effects of Sporting Compression Garments on Cardiovascular Function, Thermoregulatory Function, and Exercise Performance." *European Journal of Applied Physiology* (2012) 112 (5): 1783–1795.

Martin, J. S., A. R. Borges, and D. T. Beck. "Peripheral Conduit and Resistance Artery Function Are Improved Following a Single, 1-h Bout of Peristaltic Pulse External Pneumatic Compression." *European Journal of Applied Physiology* (2015) 115 (9): 2019–2029.

McAinch, A. J., M. A. Febbraio, J. M. Parkin, S. Zhao, K. Tangalakis, L. Stojanovska, and M. F. Carey. "Effect of Active Versus Passive Recovery on Metabolism and Performance During Subsequent Exercise." *International Journal of Sport Nutrition and Exercise Metabolism* (2004) 14 (2): 185–196.

Mika, A., P. Mika, B. Fernhall, and V. B. Unnithan. "Comparison of Recovery Strategies on Muscle Performance After Fatiguing Exercise." *American Journal of Physical Medicine & Rehabilitation* (2007) 86 (6): 474–481.

Miyamoto, N., K. Hirata, N. Mitsukawa, T. Yanai, and Y. Kawkami. "Effect of Pressure Intensity of Graduated Elastic Compression Stocking on Muscle Fatigue Following Calf-Raise Exercise." *Journal of Electromyography and Kinesiology* (2011) 21 (2): 249–254.

Montgomery, P. G., D. B. Pyne, W. G. Hopkins, J. C. Dorman, K. Cook, and C. L. Minhan. "The Effect of Recovery Strategies on Physical Performance and Cumulative Fatigue in Competitive Basketball." *Journal of Sports Sciences* (2008) 26 (11): 1135–1145.

Nicholas, C. W., P. A. Green, R. D. Hawkins, and C. Williams. "Carbohydrate Intake and Recovery of Intermittent Running Capacity." *International Journal of Sport Nutrition and Exercise Metabolism* (1997) 7 (4): 251–260.

Noakes, T. D. "Drinking Guidelines for Exercise: What Evidence Is There That Athletes Should Drink 'as Much as Tolerable', 'to Replace the Weight Lost During Exercise' or 'Ad Libitum'?" *Journal of Sports Sciences* (2007) 25 (7): 781–796.

Noakes, T. D. "Hydration in the Marathon: Using Thirst to Gauge Safe Fluid Replacement." *Sports Medicine* (2007) 37 (4–5): 463–466.

Parkin, J. A., M. F. Carey, I. K. Martin, L. Stojanovska, and M. A. Febbraio. "Muscle Glycogen Storage Following Prolonged Exercise: Effect of Timing of Ingestion of High Glycemic Index Food." *Medicine and Science in Sports and Exercise* (1997) 29 (2): 220–224.

Penev, P. D. "Association Between Sleep and Morning Testosterone Levels in Older Men." *Sleep* (2007) 30 (4): 427–432.

Pennings, B., R. Koopman, M. Beelen, J. M. G. Senden, W. H. M. Saris, and L. J. C. van Loon. "Exercising Before Protein Intake Allows for Greater Use of Dietary Protein-Derived Amino Acids for De Novo Muscle Protein Synthesis in Both Young and Elderly Men." *American Journal of Clinical Nutrition* (2011) 93 (2): 322–331.

Perez-Schindler, J., D. L. Hamilton, D. R. Moore, K. Baar, and A. Philp. "Nutritional Strategies to Support Concurrent Training." *European Journal of Sport Science* (2015) 15 (1): 41–52.

Phillips, S. M. "A Brief Review of Critical Processes in Exercise-Induced Muscular

Hypertrophy." *Sports Medicine* (2014) 44 (S1): S71–S77

Pigeon, W. R., M. Carr, C. Gorman, and M. L. Perlis. "Effects of a Tart Cherry Juice Beverage on the Sleep of Older Adults with Insomnia: A Pilot Study." *Journal of Medicine and Food* (2010) 13 (3): 579–583.

Res, P. T., B. Groen, B. Pennings, M. Beelen, G. A. Wallis, A. P. Gijsen, J. M. Senden, and L. J. Van Loon. "Protein Ingestion Before Sleep Improves Postexercise Overnight Recovery." *Medicine and Science in Sports and Exercise* (2012) 44 (8): 1560–1569.

Reynolds, A. C., J. Dorrian, P. Y. Liu, H. P. Van Dongen, G. A. Wittert, L. J. Harmer, and S. Banks. "Impact of Five Nights of Sleep Restriction on Glucose Metabolism, Leptin and Testosterone in Young Adult Men." *PLoS One* (2012) 7 (7): e41218.

Riman, D., L. Messonier, J. Castells, X. Devillard, and P. Calmels. "Effects of Compression Stockings During Exercise and Recovery on Blood Lactate Kinetics." *European Journal of Applied Physiology* (2010) 110 (2): 425–433.

Sands, W. A., J. R. McNeal, S. R. Murray, and M. H. Stone. "Dynamic Compression Enhances Pressure-to-Pain Threshold in Elite Athlete Recovery: Exploratory Study." *Journal of Strength and Conditioning Research* (2015) 29 (5): 1263–1272.

Sawka, M. N., S. J. Montain, and W. A. Latzka. "Hydration Effects on Thermoregulation and Performance in the Heat." *Comparative Biochemistry and Physiology Part A, Molecular & Integrative Physiology* (2001) 128 (4): 679–690.

Scanlon, A. T., B. J. Dascombe, P. R. Reaburn, and M. Osborne. "The Effects of Wearing Lower-Body Compression Garments During Endurance Cycling." *International Journal of*

Sports Physiology and Performance (2008) 3 (4): 424–438.

Seiler, S., O. Haugen, and E. Kuffel. "Autonomic Recovery After Exercise in Trained Athletes: Intensity and Duration Effects." *Medicine and Science in Sports and Exercise* (2007) 39 (8): 1366–1373.

Sperlich, B., M. Haegele, S. Achtzehn, J. Linville, H. C. Holmberg, and J. Mester. "Different Types of Compression Clothing Do Not Increase Sub-maximal and Maximal Endurance Performance in Well-Trained Athletes." *Journal of Sports Sciences* (2010) 28 (6): 609–614.

Suzuki, M. "Glycemic Carbohydrates Consumed with Amino Acids or Protein Right After Exercise Enhance Muscle Formation." *Nutrition Review* (2003) 61 (5 Pt 2): S88–S94.

Symons, T. B., M. S. Moore, and R. R. Wolfe. "A Moderate Serving of High-Quality Protein Maximally Stimulates Muscle Protein Synthesis in Young and Elderly Subjects." *Journal of the American Dietetic Association* (2009) 109 (9): 1582–1586.

Tipton, K. D., A. A. Ferrando, S. M. Phillips, D. Doyle Jr, and R. R. Wolfe. "Postexercise Net Protein Synthesis in Human Muscle from Orally Administered Amino Acids." *American Journal of Physiology* (1999) 276 (4 Pt 1): E628–E634.

Tomlin, D. L., and H. A. Wenger. "The Relationship Between Fitness and Recovery from High Intensity Intermittent Exercise." *Sports Medicine* (2001) 31 (1): 1–11.

Tseng, C. Y., J. P. Lee, Y. S. Tsai, S. D. Lee, C. L. Kao, T. C. Liu, C. Lai, M. B. Harris, and C. H. Kuo. "Topical Cooling (Icing) Delays Recovery from Eccentric Exercise-Induced Muscle Damage." *Journal of Strength and Conditioning Research* (2013) 27 (5): 1354–1361.

Tucker, T. J., D. R. Slivka, J. S. Cuddy, W. S. Hailes, and B. C. Ruby. "Effect of Local Cold Application on Glycogen Recovery." *Journal of Sports Medicine and Physical Fitness* (2012) 52 (2): 158–164.

Vaile, J., S. Halson, N. Gill, and B. Dawson. "Effect of Hydrotherapy on Recovery from Fatigue." *International Journal of Sports Medicine* (2008) 29 (7): 539–544.

Vaile, J., S. Halson, N. Gill, and B. Dawson. "Effect of Cold Water Immersion on Repeat Cycling Performance and Thermoregulation in the Heat." *Journal of Sports Sciences* (2008) 26 (5): 431–440.

Valtin, H. " 'Drink at Least Eight Glasses of Water a Day.' Really? Is There Scientific Evidence for '8 x 8'?" *American Journal of Physiology. Regulatory, Integrative and Comparative Physiology* (2002) 283 (5): R993–R1004.

Van Cauter, E., R. Leproult, and L. Plat. "Age-Related Changes in Slow-Wave Sleep and REM Sleep and Relationship with Growth Hormone and Cortisol Levels in Healthy Men." *Journal of the American Medical Association* (2000) 284 (7): 861–868.

VanHelder, T., and M. W. Radomski. "Sleep Deprivation and the Effect on Exercise Performance." *Sports Medicine* (1989) 7 (4): 235–247.

Van Loon, L. J., M. Kruijshoop, H. Verhagen, W. H. Saris, and A. J. Wagenmakers. "Ingestion of Protein Hydrolysate and Amino Acid-Carbohydrate Mixtures Increases Postexercise Plasma Insulin Responses in Men." *Journal of Nutrition* (2000) 130 (10): 2508–2513.

Versey, N. G., S. L. Halson, and B. T. Dawson. "Effect of Contrast Water Therapy Duration on Recovery of Running Performance." *International Journal of Sports Physiology and Performance* (2012) 7 (2): 130–140.

Wiener, A., J. Mizrahi, and O. Verbitsky. "Enhancement of Tibialis Anterior Recovery by Intermittent Sequential Pneumatic Compression of the Legs." *Basic Applied Myology* (2001) 11 (2): 87–90.

Wilcox, I., J. Cronin, and W. Hing. "Physiological Response to Water Immersion: A Method for Sport Recovery?" *Sports Medicine* (2006) 6 (9): 747–765.

Zelikovski, A., C. L. Kaye, G. Fink, S. A. Spitzer, and Y. Shapiro. "The Effects of the Modified Intermittent Sequential Pneumatic Device (MISPD) on Exercise Performance Following an Exhaustive Exercise Bout." *British Journal of Sports Medicine* (1993) 27 (4): 255–259.

Chapter 12: Speed Skills

Ardigo, L. P., C. LaFortuna, A. E. Minetti, P. Mognoni, and F. Saibene. "Metabolic and Mechanical Aspects of Foot Landing Type, Forefoot and Rearfoot Strike, in Human Running." *Acta Physiologica Scandinavica* (1995) 155 (1): 17–22.

Beneke, R., and M. Hutler. "The Effects of Training on Running Economy and Performance in Recreational Athletes." *Medicine and Science in Sports and Exercise* (2005) 37 (10): 1794–1799.

Garside, I., and D. A. Doran. "Effects of Bicycle Frame Ergonomics on Triathlon 10-km Running Performance." *Journal of Sports Sciences* (2000) 18 (10): 825–833.

Hasegawa, H., T. Yamauchi, and W. J. Kraemer. "Foot Strike Patterns of Runners at the 15-km Point During an Elite-Level Half Marathon." *Journal of Strength and Conditioning Research* (2007) 21 (3): 888–893.

Lucia, A., J. Oliván, J. Bravo, M. Gonzalez-Freire, and C. Foster. "The Key to Top-Level Endurance Running Performance: A Unique

Example." *British Journal of Sports Medicine* (2008) 42 (3): 172–174.

Nummela, A., T. Keranen, and L. O. Mikkelsson. "Factors Related to Top Running Speed and Economy." *International Journal of Sports Medicine* (2007) 28 (8):655–661

Paavolainen, L., A. Nummela, H. Rusko, and K. Hakkinen. "Neuromuscular Characteristics and Fatigue During 10-km Running." *International Journal of Sports Medicine* (1999) 20 (8): 516–521.

Peeling, P., and G. Landers. "Swimming Intensity During Triathlon: A Review of Current Research and Strategies to Enhance Race Performance." *Journal of Sports Sciences* (2009) 27 (10): 1079–1085.

Price, D., and B. Donne. "Effect of Variation in Seat Tube Angle at Different Seat Heights on Submaximal Cycling Performance in Man." *Journal of Sports Sciences* (1997) 15: 395–402.

Saunders, P. U., D. B. Pyne, R. D. Telford, and J. A. Hawley. "Factors Affecting Running Economy in Trained Distance Runners." *Sports Medicine* (2004) 34 (7): 465–485.

Steudel-Numbers, K. L., T. D. Weaver, and C. M. Wall-Scheffler. "The Evolution of Human Running: Effects of Changes in Lower-Limb Length on Locomotor Economy." *Journal of Human Evolution* (2007) 53 (2): 191–196.

Chapter 13: Muscular Force

Ahmad, C. S., A. M. Clark, N. Heilmann, J. S. Schoeb, T. R. Gardner, and W. N. Levine. "Effect of Gender and Maturity on Quadriceps-to-Hamstring Strength Ratio and Anterior Cruciate Ligament Laxity." *American Journal of Sports Medicine* (2006) 34 (3): 370–374.

Aspenes, S. T., and T. Karlsen. "Exercise-Training Intervention Studies in Competitive Swimming." *Sports Medicine* (2012) 42 (6): 527–543.

Baar, K. "Using Molecular Biology to Maximize Concurrent Training." *Sports Medicine* (2015) 44 (Supplement 2): S117–S125.

Barnes, K. R., W. G. Hopkins, M. R. McGuigan, M. E. Northuis, and A. E. Kilding. "Effects of Resistance Training on Running Economy and Cross-Country Performance." *Medicine and Science in Sports and Exercise* (2013) 45 (12): 2322–2331.

Behm, D. G., D. Cappa, and G. A. Power. "Trunk Muscle Activation During Moderate and High-Intensity Running." *Applied Physiology, Nutrition, and Metabolism* (2009) 34 (6): 1008–1016.

Behm, D. G., and D. G. Sale. "Intended Rather Than Actual Movement Velocity Determines Velocity-Specific Training Response." *Journal of Applied Physiology* (1993) 74 (1): 359–368.

Coombs R., and G. Garbutt. "Developments in the Use of the Hamstring/Quadriceps Ratio for the Assessment of Muscle Balance." *Journal of Sports Science and Medicine* (2002) 1 (3): 56–62.

Cormie, P., M. R. McGuigan, and R. U. Newton. "Developing Maximal Neuromuscular Power: Part 1—Biological Basis of Maximal Power Production." *Sports Medicine* (2011) 41 (1): 17–38.

Cormie, P., M. R. McGuigan, and R. U. Newton. "Developing Maximal Neuromuscular Power: Part 2—Training Considerations for Improving Maximal Power Production." *Sports Medicine* (2011) 41 (2): 125–146.

Damasceno, M. V., A. E. Lima-Silva, L. A. Pasqua, V. Tricoli, M. Duarte, D. J. Bishop, and R. Bertuzzi. "Effects of Resistance Training on Neuromuscular Characteristics and Pacing

During 10-km Running Time Trial." *European Journal of Applied Physiology* (2015) 115 (7): 1513–1522.

Davies, T., R. Orr, M. Halaki, and D. Hackett. "Effect of Training Leading to Repetition Failure on Muscular Strength: A Systematic Review and Meta-Analysis." *Sports Medicine* (2016) 46 (4): 487–502.

Ebben, W. P., M. L. Fauth, L. R. Garceau, and E. J. Petrushek. "Kinetic Quantification of Plyometric Exercise Intensity". *Journal of Strength and Conditioning Research* (2011) 25 (12): 3288–3298.

Ebben, W. P., A. G. Kindler, K. A. Chirdon, N. C. Jenkins, A. J. Polichnowski, and A. V. Ng. "The Effect of High-Load vs. High-Repetition Training on Endurance Performance." *Journal of Strength and Conditioning Research* (2004) 18 (3): 513–517.

Garrido, N., D. A. Marinho, V. M. Reis, R. van den Tillaar, A. M. Costa, A. J. Silva, and M. C. Marques. "Does Combined Dry Land Strength and Aerobic Training Inhibit Performance of Young Competitive Swimmers?" *Journal of Sports Science and Medicine* (2010) 9 (2): 300–310.

Girold, S., D. Maurin, B. Dugué, J. C. Chatard, and G. Millet. "Effects of Dry-Land vs. Resisted- and Assisted-Sprint Exercises on Swimming Sprint Performances." *Journal of Strength and Conditioning Research* (2007) 21 (2): 599–605.

Goto, K., M. Nagasawa, O. Yanagisawa, T. Kizuka, N. Ishii, and K. Takamatsu. "Muscular Adaptations to Combinations of High- and Low-Intensity Resistance Exercises." *Journal of Strength and Conditioning Research* (2004) 18 (4): 730–737.

Hasegawa, H., T. Yamauchi, and W. J. Kraemer. "Foot Strike Patterns of Runners at the 15K Point During an Elite-Level Half Marathon." *Journal of Strength and Conditioning Research* (2007) 21 (3): 888–893.

Johnson, R. E., T. J. Quinn, R. Kertzer, and N. B. Vroman. "Strength Training in Female Distance Runners: Impact on Running Economy." *Journal of Strength and Conditioning Research* (1997) 11 (4): 224–229.

Jung, A. P. "The Impact of Resistance Training on Distance Running Performance." *Sports Medicine* (2003) 33 (7): 539–552.

Karsten, B., L. Stevens, M. Colpus, E. Larumbe-Zabala, and F. Naclerio. "The Effects of a Sports Specific Maximal Strength and Conditioning Training on Critical Velocity, Anaerobic Running Distance and 5-km Race Performance." *International Journal of Sports Physiology and Performance* (2016) 11 (1): 80–85.

Kokkonen, J., A. G. Nelson, and A. Cornwell. "Acute Muscle Stretching Inhibits Maximal Strength Performance." *Research Quarterly in Exercise and Sport* (1998) 69 (4): 411–415.

Lauersen, J. B., D. M. Bertelsen, and L. B. Andersen. "The Effectiveness of Exercise Interventions to Prevent Sports Injuries: A Systematic Review and Meta-analysis of Randomised Controlled Trials." *British Journal of Sports Medicine* (2014) 48 (11): 871–877.

Lee, B. C., and S. M. McGill. "Effect of Long-Term Isometric Training on Core/Torso Stiffness." *Journal of Strength and Conditioning Research* (2015) 29 (6): 1515–1526.

Levenhagen, D. K., J. D. Gresham, M. G. Carlson, D. J. Maron, M. J. Borel, and P. J. Flakoll. "Postexercise Nutrient Intake Timing in Humans Is Critical to Recovery of Leg Glucose and Protein Homeostasis." *American Journal of Physiology. Endocrinology and Metabolism* (2001) 280 (6): E982–E993.

Markovic, G., I. Jukic, D. Milanovic, and D. Metikos. "Effects of Sprint and Plyometric Training on Muscle Function and Athletic Performance." *Journal of Strength and Conditioning Research* (2007) 21 (2): 543–549.

Markovic, G., and P. Mikulic. "Neuro-musculoskeletal and Performance Adaptations to Lower-Extremity Plyometric Training." *Sports Medicine* (2010) 40 (10): 859–895.

McDaniel, J., A. Subudhi, and J. C. Martin. "Torso Stabilization Reduces the Metabolic Cost of Producing Cycling Power." *Canadian Journal of Applied Physiology* (2005) 30 (4): 433–441.

Mikkola, J., H. Rusko, A. Nummela, T. Pollari, and K. Häkkinen. "Concurrent Endurance and Explosive Type Strength Training Improves Neuromuscular and Anaerobic Characteristics in Young Distance Runners." *International Journal of Sports Medicine* (2007) 28 (7): 602–611.

Mikkola, J., V. Vesterinen, R. Taipale, B. Capostagno, K. Häkkinen, and A. Nummela. "Effect of Resistance Training Regimens on Treadmill Running and Neuromuscular Performance in Recreational Endurance Runners." *Journal of Sports Sciences* (2011) 29 (13): 1359–1371.

Millet, G. P., B. Jaouen, F. Borrani, and R. Candau. "Effects of Concurrent Endurance and Strength Training on Running Economy and VO(2) Kinetics." *Medicine and Science in Sports and Exercise* (2002) 34 (8): 1351–1359.

Mitchell, C. J., T. A. Churchward-Venne, D. W. West, N. A. Burd, L. Breen, S. K. Baker, and S. M. Phillips. "Resistance Exercise Load Does Not Determine Training-Mediated Hypertrophic Gains in Young Men." *Journal of Applied Physiology* (2012) 113 (1): 71–77.

Nummela, A., T. Keranen, and L. O. Mikkelsson. "Factors Related to Top Running Speed and

Economy." *International Journal of Sports Medicine* (2007) 28 (8): 655–661.

Paavolainen, L., K. Häkkinen, I. Hämäläinen, A. Nummela, and H. Rusko. "Explosive-Strength Training Improves 5-km Running Time by Improving Running Economy and Muscle Power." *Journal of Applied Physiology* (1999) 86 (5): 1527–1533.

Paavolainen, L., A. Nummela, H. Rusko, and K. Hakkinen. "Neuromuscular Characteristics and Fatigue During 10K Running." *International Journal of Sports Medicine* (1999) 20 (8): 516–521.

Phillips, S. M. "A Brief Review of Critical Processes in Exercise-Induced Muscular Hypertrophy." *Sports Medicine* (2014) 44 (Supplement 1): S71–S77.

Ramírez-Campillo, R., C. Alvarez, C. Henríquez-Olguín, E. B. Baez, C. Martínez, D. C. Andrade, and M. Izquierdo. "Effects of Plyometric Training on Endurance and Explosive Strength Performance in Competitive Middle- and Long-Distance Runners." *Journal of Strength and Conditioning Research* 2014: 28 (1): 97–104.

Rasmussen, B. B., K. D. Tipton, S. L. Miller, S. E. Wolf, and R. R. Wolfe. "An Oral Essential Amino Acid-Carbohydrate Supplement Enhances Muscle Protein Anabolism After Resistance Exercise." *Journal of Applied Physiology* (2000) 88 (2): 386–392.

Ronnestad, B. R., E. A. Hansen, and T. Raastad. "In-Season Strength Maintenance Training Increases Well-Trained Cyclists' Performance." *European Journal of Applied Physiology* (2010) 110 (6): 1269–1282.

Ronnestad, B. R., and I. Mujika. "Optimizing Strength Training for Running and Cycling Performance: A Review." *Scandinavian Journal of Medicine & Science in Sports* (2014) 24 (4): 603–612.

Rumpf, M. C., R. G. Lockie, J. B. Cronin, and F. Jalilvand. "The Effect of Different Sprint Training Methods on Sprint Performance Over Various Distances: A Brief Review." *Journal of Strength and Conditioning Research* (2016) 30 (6):1767–1785.

Saunders, P. U., R. D. Telford, D. B. Pyne, E. M. Peltola, R. B. Cunningham, C. J. Gore, and J. A. Hawley. "Short-Term Plyometric Training Improves Running Economy in Highly Trained Middle and Long Distance Runners." *Journal of Strength and Conditioning Research* (2006) 20 (4): 947–954.

Sedano, S., P. J. Marín, G. Cuadrado, and J. C. Redondo. "Concurrent Training in Elite Male Runners: The Influence of Strength Versus Muscular Endurance Training on Performance Outcomes." *Journal of Strength and Conditioning Research* (2013) 27 (9): 2433–2443.

Seger, J. Y., B. Arvidsson, and A. Thorstensson. "Specific Effects of Eccentric and Concentric Training on Muscle Strength and Morphology in Humans." *European Journal of Applied Physiology and Occupational Physiology* (1998) 79 (1): 49–57.

Sforzo, G. A., and P. R. Touey. "Manipulating Exercise Order Affects Muscular Performance During a Resistance Exercise Training Session." *Journal of Strength and Conditioning Research* (1996) 10 (1): 20–24.

Simão, R., B. F. de Salles, T. Figueiredo, I. Dias, and J. M. Willardson. "Exercise Order in Resistance Training." *Sports Medicine* (2012) 42 (3): 251–265.

Skovgaard, C., P. M. Christensen, S. Larsen, T. R. Andersen, M. Thomassen, and J. Bangsbo. "Concurrent Speed Endurance and Resistance Training Improves Performance, Running Economy, and Muscle NHE1 in Moderately Trained Runners." *Journal of Applied Physiology* (2014) 117 (10): 1097–1109.

Spurrs, R. W., A. J. Murphy, and M. L. Watsford. "The Effect of Plyometric Training on Distance Running Performance." *European Journal of Applied Physiology* (2003) 89 (1): 1–7.

Støren, O., J. Helgerud, E. M. Støa, and J. Hoff. "Maximal Strength Training Improves Running Economy in Distance Runners." *Medicine and Science in Sports and Exercise* (2008) 40 (6): 1087–1092.

Sunde, A., O. Støren, M. Bjerkaas, M. H. Larsen, J. Hoff, and J. Helgerud. "Maximal Strength Training Improves Cycling Economy in Competitive Cyclists." *Journal of Strength and Conditioning Research* (2010) 24 (8): 2157–2165.

Tanaka, H., D. L. Costill, R. Thomas, W. J. Fink, and J. J. Widrick. "Dry-Land Resistance Training for Competitive Swimming." *Medicine and Science in Sports and Exercise* (1993) 25 (8): 952–959.

Tanaka, H., and T. Swensen. "Impact of Resistance Training on Endurance Performance. A New Form of Cross-Training?" *Sports Medicine* (1998) 25 (3): 191–200.

Tipton, K. D., B. B. Rasmussen, S. L. Miller, S. E. Wolf, S. K. Owens-Stovall, B. E. Petrini, and R. R. Wolfe. "Timing of Amino Acid-Carbohydrate Ingestion Alters Anabolic Response of Muscle to Resistance Exercise." *American Journal of Physiology. Endocrinology and Metabolism* (2001) 281 (2): E197–E206.

Turner, A. M., M. Owings, and J. A. Schwane. "Improvement in Running Economy After 6 Weeks of Plyometric Training." *Journal of Strength and Conditioning Research* (2003) 17 (1): 60–67.

Willardson J. M. "A Brief Review: Factors Affecting the Length of the Rest Interval Between Resistance Exercise Sets." *Journal of Strength and Conditioning Research* (2006) 20 (4): 978–984.

Yamamoto, L. M., R. M. Lopez, J. F. Klau, E. J. Casa, W. J. Kraemer, and C. M. Maresh. "The Effects of Resistance Training on Endurance Running Performance Among Highly Trained Runners: A Systematic Review." *Journal of Strength and Conditioning Research* (2008) 22 (6): 2036–2044.

Chapter 14: The Training Diary

Atkinson, G., O. Peacock, and L. Passfield. "Variable Versus Constant Power Strategies During Cycling Time-Trials: Prediction of Time Savings Using an Up-to-Date Mathematical Model." *Journal of Sports Sciences* (2007) 25 (9): 1001–1009.

Billat, V. L., J. Slawinski, M. Danel, and J. P. Koralsztein. "Effect of Free Versus Constant Pace on Performance and Oxygen Kinetics in Running." *Medicine and Science in Sports and Exercise* (2001) 33 (12): 2082–2088.

Cherry, P. W., H. K. Lakomy, M. E. Nevill, and R. J. Fletcher. "Constant External Work Cycle Exercise—The Performance and Metabolic Effects of All-Out and Even-Paced Strategies." *European Journal of Applied Physiology and Occupational Physiology* (1997) 75 (1): 22–27.

de Koning, J. J., C. Foster, A. Bakkum, S. Kloppenburg, C. Thiel, T. Joseph, J. Cohen, and J. P. Porcari. "Regulation of Pacing Strategy During Athletic Competition." *PLoS One* (2011) 6 (1): e15863.

Foster, C., A. C. Snyder, N. N. Thompson, M. A. Green, M. Foley, and M. Schrager. "Effect of Pacing Strategy on Cycle Time Trial Performance." *Medicine and Science in Sports and Exercise* (1993) 25 (3): 383–388.

González-Alonso, J., C. Teller, S. L. Andersen, F. B. Jensen, T. Hyldig, and B. Nielsen. "Influence of Body Temperature on the Development of Fatigue During Prolonged Exercise in the Heat." *Journal of Applied Physiology* (1999) 86 (3): 1032–1039.

Suriano, R., F. Vercruyssen, D. Bishop, and J. Brisswalter. "Variable Power Output During Cycling Improves Subsequent Treadmill Run Time to Exhaustion." *Journal of Science and Medicine in Sport* (2007) 10 (4): 244–251.

Swain, D. P. "A Model for Optimizing Cycling Performance by Varying Power on Hills and in Wind." *Medicine and Science in Sports and Exercise* (1997) 29 (8): 1104–1108.

INDEX

A page number followed by t or s indicates a table or sidebar, respectively.

ABOUT THE AUTHOR

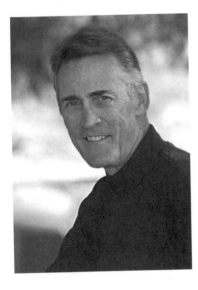

Joe Friel was one of the first triathlon coaches in the United States. He began racing triathlons and training triathletes in 1983. He also launched what is widely considered the first triathlon store in the world in 1984. In 1997, he was a founding member of the USA Triathlon National Coaching Commission and also served as cochairman.

Joe has a master's degree in exercise science, so his training methods are grounded in the principles of science, and they have been further polished and enhanced by more than 30 years of personal coaching experience. The athletes he has coached range from novices to elite amateurs to professionals to Olympians. He is a frequent presenter at athletic seminars and coaching conferences. Sports federations from various countries often ask him to update their national coaches on current best practices in training. Joe occasionally leads camps for athletes around the world and advises top endurance athletes and coaches in several sports. He also consults with companies in the sports equipment industry.

Joe has written numerous books on training for endurance sports, including his best-selling *Training Bible* books for triathletes, cyclists, and mountain bikers. He is also a frequent contributor to such magazines as *VeloNews*, *Bicycling*, *Triathlete*, and *220 Triathlon*.

In 1999, Joe cofounded TrainingPeaks (www.TrainingPeaks.com), today considered the world's leading provider of training software for endurance athletes.

As a multisport athlete, Joe has competed in hundreds of events, including national and world championships; has been selected as an All-American age-group athlete several times; and is a USA Triathlon (USAT) regional multisport champion. Joe lives and trains in Scottsdale, Arizona, during the winter and in Boulder, Colorado, during the summer.

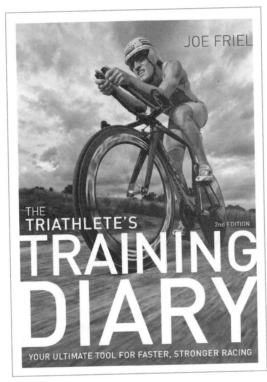
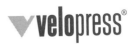